Notable Names

in

Anaesthesia

NOTABLE NAMES
IN
ANAESTHESIA

EDITED BY

J. ROGER MALTBY
MB, BChir, FRCA, FRCPC

Professor of Anesthesia, University of Calgary
and Staff Anesthesiologist,
Foothills Medical Centre, Calgary, Alberta, Canada

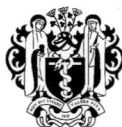

The ROYAL
SOCIETY *of*
MEDICINE
PRESS *Limited*

©2002 Royal Society of Medicine Press Ltd
1 Wimpole Street, London W1G 0AE, UK
207 E Westminster Road, Lake Forest, IL 60045, USA
www.rsmpress.co.uk

British Library Cataloguing in Publication Data
A catalogue record for this book is available from the British Library

ISBN 1-85315-512-8

Cover images of William Thomas Green Morton and John Snow reproduced with kind permission from the Wood Library–Museum, Park Ridge, IL and the London School of Hygiene and Tropical Medicine respectively.

Typeset by Robographics, Erskine
Printed by Bell & Bain Ltd, Glasgow

Contents

Contributors

J. Antonio Aldrete
Professor of Anesthesiology, University of South Florida, School of Medicine, Tampa, Florida, USA

James A. Bain
Professor Emeritus of Anesthesia, University of Western Ontario, London, Ontario, Canada

Jonathan C. Berman
Staff Anesthesiologist, North Suburban Medical Center, Assistant Professor of Anesthesiology, University of Colorado, Denver, Colorado, USA

Archie I.J. Brain
Honorary Consultant Anaesthetist, Royal Berkshire Hospital, Reading, Berkshire and Honorary Research Fellow, Institute of Laryngology, University of London, UK

Philip R. Bromage
Post-retirement Professor of Anesthesia, McGill Department of Anesthesia, Montreal, Quebec, Canada

Ronald S. Cormack
Former Consultant Anaesthetist, Northwick Park Hospital, Harrow, Middlesex, UK

Harold T. Davenport
Former Consultant Anaesthetist, Northwick Park Hospital, Harrow, Middlesex, UK

Michael A. Denborough
Emeritus Professor, John Curtin School of Medical Research, Australian National University, Canberra ACT, Australia

Hans G. Epstein
Former University Physicist, Nuffield Department of Anaesthetics, Oxford, UK

T. Cecil Gray
Professor Emeritus of Anaesthesia, University of Liverpool, Liverpool, Merseyside, UK

Danielle L. Huggard-Nelson
Resident in Pediatrics, Faculty of Medicine, University of Calgary, Calgary, Alberta, Canada

John S. Inkster
Former Senior Consultant Anaesthetist, Children's Hospital, Newcastle upon Tyne, UK

J. Alastair Lack
Consultant Anaesthetist, Salisbury Hospital, Salisbury, Wiltshire, UK

John R. Lehane
Consultant Anaesthetist, Nuffield Department of Anaesthetics, Oxford, UK

S. Rao Mallampati
Staff Anesthesiologist, Brigham and Women's Hospital and Assistant Professor of Anesthesia, Harvard Medical School, Boston, Massachusetts, USA

J. Roger Maltby
Professor of Anesthesia, University of Calgary and Staff Anesthesiologist, Foothills Medical Centre, Calgary, Alberta, Canada

William W. Mapleson,
Professor Emeritus of the Physics of Anaesthesia, Department of Anaesthetics and Intensive Care Medicine, University of Wales College of Medicine, Cardiff, UK

Ronald S. Melzack
Professor Emeritus of Psychology, McGill University, Montreal, Quebec, Canada

Lucien E. Morris
Founding Chair and Professor Emeritus of Anesthesiology, Medical College of Ohio, Toledo, Ohio, USA

John F. Nunn
Emeritus Consultant Anaesthetist, Northwick Park Hospital, Harrow, Middlesex, UK

Wallace H. Ring
Clinical Professor of Anesthesiology (retired), University of Utah and Staff Anesthesiologist (retired), Primary Children's Hospital, Salt Lake City, Utah, USA

G. Jackson Rees
Former Consultant Anaesthetist, Royal Liverpool and Alder Hey Children's Hospital, Liverpool, Merseyside, UK

Leslie Rendell-Baker
Professor Emeritus of Anesthesiology, Mount Sinai School of Medicine, New York City, New York, USA

Göran Settergren
Associate Professor (docent), Department of Cardiothoracic Anaesthetics and Intensive Care, Karolinska Institute, Stockholm, Sweden

John W. Severinghaus
Professor Emeritus of Anesthesiology, Senior Staff Emeritus, Cardiovascular Research Institute, University of California San Francisco, San Francisco, California, USA

David J. Steward
Professor of Clinical Anesthesiology (retired), Keck School of Medicine, University of Southern California and Former Head of Department of Anesthesiology, Children's Hospital Los Angeles, Los Angeles, California, USA

H. Jeremy C. Swan
Professor Emeritus of Medicine, University of California, Los Angeles and Former Chief of Cardiology, Cedars Sinai Medical Center, Los Angeles, California, USA

Preface

My interest in eponyms in medicine began during my clinical years as a student at the London Hospital Medical College (1958–61). When my fellow students or I mentioned a named disease, operation or instrument, several of our consultants expected us to have some knowledge of the eponym. Footnotes in Bailey and Love's *A Short Practice of Surgery* (Arnold) were invaluable and Bailey and Bishop's illustrated *Notable Names in Medicine and Surgery* (H.K. Lewis) provided short biographies for more leisurely reading. Many years later, as an anaesthetist, I returned to the latter book to see how many eponymous anaesthetists were included. There were none. *Notable Names in Anaesthesia* attempts to fill this void.

Anaesthetists use proper names or eponyms in operating theatres to identify items of equipment, such as spinal needles (Quincke, Whitacre), laryngoscope blades (Macintosh, Miller), intravenous solutions (Hartmann's, lactated Ringer's), techniques (Bier's technique of intravenous regional anaesthesia, Sellick's manoeuvre), complications (Mendelson's syndrome) and scoring systems (Aldrete, Apgar). Eponymous lectures at national and international meetings are named after anaesthetists who made extra-ordinary contributions to the development of anaesthesia (Griffith, Hewitt, Koller, Labat, Rovenstine, Snow) while anaesthesia museums are named after those who established the original collections (Kaye, King, Wood).

Although this book is historical, it is not a history of anaesthesia. Its purpose is to bring to life the people behind the names – who they were; when and where they worked; why and how they invented equipment or scoring systems; and why some are recognized as great leaders. Readers may be disappointed not to find the names of some chemists, pharmacologists and anaesthetists who also made major contributions. The reason for their omission is usually that either their names did not become eponymous or that the equipment or technique that bore their names has become obsolete. Many of these names are found in Faulconer and Key's *Foundations of Anesthesiology* (Thomas), or in other sources on the history of anaesthesia.

The title of *Notable Names in Anaesthesia*, rather than 'notable anaesthetists', was chosen so that the names of surgeons, other medical specialists, equipment manufacturers, a physicist, an English eccentric and a medicolegal case of interest to anaesthetists could be included. Many of the names will be familiar to British and North American anaesthetists who are currently practising or are in training, or who practised in the second half of the 20th century.

The lives of these notable names cover nearly 200 years, from pre-anaesthetic days to the present. The reader is given an insight into how anaesthesia began and was practised in the 19th century; the formation of societies of anaesthetists and the initiation of formal training in the first half of the 20th century; and the explosion of science and emphasis on safety in the second half of the 20th century.

Some of those who supplied information or wrote their own stories also made amusing comments. One of them explained that his response would be slow because his eyesight was failing from macular degeneration. When I mentioned that another of the contributors also had macular degeneration, he quickly responded that perhaps the title of the book should be *Degenerates in Anaesthesia*! Another requested close attention to the two pictures that he sent so that his portrait would not be confused with that of his experimental pig!

Transatlantic English always poses problems, but particularly in the specialty of anaesthesia. Unfortunately, it is not only the spelling but also the meaning of the same word that is different. In this book, the British spelling is used for 'anaesthesia' The word 'anaesthetist' is used for either 'anesthetist' or 'anesthesiologist', except in titles such as the American Society of Anesthetists (Anesthesiologists since 1945) or Professor of Anesthesiology.

Not every reader will agree with my selection of notable names. Others could have been included and perhaps someone else will write about them and about new ones, which will almost certainly appear.

J. Roger Maltby
January 2002

Acknowledgements

Many individuals made helpful suggestions on the selection of notable names to be included in this book. All the suggestions were considered but I take full responsibility for the final selection.

A major part of my research was made possible by six months sabbatical leave from the University of Calgary (1999–2000), combined with a grant from the Medical History Fund of the Alberta Medical Foundation and a Paul M. Wood Fellowship at the Wood Library–Museum, Park Ridge, Illinois. Special thanks for assistance and encouragement go to Patrick Sim, librarian; Judith Robins, archivist; Karen Bieterman, assistant librarian; Carole Siragusa, secretary; and George Bause, honorary museum curator of the Wood Library–Museum; and to Trish Willis, archivist; Geoffrey Hall-Davies, honorary curator; David Wilkinson, former honorary archivist; and Neil Adams, honorary archivist of the Association of Anaesthetists of Great Britain and Ireland.

Denise Upton and Sulakhan Chopra of the Health Sciences Library, University of Calgary, provided frequent assistance in locating references, often with amused comments that hardly any other library users sought publications older than 10 years, let alone 100 years. Valerie Repper of the Department of Anesthesia, Foothills Medical Center, Calgary provided secretarial assistance in the preparation of illustrations.

Finally, I wish to thank the Royal Society of Medicine Press, the publishers, for their friendly advice and guidance during every stage of preparation of this book.

Abbreviations

AAGBI	Association of Anaesthetists of Great Britain and Ireland
AB	Bachelor of Arts (USA)
AM	Master of Arts (USA)
ASA	American Society of Anesthesiologists
ASRA	American Society of Regional Anesthesia
BA	Bachelor of Arts (UK)
BCh, BChir, BS	Bachelor of Surgery, graduating medical degree (UK)
BS	Bachelor of Science (USA)
CBE	Commander of the order of the British Empire
CRCPC	Certification of the Royal College of Physicians and Surgeons of Canada (until 1972)
DA	Diploma in Anaesthetics (UK)
DM	Higher degree of Doctor of Medicine, Oxford University (UK)
ESRA	European Society of Regional Anesthesia
FFARCS	Fellow of the Faculty of Anaesthetists of the Royal College of Surgeons of England
FFARCSI	Fellow of the Faculty of Anaesthetists of the Royal College of Surgeons in Ireland
FRCA	Fellow of the Royal College of Anaesthetists (formerly FFARCS)
FRCOG	Fellow of the Royal College of Obstetricians and Gynaecologists (UK)
FRCP	Fellow of the Royal College of Physicians (of London)
FRCPC	Fellow of the Royal College of Physicians and Surgeons of Canada
FRCS	Fellow of the Royal College of Surgeons (of England)
FRS	Fellow of the Royal Society
LRCP	Licentiate of the Royal College of Physicians, graduating diploma (UK)
LSA	Licentiate of the Society of Apothecaries, registerable qualification, now LMSSA (UK)
MB	Bachelor of Medicine, graduating medical degree (UK)
MD	Higher degree of Doctor of Medicine (UK)
MD	Graduating degree of Doctor of Medicine (USA)
MRCS	Member of the Royal College of Surgeons of England, graduating diploma (UK)
MRCP	Member of the Royal College of Physicians (higher, specialist qualification)
OBE	Officer of the order of the British Empire
UK	United Kingdom of Great Britain and Northern Ireland
US, USA	United States of America
WFSA	World Federation of Societies of Anaesthesiologists
WLM	Wood Library–Museum of Anesthesiology

ALDRETE POSTANAESTHETIC RECOVERY SCORE

Jorge Antonio Aldrete (1937–)

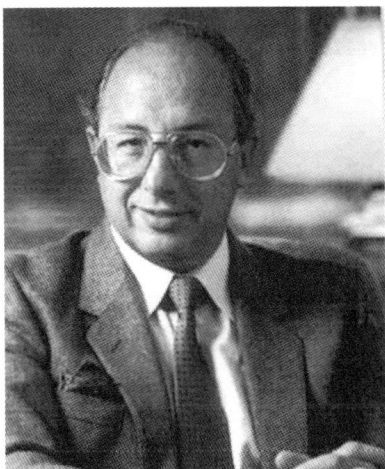

Antonio Aldrete was born in Mexico City, Mexico in 1937 and graduated from the medical school of the National University of Mexico in 1960. After a one-year internship and two years of surgical training, he was enticed towards anaesthesia by the popularity of cardiopulmonary resuscitation. He took a residency in anaesthesia at Case Western Reserve University in Cleveland, Ohio under Robert Hingson. He then moved to the Veterans Administration Hospital in Denver, Colorado to be the anaesthetist for the University of Colorado's pioneering liver transplant team. The team was headed by Tom Starzl who performed the first human liver transplant in 1963.

Aldrete was appointed Chief of Anesthesia in 1967. The recovery room had only one graduate nurse, Ruth Herring, who was very experienced and proficient. However, she had been in the civil service since the Second World War and was therefore eligible for frequent time off. As long as she was there, everyone was safe, but in her absence, the nursing office sent any new recruit who was not needed or wanted elsewhere. Panic calls came regularly and, occasionally, serious problems were not recognized on time. It became evident that, regardless of who was in the recovery room, there was a need to standardize nursing surveillance and records.

Aldrete had the idea of creating a simple point score system for patients arriving in the recovery room after anaesthesia (Figure 1). It was analogous to the Apgar score for neonates – easy to learn, and quick to record. Its purpose was to ensure that nurses observed and recorded important clinical signs of patients at regular intervals, to provide objective information on their physical condition.

The proposed recovery room score had a rating of 0, 1 or 2 for five clinical signs: activity, respiration, circulation, consciousness and colour. A score of 10 indicated a patient in the best possible condition. This was enthusiastically endorsed by Robert Virtue who was in charge of the residency training programme at the time. After a pilot project on 30 patients proved effective, a larger population of patients was studied. The American Society of Anesthesiologists set up a preceptorship programme to attract more students into the specialty. A sophomore medical student named

Figure 1. Original Aldrete postanaesthetic recovery score

		arrival	1 hour	2 hour	3 hour
Activity					
Moves 4 extremities voluntarily or on command	= 2				
Moves 2 extremities voluntarily or on command	= 1				
Moves 0 extremities voluntarily or on command	= 0				
Respiration					
Able to deep breathe and cough freely	= 2				
Dyspnoea or limited breathing	= 1				
Apnoeic	= 0				
Circulation					
BP ± 20% of preanaesthetic level	= 2				
BP ± 20-50% of preanaesthetic level	= 1				
BP ± 50% of preanaesthetic level	= 0				
Consciousness					
Fully awake	= 2				
Arousable on calling	= 1				
Not responding	= 0				
Colour					
Pink	= 2				
Pale, dusky, blotchy, jaundiced, other	= 1				
Cyanotic	= 0				
	Totals				

Diane Kroulik was recruited for the project in the summer of 1968. She eventually trained in anaesthesia and entered private practice in Arizona. Kroulik evaluated most of the patients at the Veterans Administration Hospital, and colleagues in Montana and Wyoming collaborated to include women patients in private practice.

Anesthesiology rejected the manuscript detailing the scoring system, since some of the reviewers felt that the score 'did not have clinical application'. The manuscript was revised and sent to *Anesthesia and Analgesia*, which immediately realised its potential, accepted it for publication and arranged a presentation at the next Congress of the International Anesthesia Research Society in 1970. The official commentator was Hingson, who recognized and praised the future value of the postanaesthetic recovery (PAR) or Aldrete score in clinical practice.

By 1980, the Joint Commission of Accreditation of Hospitals implemented the requirement for criteria, including a recommendation for use of the Aldrete PAR score, to allow discharge from postanaesthetic care units. When pulse oximetry became available, oxygen saturation replaced colour with the following scores:

Able to maintain O_2 saturation >92% on room air   = 2
Needs O_2 inhalation to maintain O_2 saturation >90% on room air = 1
O_2 saturation <90% even with O_2 supplement   = 0

The increasing popularity of ambulatory surgery made it evident that a more detailed assessment was required to assure 'street fitness'. The 0–2 score for five indices of wound dressing, pain, ambulation, fasting–feeding and urine output have proved satisfactory. Proposed modifications of the Aldrete score demonstrate its flexibility. They are applicable to patients of all ages and in hospitals or freestanding ambulatory surgery centres. For patients having 'conscious sedation', the Aldrete score has been proposed as the determining factor in whether or not to transport patients from the operating room directly to the discharge units in the so-called 'fast track system' that bypasses postanaesthetic recovery rooms altogether.

Aldrete has made many contributions to anaesthesia in his hospital and academic appointments. He was the anaesthetist for the first 180 liver transplants in Denver and was Professor and Chairman at the University of Colorado Health Sciences Center, Denver from 1975–80. He was Professor of Anesthesiology at the University of Alabama Hospitals, Birmingham 1980–86; Chairman, Department of Anesthesiology at Cook County Hospital, Chicago, Illinois 1986–89; and has been Professor of Anesthesiology at the University of South Florida, Tampa since 1995. He has published many papers and edited or co-edited books on a wide range of topics (eg malignant hyperthermia, low flow and closed system anaesthesia, emotional and psychological responses to anaesthesia and surgery, theory and practice of anaesthesia, cost of anaesthesia, chronic pain and arachnoiditis) in both English and Spanish.

Aldrete was the leader of a medical group that assisted the Mexican Red Cross after the 1985 earthquake, and he led the transfer of medical supplies and equipment from the Colorado Medical Society to the Secretaria de Salubridad in Mexico after the destruction of hospitals at that time. He was also the leader of a medical group to assist the Salvadorean Red Cross after the 1986 earthquake. During his free time he has enjoyed coaching teenage soccer teams and doing extensive research on the original contributions to anaesthesia by Latin Americans, and pain relief in pre-Columbian times.

Further Reading

Aldrete JA. Modifications to the postanesthesia score for use in ambulatory surgery. *Journal of PeriAnesthesia Nursing* 1998; 13: 148-55.

Aldrete JA. The post-anesthesia recovery score revisited. *Journal of Clinical Anesthesia* 1995; 7: 89-91.

Aldrete JA, Kroulik D. A postanesthetic recovery score. *Anesthesia and Analgesia* 1970; 49: 924-33.

APGAR SCORE

Virginia Apgar (1909–1974)

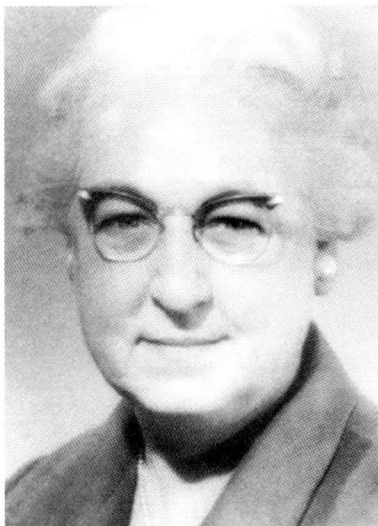

Virginia Apgar was born in Westfield, New Jersey in 1909. Her father worked in sales and insurance positions and had a passion for science. He kept a well-equipped laboratory in their basement and had a homemade telescope, but was not wealthy. She supported herself through Mount Holyoke College in Massachusetts by scholarships, supplemented by odd jobs that included catching stray cats for the zoology laboratory.

Her first choice of medical school would have been Harvard in Boston, Massachusetts but Harvard did not admit women in 1929. Instead she enrolled at Columbia University College of Physicians and Surgeons in New York City. The stock market crash worsened her family's already precarious financial situation, and she had to borrow money from a family friend. Apgar graduated in 1933, fourth in her class of 73, four of whom were women.

Towards the end of her second year as a surgical resident at Columbia Presbyterian Hospital, despite making excellent progress, the Chairman of Surgery encouraged her to change to anaesthesia. New York already had too many surgeons, and patients expected to have a male surgeon. His four previous female residents had been unable to establish surgical practices. He knew that Apgar's family was not wealthy, that she was already in debt and that, not being married, she would have to support herself.

Her anaesthesia training was typical for that era. She spent nearly one year with the nurse anaesthetists at the Columbia Presbyterian Hospital, followed by six months with Ralph Waters at the University of Wisconsin in Madison. Residents' quarters in Madison were exclusively for men, so she had difficulty finding housing and was forced to move three times. Apgar continued her training with Emery Rovenstine at Bellevue Hospital in New York, this time living in maids' quarters at the clinic.

She returned to Columbia as the first Director of the Division of Anesthesiology from 1938 to 1949. When Emanuel Papper was appointed Chairman in 1949, Apgar was the first woman to be a full Professor at Columbia and she entered the new field of obstetrical anaesthesia. In the same year, she was in the hospital cafeteria having breakfast with some medical students when one of them asked how she would evaluate a newborn. She

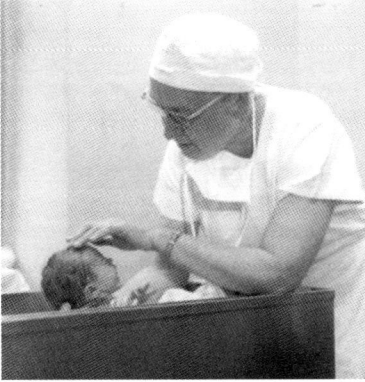

Figure 1. Apgar assessing a newborn baby. (Archives & Special Collections, Columbia University Health Sciences Division. Photograph by Elizabeth Wilcox.)

reached for a piece of paper, scribbled down a scoring system of 0, 1 or 2 for each of five signs, (Table 1 and Figure 1), then hurried to the labour ward to test it.

The maximum score was 10; heart rate and respiratory effort were the most important signs and colour was the least reliable. Apgar rejected relative weighting of the signs because more time would be spent on calculations instead of on the baby's well-being. With the score, less than one minute was needed to assess the status of the newborn. In 1962, Joe Butterfield, a paediatrician from Denver, Colorado used the letters of Apgar's name as an acronym for medical students: Appearance (colour), Pulse (heart rate), Grimace (reflex irritability), Activity (muscle tone), Respiration (respiratory effort).

Apgar was a pioneer in both clinical and research aspects of obstetrical anaesthesia. Fifty years ago, little attention was given to the newborn baby. She and her paediatric colleagues demonstrated that acidosis and hypoxia in newborns were not normal, as previously believed, and should be actively treated. She was the first person to catheterize the umbilical artery of a newborn, albeit by accident. Recognizing the significance and importance of what she had done, she and her colleagues then taught the technique to visiting neonatologists.

In 1959 she took her Master of public health degree (MPH) at The John Hopkins University in Baltimore, Maryland to improve her knowledge of biostatistics for research in obstetrical anaesthesia. She was increasingly interested in genetics and birth defects and became Clinical Professor of Paediatrics (Teratology) at Cornell University Medical College in Ithaca, New York. She held several executive positions in the National Foundation–March of Dimes from 1959 until her death in 1974.

Although privately Apgar acknowledged the limitations put on women in medicine, publicly she was reserved on this topic. In her personal correspondence she referred to her frustration about salary differences between male and female physicians and her exclusion from 'stag' dinners that followed scientific meetings at which she herself had been an invited speaker.

Table 1. The Apgar scoring system

Sign	0	1	2
Heart Rate	Absent	Slow (<100)	>100
Respiratory Effort	Absent	Weak cry: hypoventilation	Good: strong cry
Muscle Tone	Limp	Some flexion of the extremities	Well flexed
Reflex Irritability	No response	Some motion	Cry
Colour	Blue: pale	Body pink: extremities blue	Completely pink

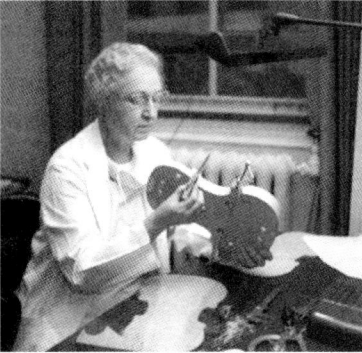

Figure 2. Apgar building her viola (Archives & Special Collections, Columbia University Health Sciences Division. Photograph by Elizabeth Wilcox..)

Apgar overcame many restrictions to lead a very successful career in anaesthesia.

Apgar did not marry but remained close to her family and led an active social life with many friends. She was an avid baseball fan and a member of the American Philatelic Society. She enjoyed fishing, gardening and golfing and took flying lessons after the age of 50. Apgar was a gifted and dedicated musician from childhood, and played in symphony orchestras. In 1956, a high school science teacher and musician, Carleen Hutchings, had a violin with her during a preoperative visit. She had made the violin herself and invited Apgar to play it. This chance meeting led Apgar to join Hutchings in studies on how musical instruments produce sound. Later, Apgar learned from Hutchings how to make her own instruments and she handcrafted a violin, mezzo violin, cello and viola (Figure 2). In 1995, a group of paediatricians, led by Joe Butterfield, bought the set of four instruments and donated them to Columbia University.

Apgar received numerous awards and distinctions, including the Gold Medal for Distinguished Achievement in Medicine, Columbia University College of Physicians and Surgeons, and the Distinguished Service Award of the American Society of Anesthesiologists in 1961. Twenty years after her death, the US postal service honoured her with a 20-cent stamp (Figure 3) in the 'Great Americans' series. In 1995 she was elected to the National Women's Hall of Fame in Seneca Falls, New York. Primarily, Apgar is remembered throughout the world for ensuring immediate assessment and care of newborn babies.

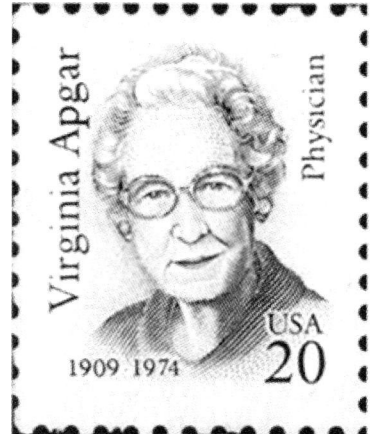

Figure 3. Virginia Apgar US postage stamp in the 'Great Americans series'.

Acknowledgement

Portrait photograph reproduced with kind permission from the Wood Library–Museum of Anesthesiology, Park Ridge, IL, USA.

Further reading

Apgar V. A proposal for a new method of evaluation of the newborn infant. *Anesthesia and Analgesia* 1953; 32: 260-7.

Butterfield J, Covey MJ. Practical epigram of the Apgar score. *Journal of the American Association* 1962; 181: 353.

Calmes SH. Virginia Apgar: a woman physician's career in a developing specialty. *Journal of American Medical Women's Association* 1984; 39: 184-8.

Ayre's T-piece

Thomas Philip Ayre (1902–1979)

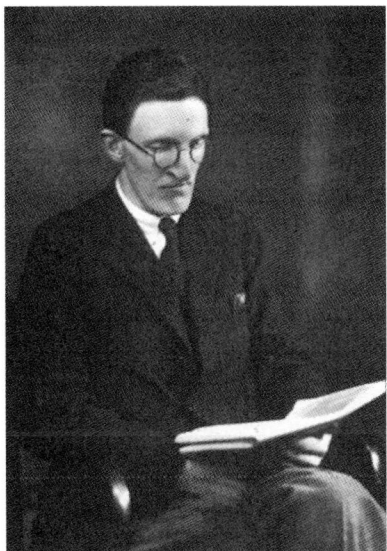

Philip Ayre was born in 1902. He graduated in medicine (MRCS, LRCP) in 1933, by which time he had already administered about 2000 anaesthetics. He joined the staff of Newcastle General Hospital, Newcastle upon Tyne in 1934, where he anaesthetized for the surgeon William Wardill. He joined the Royal Victoria Infirmary and its associated Babies' Hospital a year or two later. It was to Wardill that the paediatrician, Sir James Spence, sent all his surgical cases, including harelip and cleft palate deformities.

Ayre was a brilliant pioneer anaesthetist. Before the days of muscle relaxants, few anaesthetists practised tracheal intubation and fewer still specialized in paediatric anaesthesia, however, Ayre was involved in both. He described paediatric anaesthesia in those days as 'a protracted and sanguine battle between surgeon and anaesthetist with the poor unfortunate baby as the battlefield'.

In 1937, Ayre invented a simple metal T-piece. This was a revolutionary concept that overcame most of the difficulties that he was encountering when providing anaesthesia for small babies. During his final year as a student, he had visited St Bartholomew's Hospital in London, where he watched Henry Boyle using a Clausen–Evans airway – an oropharyngeal airway that had an in-built, fresh gas flow tube (Figure 1). Ayre remembered this, removed the metal T-piece component and fitted it directly into a Magill endotracheal tube. He simplified the T-piece and attached 6–10 inches (15–25 cm) of open-ended straight red rubber tubing to the distal end as a reservoir for fresh gases

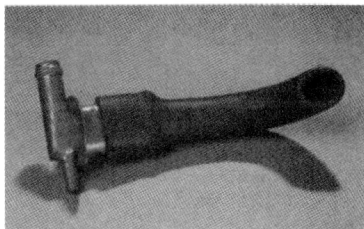

Figure 1. Clausen–Evans airway. (Reproduced with kind permission from the Association of Anaesthetists of Great Britain and Ireland.)

(Figure 2). There were no valves or reservoir bag, so dead space and resistance to breathing were minimized. He recommended a fresh gas flow of twice the child's minute volume, and that the volume of the reservoir tube should be one-third of the tidal volume (Table 1). A strand of fine gauze, fixed to the open end of the reservoir tube, waved to and fro with spontaneous respiration. Later, controlled ventilation was achieved by intermittent

Table 1. Fresh gas flow and reservoir tube volume

Age	Fresh gas flow (L min^{-1})	Reservoir tube (mL)
0–3 months	3–4	6–12
3–6 months	4–5	12–18
6–12 months	5–6	18–24
1–2 years	6–7	24–42
2–4 years	7–8	42–60
4–8 years	8–9	60–72

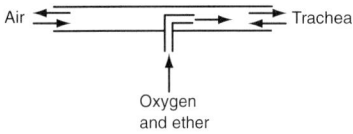

Figure 2. Ayre's T-piece system. (Reproduced with permission from *A Synopsis of Anaesthesia*, 4th edn, John Wright, 1964: 98.)

occlusion of the open end by the anaesthetist's thumb.

The fresh gas inflow tube of the original T-piece passed into the lumen where it turned 90° (Figure 3). These were manufactured by Charles King in London. Ayre quickly discovered that the general condition of the infant was always better when the gas was directed towards the patient. He thought that this was because there was a degree of assistance to inspiration. His observation was correct, but it is now realized that he was unwittingly creating a degree of positive end-expiratory pressure. In this way the functional residual capacity was being maintained to the great benefit of the patient.

Early in the Second World War, the Babies' Hospital was evacuated from Newcastle to Blagdon Hall (a large country house near Seaton Burn in Northumberland). This was the family seat of Lord Ridley. Lady Ridley, who was not qualified in medicine or nursing, was involved in the welfare of sick children and was a friend of Sir James Spence. For about two years, Wardill and Ayre, with Lady Ridley assisting and acting as theatre sister, sporadically repaired harelip and cleft palate deformities in a bathroom at Blagdon Hall.

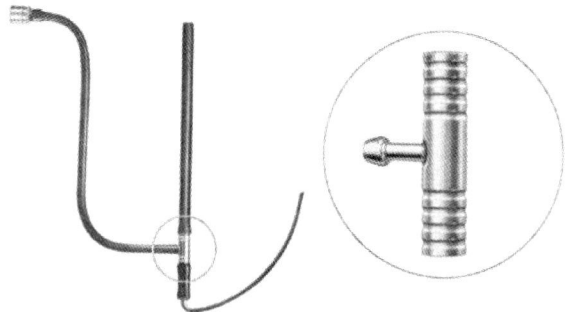

Figure 3. Curved fresh gas inflow tube within the lumen of an early T-piece. (Reproduced from *British Journal of Surgery* 1937; 25: 131–2, with permission from Blackwell Sciences.)

Modifications of Ayre's T-piece system continue to be used in paediatric anaesthesia. In Liverpool in 1950, Jackson Rees added an open-ended bag to the expiratory limb that facilitated manual controlled ventilation. In London, Ontario in 1972, James Bain and Wolfgang Spoerel (1923–89) introduced a coaxial circuit for use in both adults and children. Ayre and others also used the T-piece system for adult neurosurgery to minimize vascular congestion. Fresh gas flows of 12–15 litres per minute were used.

Ayre was a splendid teacher, administrator, adviser and an acute observer of life. His spontaneous humour and wit were shown in his earlier years at Newcastle as organizer of the memorable annual students' concerts, and in later years in his professional writing. Philip Ayre spent all of his working life in the Newcastle region, and for over 45 years anaesthetized at most of the city's hospitals. He was Head of the Department of Anaesthetics at Newcastle General Hospital from 1950 until his official retirement in 1966.

His sense of humour, combined with remarkable courage, enabled Ayre to endure and overcome great personal tragedies in his lifetime. He coped with personal disadvantages – he had alopecia and wore a wig, and the repair of his own harelip and cleft palate was bad enough to be obvious and to make his speech almost unintelligible. The honking sound, which was his attempt at speech, fascinated his young patients and mesmerized them so much that they became unaware of the vapours that were enveloping them. His domestic life was tragic; his only son drowned in a fire service water tank and his daughter was disabled from birth. His wife was one of the earliest mitral valvotomy patients and she did not survive for long after surgery. He died from a massive myocardial infarction at the age of 78.

Ayre was elected to be an honorary member of The Association of Anaesthetists of Great Britain and Ireland in 1972. In 1974, The North of England Society of Anaesthetists presented him with a gold replica of his original T-piece, with the bent gas flow tube; it is now in the safekeeping of the Royal College of Anaesthetists. The Society also created the Philip Ayre Medal for presentation on rare occasions to an eminent anaesthetist. In this way the name of Thomas Philip Ayre will long be remembered in the northeast of England.

Acknowledgement

Portrait photograph reproduced with kind permission from the Wood Library–Museum of Anesthesiology, Park Ridge, IL, USA.

Further Reading

Ayre P. Anaesthesia for hare-lip and cleft palate operations on babies. *British Journal of Surgery* 1937; **25**: 131-2.
Ayre P. Theme and variations (On a T-Piece). *Anaesthesia* 1967; **22**: 359.
J.G.M. Thomas Philip Ayre [Obituary]. *Lancet* 1980; **1**: 106.

BAIN COAXIAL BREATHING SYSTEM

James Bain (1934–)

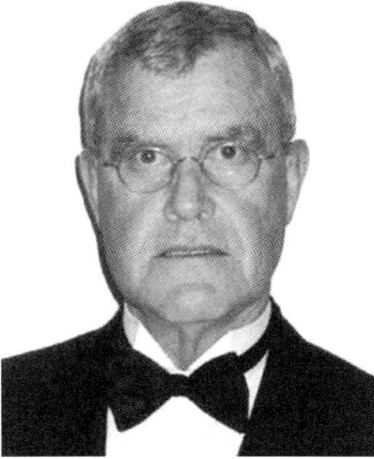

Jim Bain was born in Listowel, Ontario in 1934. He graduated from medical school at the University of Western Ontario in London, Ontario and took his anaesthesia training in Toronto and London from 1960 to 1964.

Bain joined Wolfgang Spoerel, Professor and Chairman at the University of Western Ontario, at the Victoria Hospital, London, Ontario in 1965. The standard anaesthetic circuit was the circle system with heavy black rubber tubing. Spoerel recognized that this was clumsy for plastic surgical procedures around the face and he modified Ayre's T-piece by using a three-inch length of Tygon tubing with a side hole. This worked well with patients who breathed spontaneously, although monitoring of ventilation was difficult because of the absence of a reservoir bag. Assisted and automatic ventilation were impossible.

Bain therefore designed a lightweight system for head and neck surgery that would allow both the surgeon and the anaesthetist to have their own space while sharing the airway. His system would have a reservoir bag so that the anaesthetist could visually monitor spontaneous respiration and provide assisted or controlled ventilation when necessary. Lightweight material was important because his plastic surgeon did not like adhesive tape on the face. The Mapleson D configuration fulfilled most of these criteria so Bain turned the system inside out and lengthened it to create a lightweight coaxial anaesthesia system (Figure 1). With the help of Henry Letanche, an anaesthesia department technician, Bain constructed a prototype circuit in one afternoon.

The outer tube was a six-foot length of 22 mm lightweight corrugated plastic tubing, and the inner tube was six feet of oxygen tubing. The end pieces were green Bird connectors (22 mm OD and 15 mm ID). An orthopaedic drill was used to make a hole in the distal Bird connector for the oxygen tubing. Black silk

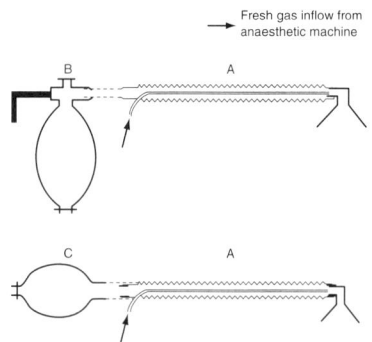

Figure 1. Bain breathing circuit (modified Mapleson D coaxial system).
(Upper) The adult breathing tube is attached to a bag mount with reservoir bag and a spring-loaded valve with a simple bracket for attachment to the anaesthetic machine (B). (Lower) Paediatric system with open-tailed bag (C). (Reproduced from *Canadian Anaesthetists' Society Journal* 1972; 19: 426–35.)

sutures held the inner tube, and collodion was used to plug leaks. The newly constructed system was light and convenient and worked well.

Bain began construction of the system in 1971, and was soon producing it in large numbers in his hospital's respiratory therapy department. He and Spoerel conducted clinical studies on these home-made circuits and, in 1972, presented their results to the Canadian Society of Plastic Surgeons in Toronto and at the Canadian Anaesthetists' Society annual meeting in Halifax, Nova Scotia. Later that year they published a description of 'A streamlined anaesthetic circuit'.

Around this time, a sales representative for Respiratory Care Incorporated in Chicago (the company that supplied the lightweight corrugated tubing) inquired of Bain what he was doing with it all. The representative arranged for a commercial prototype of the system to be made with a view to commercial manufacture and sales. Meanwhile, Bain took the system to his university in a brown bag for possible patenting. He was told, 'Young man, this is just a bunch of plastic!' Prompted by a telephone call about patent rights, he realized this was indeed an invention that could be patented. He quickly filed documents through a private patent attorney, who suggested calling it the 'Bain breathing circuit' or BBC.

Bain anaesthetized many teenage children with the Jackson Rees modification of the Mapleson D system for Harrington's spinal instrumentation when he was an anaesthesia resident at the Hospital for Sick Children in Toronto in 1964. The recommended fresh gas flow for that system was three times the minute ventilation, and invariably the $PaCO_2$ with manual controlled ventilation was low (20–35 mmHg). That experience prompted him to reduce fresh gas inflows in his new system. He found that the $PaCO_2$ was within the normal range with a 7-litre fresh gas flow in adults (approximately minute ventilation) with both spontaneous and controlled ventilation. Even at 5.5 litres (approaching alveolar ventilation) the $PaCO_2$ levels were acceptable. The system was popular with his plastic surgeon, Robert McFarlane, and Bain's colleagues also started using it for head and neck cases (Figures 2 and 3).

Bain gives Spoerel credit for being instrumental in the success of the system. The new University Hospital in London, Ontario opened in 1972–73 and each operating theatre was fitted with a redesigned anaesthesia machine without CO_2 absorbers and with only Bain circuits. Spoerel's faith was greater than Bain's. The Bain system soon became popular across Canada and in other countries. This was in the decade before pulse oximetry and capnography became widely available. An advantage over the circle absorption system was that adequate CO_2 elimination was predictable if minute volume exceeded a fresh gas flow of 70 ml/kg with controlled ventilation and a fresh gas flow of 100 ml/kg during spontaneous respiration.

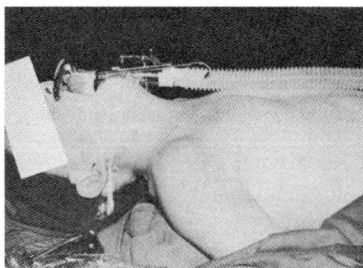

Figure 2. Bain system for repair of cleft palate. (Reproduced from *Canadian Anaesthetists' Society Journal* 1972; 19: 426–35.)

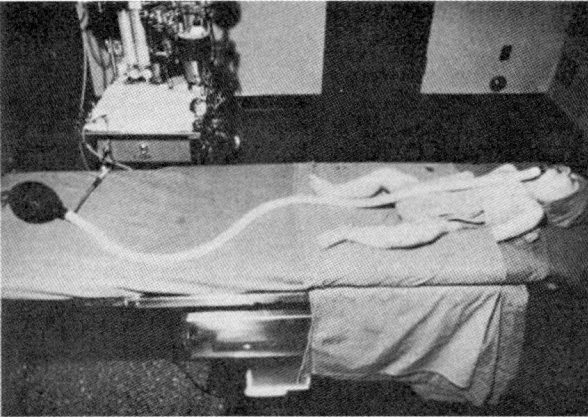

Figure 3. Paediatric Bain system remote from anaesthesia machine, attached only by gas inflow line. (Reproduced from *Canadian Anaesthetists' Society Journal* 1972; 19: 426–35.)

The outer tubing of some of the early Bain systems was black and therefore opaque. Proximal disconnection of the inner tubing could not be detected by visual inspection. When this occurred, the fresh gas entered the machine end of the outer tubing instead of the patient end, adding 500 ml dead space and producing severe hypercarbia. In 1975, Simon Pethick, an anaesthesia resident in Calgary, Alberta described the use of the oxygen flush button to ensure that the proximal connection of the inner tube was intact. Oxygen flush causes a high velocity flow in the inner tube, so that with the distal end open, the Venturi effect lowers the pressure in the outer tube and causes the reservoir bag to collapse completely. Conversely, if the inner tube is disconnected from its proximal mount, the reservoir bag will inflate slightly. The Foëx–Crampton Smith manoeuvre involves occlusion of the patient end of the inner tube with a finger or syringe – the rotameters will dip owing to back pressure if the system is intact.

The Bain system is wasteful of nitrous oxide and volatile agents. This was especially noticeable as new, more expensive agents were introduced. Atmospheric pollution from scavenged gases became a concern, as did the amount of plastic waste produced from these single use circuits. Anaesthetists returned to using the circle system with carbon dioxide absorption and lightweight corrugated tubing. As pulse oximetry and capnography became standard in the 1980s and anaesthetic agent monitors became standard in the 1990s, low-flow anaesthesia was implemented. Nevertheless, the Bain system remains popular in India and other countries where these monitors are not widely available, and with some paediatric anaesthetists.

Further reading

Bain JA, Spoerel WE. A streamlined anaesthetic system. *Canadian Anaesthetists' Society Journal* 1972; **19**: 426–35.

Foëx P, Crampton Smith A. A test for co-axial circuits. The Foëx-Crampton Smith manoeuvre. *Anaesthesia* 1977; **32**: 294.

Pethick SL. Pressure test for Bain anaesthesia circuit. *Canadian Anaesthetists' Society Journal* 1975; **22**: 115.

BEECHER AND TODD REPORT

Henry Knowles Beecher (1904-1976)

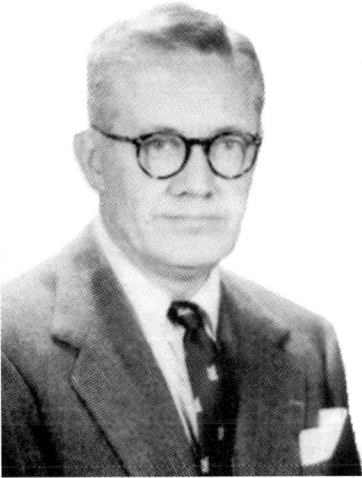

Henry K. Beecher was born Henry Knowles Unangst in Wichita, Kansas in 1904. His German surname, Unangst, means 'without fear'. He worked and borrowed money to study physical chemistry at the University of Kansas where he graduated with an AB in 1926 and an AM in 1927. His goal was a PhD in chemistry at the Sorbonne in Paris, France but he was persuaded to study medicine instead. Before entering Harvard Medical School in Boston, Massachusetts he changed his name to Beecher, since he was related through his maternal grandmother to Henry Ward Beecher (1813-87), the famous 19th century American slavery abolitionist.

Beecher became interested in respiratory physiology soon after he began medical school in 1928. He earned research fellowships in 1929, 1930 and 1931 and graduated *cum laude* in 1932. In his final year, he defined the role of aspiration of vomitus in the development of postoperative pneumonia. These achievements caught the attention of Edward Churchill, the Homans Professor of Surgery at Harvard, who became Beecher's professional mentor.

Beecher completed two years of surgical training at Massachusetts General Hospital (MGH) in Boston. He then worked in Nobel Laureate August Krogh's physiology laboratory in Copenhagen, Denmark, returning to Boston in 1936 where Churchill appointed him Anesthetist-in-Chief in the division of surgery at MGH and Instructor of Anesthesia at Harvard. Beecher wanted to receive formal training in anaesthesia but Churchill dissuaded him. The 'Henry Isaiah Dorr Professor of Research and Teaching in Anesthesia and Anesthetics' was established in 1917 and Beecher became the first incumbent in 1941. During the Second World War, he was a consultant in anaesthesia and resuscitation to the US Army in North Africa and Italy. He stepped down as head of anaesthesia at MGH in 1969 and retired from the chair in 1970, by which time he had gained departmental status for anesthesia.

During 1948-52, the US Army Medical Research and Development Board funded a study of anaesthetic-related deaths among 599,548 anaesthetics in 10 leading academic centres, with Beecher and his colleague Donald Todd (1918-98) as principal investigators. This was one of the earliest multicentre epidemiological studies in the USA. They published their controversial

'Beecher and Todd Report' as a booklet and in *Annals of Surgery* in 1954. They concluded that mortality rates were disproportionately high in the first decade of life and in elderly patients. They contrasted the inaccuracies of anaesthetist's clinical impressions with their own accurately documented facts. They also found that the death rate increased nearly six-fold, from 1:2100 to 1:370, when muscle relaxants (usually curare) were used. There was no correlation between curare-related deaths and severity of illness, major surgery, or training and experience of the anaesthetist. The deaths occurred despite effective 'bag squeezing' artificial respiration. Beecher and Todd concluded that the deaths occurred from circulatory, not respiratory, failure and that curare was inherently toxic. They believed that the high number of anaesthetic deaths, not just those related to curare, should be addressed as a public health issue. They commented that millions of dollars were spent on poliomyelitis research during the period of their study. However, in that time period, anaesthesia accounted for twice as many deaths as poliomyelitis did and similar funds were needed to identify and overcome the hazards of anaesthesia.

This was a well-conducted study that attempted to address intraoperative and postoperative mortality, yet it raised storms of protest on both sides of the Atlantic. British anaesthetists did not accept the idea that curare was inherently toxic, but attributed the curare-related deaths to their American colleagues' reluctance to administer neostigmine to reverse residual neuro-muscular blockade. Some of the American opposition may reflect the attitude of independent private practitioners to academic criticism, especially when the senior author (Beecher) had no anaesthetic training and chose to publish the results in a surgical journal. Beecher and Todd argued in favour of the proper use of muscle relaxants as adjuvants to facilitate surgery, but not as a cover for inadequate anaesthesia, and recommended further study. However, Beecher was a consultant to the US army during the 1949–53 Korean War and, probably on his advice, the army did not approve curare during that conflict. It is possible that more men died from receiving too much thiopentone during tracheal intubation, or from deep ether for muscular relaxation, than would have died from curare. One thing is certain – Beecher and Todd demonstrated the need for studying and reducing anaesthetic-related mortality.

Beecher's investigation of the relationship between subjective psychological states and objective drug responses began during the Second World War. He noticed that the majority of badly wounded men, although they had received no morphine for hours, had so little pain that they did not want pain relief medication. This observation led to Beecher advocating the use of a placebo control in all clinical drug trials and to him being the originator of the prospective, double-blind, placebo-controlled clinical trial.

Towards the end of the 1950s, Beecher became increasingly concerned with ethical aspects of human experimentation. In 1965 he questioned the behaviour of some of his research colleagues and acknowledged that some earlier work in his own laboratory was not above reproach. His comments were ignored until 1966 when he published 22 examples of experiments on humans in which unnamed but renowned investigators had disregarded basic ethical standards outlined in the Nuremberg Code of 1947. The National Institutes of Health and the Food and Drug Administration altered their guidelines to comply. Beecher's revelations were responsible for initiating peer review of experimental protocols and ensuring that investigators obtained informed consent from participants in clinical research.

Beecher's last legacy came when, after Christiaan Barnard (1922–2001) performed the first human heart transplant in Cape Town, South Africa in December 1967, he addressed the problem of the hopelessly unconscious patient and the definition of death. Beecher chaired a committee at Harvard in 1968 to consider exactly when a person could be considered dead. The committee concluded that a persistently flat electroencephalogram was reasonable, reliable and objective. This definition of death was especially important for cadaver organ transplantation and was widely adopted.

Although Beecher had a controversial relationship with organized anaesthesia, his influence permeated the treatment of battlefield injuries, the academic approach to anaesthesia and patient safety, medical research ethics and the definition of death. His peers saw his controversial side; but Beecher pursued what he believed to be right.

Acknowledgement

Portrait photograph reproduced with kind permission from the Wood Library–Museum of Anesthesiology, Park Ridge, IL, USA.

Further Reading

Bacon DR. An enduring controversy: Henry K. Beecher and curare. *Bulletin of Anesthesia History* 2001; **19 (4):** 8–10.

Beecher HK. Ethics and clinical research. *New England Journal of Medicine* 1966; **274:** 1354–60.

Beecher HK, Todd DP. A study of the deaths associated with anesthesia and surgery. *Annals of Surgery* 1954; **140:** 2–34.

BERMAN AIRWAY

Robert Alvin Berman (1914–1999)

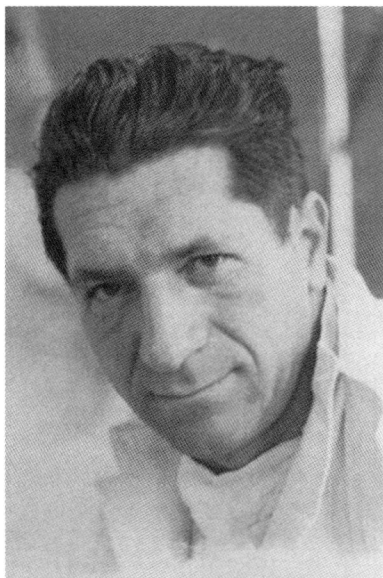

Robert Berman was born in Brooklyn, New York in 1914. He graduated from the University of North Carolina, Chapel Hill in 1936, where he also attended medical school. During his first year, while he was questioning the method of teaching in the anatomy curriculum, the Dean told him that it was often hard to place Jewish students in other medical schools after they finished the two-year curriculum. Berman made it easy – he left and enrolled at the University of Sheffield in Yorkshire, England. This rebellious spirit, defiant attitude and sharp tongue would always be a hallmark of his. The Second World War broke out while he was home in 1939; visas were revoked and he could not return to England. He eventually went to medical school in Chicago, Illinois and graduated in 1943. Upon completion of his internship at Israel Zion Hospital in New York City, he returned to Chicago to set up a general medical practice supplemented by work as a hotel doctor at the Palmer House Hotel. A two-year posting in the US Coast Guard Public Health Service during the war interrupted his plans.

No one mentor or incident led to his choice of anaesthesia as a career, but he recognized that the developing specialty used applied basic sciences and had great potential. He started his residency at Brooklyn Jewish Hospital in Brooklyn, New York but left the programme owing to a difference of opinion with the chairman of the department. He completed his anaesthesia training at Mount Sinai Hospital in New York City in 1949. By then, he had already worked on mechanical ventilation and development of airway devices, and had thought about making a heart–lung machine.

During his residency, an incident occurred that led to his development of a translucent oropharyngeal airway. He was performing a laryngoscopy when he noticed a safety pin in the pharynx. He deduced that it must have come from the channel of his opaque Guedel black rubber airway that he, like other residents, washed after each use and then carried in his pocket along with safety pins. He went home that evening, thinking how he could prevent this from happening again. He visited a neighbour, Meyer Moch, who was a plastic fabricator. He explained that if the airways could be made transparent, this accident with the safety pin should never happen.

They went to Moch's basement and pulled out some butyrate (plastic-type) tubing. They then moulded it into the shape of an airway by heating it over a flame and finishing it off with a sander. By chance, Moch had no pharyngeal reflexes and was able to place the airway in his own mouth to check the fit. Berman had his manufacturer and subject in one place! When other residents at the hospital saw the new easy-to-clean airway with no blind channel they wanted one too. Berman and his neighbour were soon making them in the basement every night to supply to his colleagues.

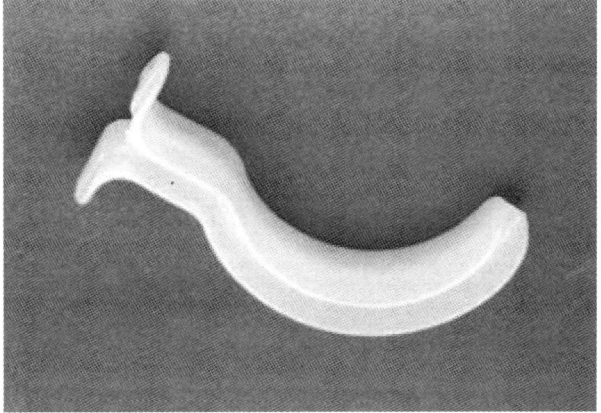

Figure 1. Berman airway. (Image courtesy of J. Berman.)

Berman left the academic environment in 1950 to become Director of Anesthesiology at the private St Joseph's Hospital in Far Rockaway, New York. He held this position for 35 years, which included every night on call. He developed the Berman airway in 1951 (Figure 1), which differed radically from the Guedel airway. The Berman airway had a central longitudinal strut with upper and lower flanges, and there is no tube in which a foreign body can lodge. Its popularity in American anaesthesia practice continues more than 50 years after its introduction.

In the late 1950s, as more attention was focused on resuscitation, Berman felt strongly that mouth-to-mouth resuscitation was unsanitary. He developed the Resuscitube and a moulded hand bellows for resuscitation that he called the Respir-Aider (Figure 2). Blood pressure cuffs are easily soiled in the operating room and he felt it was not hygienic to use them from patient to patient, so he patented a disposable plastic blood pressure cuff, Quik-Cuff, in 1957. His ideas for using plastic to produce single-use disposable items of medical equipment were at the forefront in this field. Although correct in

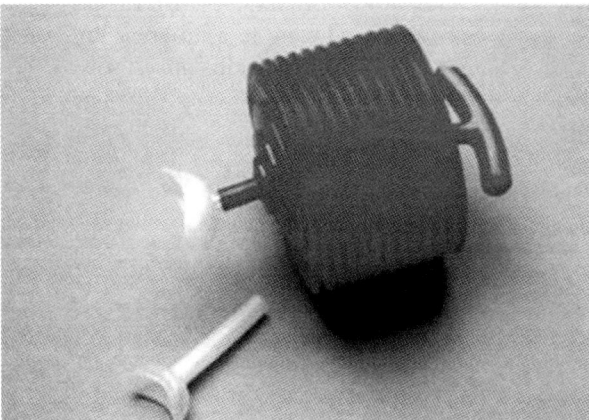

Figure 2. Respir-Aider and Resuscitube. (Image courtesy of J. Berman.)

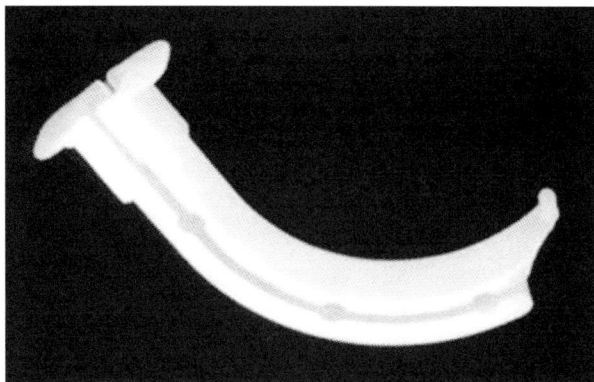

Figure 3. Berman intubating airway. (Image courtesy of J. Berman.)

theory, his innovations never had commercial success.

In the 1970s, Berman produced blow-moulded endotracheal tubes, anatomically shaped endotracheal tubes and a tapered endotracheal tube. In 1977, he resurrected an idea he had during his residency of an intubating airway. His new Berman intubating airway (Figure 3) led the way for a generation of intubating devices for blind and fibreoptic intubation. He had other ideas for airways, including an expandable airway and a balloon airway. He collaborated with the same two plastics fabricators (Meyer Moch and William Jordan) throughout his career. With advancing years, prohibitive costs and lack of a research and development team, it became harder to develop products, but he always remained active and innovative in trying to solve the problems of airway management.

Berman loved anaesthesia and published articles, letters and comments in anaesthesia journals. He was not active in the politics of either the American Society of Anesthesiologists or the New York State Society of Anesthesiologists, although he attended its postgraduate assembly on 51 out of 52 possible occasions and presented scientific exhibits there on eight occasions.

Acknowledgement

Portrait photograph courtesy of J. Berman.

Further reading

Berman RA. A method for blind oral intubation of the trachea or esophagus. *Anesthesia and Analgesia* 1977; **56**: 866–7.

Cappe B, Berman R. Airways – a new make and a new type. *Anesthesiology* 1949; **10**: 358–9.

BIER INTRAVENOUS BLOCK

August Karl Gustav Bier (1861–1949)

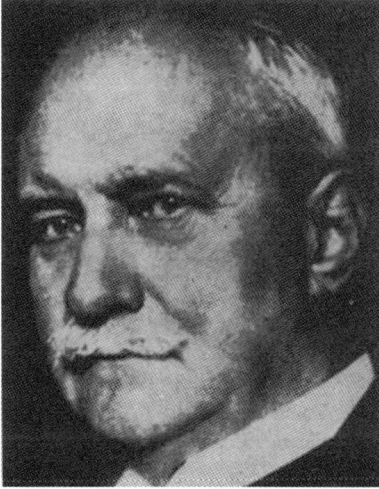

August Bier was born in Helsen, Germany in 1861. As was common in his country, he was educated at several universities and attended medical schools in Berlin, Leipzig and Kiel. When he graduated in 1886 from Kiel, he decided to devote his life to surgery. There he became an assistant to Friedrich von Esmarch and supervised the changeover from the antiseptic to the aseptic system in the operating theatres. He learned that his medical colleague Heinrich Quincke had been safely performing lumbar puncture in neurological examination since 1890, and he conceived the idea that this technique could be used to inject cocaine into the cerebrospinal fluid to produce widespread analgesia.

He knew the dangers of general anaesthesia and also the limited efficacy of local infiltration anaesthesia in major operations. He deliberately set out to 'cocainize' the spinal cord to produce analgesia over a large part of the body. He performed the first spinal anaesthetic on a 34-year-old man with disseminated tuberculosis on 16 August 1898. He placed the patient in the lateral position, performed the lumbar puncture with a very fine, hollow, styletted needle and injected 3 mL of a 0.5% solution of cocaine. He waited for 20 minutes. Sensation was lost over the lower half of the body and Bier performed a painless resection of the ankle joint.

He then described how, after successfully using the method in six patients, he allowed his junior colleague, Otto Hildebrandt (1868–1954) to inject 2 mL of 1% cocaine solution into his own (Bier's) spinal fluid. When the syringe did not fit the needle, and his cerebrospinal fluid and the cocaine leaked out, Bier terminated the experiment. He then performed a successful spinal anaesthetic on Hildebrandt, using 0.5 mL of 1% cocaine solution. Analgesia of the lower limbs occurred within eight minutes. Over the next 25 minutes, Hildebrandt did not feel pain during pinching of the skin with dental forceps, placing a burning cigar to the legs, pulling out pubic hairs and vigorous knuckle blows to the tibia. Sensation gradually returned after 45 minutes. On the following day both men had severe headaches; Hildebrandt also had painful, bruised legs but was able to work. Both took several days to recover fully.

Leonard Corning (1855–1923), a New York neurologist, had published a single case report in 1885, but this was most likely to be epidural analgesia.

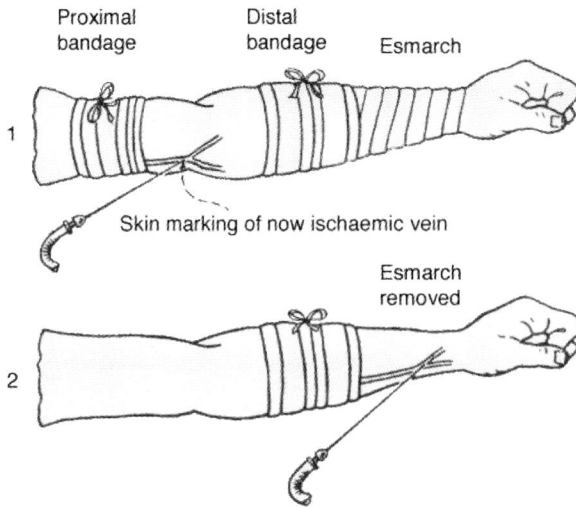

Figure 1. Bier's technique with tourniquets above and below the elbow. (Reproduced from *The art of anaesthesia*, 2nd edn 1919, with permission from Lippincott Williams & Wilkins.)

He had treated a man who suffered from spinal weakness, seminal incontinence and masturbation addiction by injecting 1.8 mL of 3% cocaine solution between the spinous processes of T11 and T12. When there was no effect after six to eight minutes he repeated the injection. After a further 10 minutes, the patient's legs 'felt sleepy', were analgesic and remained that way for at least one hour. Corning wondered if the technique might "find application as a substitute for etherization for genito-urinary or other branches of surgery" but, like Humphry Davy with nitrous oxide, he did not pursue the idea.

In 1903, Bier became Professor of Surgery at Bonn. In 1907, he succeeded Ernst von Bergmann (1836–1907) as the Chair of Surgery in Berlin. He remained in that position as a great surgeon, an inspiring lecturer and successful investigator until he retired in 1932.

In 1908, Bier described intravenous procaine analgesia (Bier's block) for resections of joints, transplantations of tendons and extensive debridements that could not be performed under infiltration anaesthesia. His first case was the resection of an elbow in a girl. He used an Esmarch bandage to exsanguinate the arm from the extremity of the fingers to above the elbow, and placed tourniquets four finger breadths above and below the elbow. He then dissected the median cubital vein under infiltration anaesthesia (Figure 1), inserted a cannula pointing distally, sutured it in place, ligated the vein proximally and injected 100 mL of 0.25% procaine through the cannula from an ordinary syringe. Analgesia of the stiff, painful elbow was immediate. The girl complained of pain during periosteal elevation but not during 15 minutes of sawing of the bones or scraping of fistulous tracts. Bier described several more cases in detail. Anaesthesia was not always complete nor immediate. Ether was necessary in one unruly man who afterwards said he felt no pain but became nervous. Bier recommended supplementary ether narcosis or scopolamine–morphine twilight sleep for both nervous and excited patients.

Many reports followed in 1909, but the technique then seems to have been largely forgotten until it was revived in 1946 by Flavio Kroeff-Pires

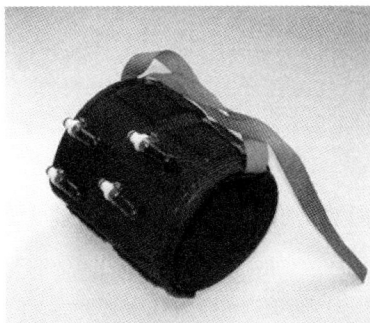

Figure 2. Double cell tourniquet.

in Porto Alegre, Brazil, using 0.5% procaine, and in 1963 by C.M. Holmes, a New Zealander on a Nuffield Dominion Fellowship at Oxford, UK. Holmes used a Gordh needle instead of Bier's cut-down cannula, 40 mL of 0.5% lignocaine instead of procaine and, occasionally, he placed a second tourniquet just below the first over the analgesic area and removed the original one. The following year, J.R. Hoyle introduced a more convenient tourniquet with two narrow cuffs (Figure 2).

Bier had an original and penetrating intellect. In 1892, he successfully treated tuberculous bones and joints with the Esmarch bandage and passive hyperaemia. He was elected to the Fellowship of the Royal College of Surgeons of England in 1913 and became a Privy Councillor with the title of Geheimrat in Germany. He made original contributions to the treatment of amputation stumps, blood transfusion and vascular surgery during the First World War, and invented the steel helmet for German troops.

Bier was also an accomplished classical scholar. In later life, he deviated from the paths of orthodox science and became interested in Heraclite's philosophy of contrasts living in harmony. He planted 750 hectares of mixed forest on his Sauen estate that would eventually become an intricate ecosystem. Nearly one hundred years later, this three-layer mixed forest has improved soil, air, microclimate and water retention. Foresters and ecologists now make pilgrimages to visit Sauen Forest. Bier died on his estate in the Russian zone of Germany, in 1949, aged 88.

Acknowledgement

Portrait photograph reproduced from *Anesthesia and Analgesia* 1970; **49**: 935–40, with permission from Lippincott Williams & Wilkins.

Further reading

Bier AK. Concerning a new method of local anesthesia of the extremities. *Survey of anesthesiology* 1967; **11**: 294–300. (Translated from: Bier A. Ueber einen neuen weg local anasthesia an den gliedmaasen zu erzeugren. *Archiv für Klinische Chirurgie* 1908; **86**: 1007–16.)

Bier AK. Experiments in cocainization of the spinal cord. In: Faulconer A, Keys TE (eds) *Foundations of anesthesiology, Vol II.* Springfield, IL: Charles C Thomas, 1965: 850–7. (Translated from: Bier A. Versuche über cocainisirung des rückenmarkes. *Deutsche Zeitschrift für Chirurgie* 1899; **51**: 361–9.)

Colbern EC. The Bier block for intravenous regional anesthesia: technic and literature review. *Anesthesia and Analgesia* 1970; **49**: 935–40.

JOHN J. BONICA LECTURE
John Joseph Bonica (1917–1994)

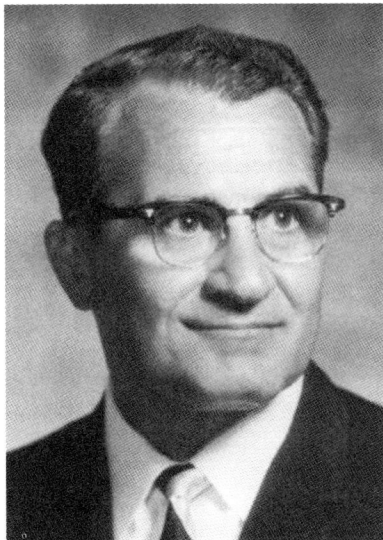

John Bonica was born in 1917 on Filicudi, one of the Aeolian islands off the northeast coast of Sicily. His father visited New York City in 1925 and settled there with his family in 1928. Following his father's death in 1932, Bonica assumed responsibility for the household. His dream was to become a physician and he shone shoes, hawked newspapers and sold fruit and vegetables to earn the money to fund his studies. In high school he took up amateur wrestling and won both city and state championships. He paid his way through Long Island University, New York and Marquette University School of Medicine in Milwaukee, Wisconsin as a professional wrestler, travelling with the carnival during the summers through small towns in the northeast USA. He used the names of 'Johnny (Bull) Walker' (Figure 1), 'Joe Bucha' and 'The Masked Marvel' to avoid recognition by his medical colleagues. He won the light heavyweight championship of Canada in 1939 and was world champion for six months in 1941. He and Emma Louise Baldetti were married in 1942.

Bonica completed a war-accelerated internship (six months) and residency in anaesthesia (18 months) at St Vincent's Hospital in New York City. He joined the US army and at the age of 27 was appointed Chief of Anesthesiology at the 7700-bed Madigan Army Hospital in Fort Lewis, Washington. He taught himself techniques of regional blocks, both for surgery and for pain relief, and used them on more than 10,000 soldiers who had been wounded in action. Their suffering was the initial stimulus for his lifelong dedication to relieving pain in others. Under orders from the surgeon general, he provided three months' anaesthesia training for 60 physicians and six months' anaesthesia training for 100 nurses in two and a half years. He also committed himself to his second pioneering effort – regional anaesthesia for obstetric pain – after his wife nearly died from open drop ether anaesthesia during the birth of their first child.

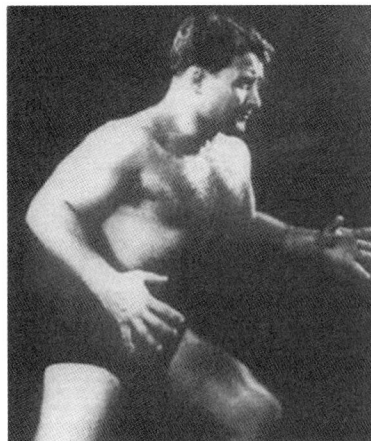

Figure 1. 'Johnny (Bull) Walker', light heavyweight wrestling champion of the world. (Image courtesy of Angela Bonica De Simone.)

In 1947, Bonica became Director of the Department of Anesthesiology at Tacoma General Hospital in Tacoma, Washington where he established the first residency training programme in anaesthesia in the state. He developed a clinical research programme to investigate the effects of regional pain relief, and established a record for obstetric analgesia techniques of zero mortality among mothers and newborns. In 1952, his department became one of the first in a private American hospital to provide a 24-hour medical anaesthesia service in obstetrics, with emphasis on continuous caudal or epidural analgesia.

In 1960, Bonica founded the Department of Anesthesiology at the University of Washington School of Medicine in Seattle, and was its Professor and Chairman for 18 years. In 1961, he opened a new multidisciplinary pain clinic with Dorothy Crowley, a nurse, and Lowell White, a neurosurgeon. Later, faculty members from orthopaedics, psychiatry, rehabilitation, surgery, family medicine, psychology and other disciplines joined the team. This model is now followed worldwide. The department became one of the most prominent in the world for regional anaesthesia techniques in surgery and obstetrics. In 1978, Bonica retired from the chair to promote worldwide research on acute and chronic pain, and to improve its treatment.

Bonica was actively involved with the American Society of Anesthesiologists (ASA) from 1952 and was president in 1966. He helped the ASA to join the World Federation of Societies of Anaesthesiologists in 1960 and was immediately elected to its Executive Committee. He became chairman of its scientific advisory committee, whose primary concern is anaesthesia education in developing countries, and planned its Latin American Anesthesiology Teaching Center in Caracas, Venezuela that opened in 1966. He was secretary-general during 1972–76 and President from 1980 to 1984.

Bonica authored or edited 41 books, contributed to 60 others and published 274 scientific articles, the majority of which were devoted to pain research and therapy, including acupuncture. In 1953, he produced the first edition of his classic *The Management of Pain* – a 1500-page book that later appeared in several languages and became the 'bible' of pain diagnosis and therapy. In it he described acute, chronic and cancer pain problems, reviewed clinical issues, and provided key information on therapeutic options. The second edition was published in 1990 (Figure 2) and the third edition was published in 2001 under the eponymous title *Bonica's Management of Pain*. He completed the second edition of *Principles and Practice of Obstetric Analgesia and Anesthesia* a few weeks before his death in 1994.

Bonica ignited public and political interest in the immense costs to society of acute and chronic pain. Bonica's wrestling career had left him with musculoskeletal problems and chronic pain punctuated by periodic severe

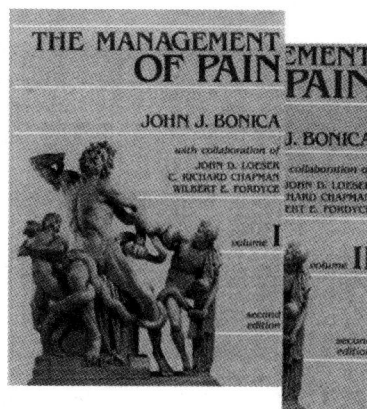

Figure 2. Two-volume second edition of *Management of Pain*.

Table 1. John J. Bonica lecturers and lecture titles

Year	Lecturer	Topic
1984	Edward R. Perl (USA)	Unravelling the story of pain.
1987	Patrick D. Wall (England)	Stability and instability of central pain mechanisms.
1990	Ronald Melzack (Canada)	The gate control theory 25 years later, new perspectives in phantom limb pain.
1993	Jean-Marie Besson (France)	The pharmacology of pain.
1996	Ronald Dubner (USA)	Neural basis of persistent pain; sensory specialization, sensory modulation, and neuronal plasticity.
1999	Erik Torebjork (Sweden)	Subpopulations of human nociceptors and their sensory correlates.

exacerbations. Pain robbed him of sleep, but he never let it interfere with his goals, his responsibilities or his self-imposed writing deadlines. He was a model of sustained courage and dedication to a humanitarian cause.

Bonica organized the First International Symposium on Pain in Seattle in 1973. This led to the creation of the International Association for the Study of Pain (IASP), and he was given the title of Founder and Honorary President. The IASP established the John J. Bonica Trainee Fellowship in 1998 to sup-

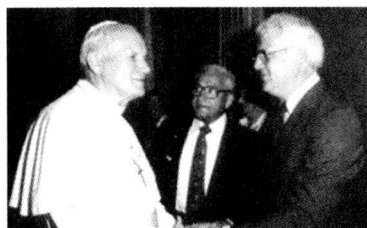

Figure 3. John Bonica and Pope John Paul II with John Liebeskind in the background. (Image courtesy of Angela Bonica De Simone.)

port training in clinical and basic science pain research, and there are eight eponymous lectureships and fellowships worldwide. Bonica's honours included the Distinguished Service Award of the American Society of Anesthesiologists in 1973; Honorary Fellowship of the Faculty of Anaesthetists of the Royal College of Surgeons of England; and Honorary Doctorate of Science Degrees from American and foreign universities. The University of Washington School of Medicine established the John J. and Emma Bonica Endowed Chair for Anesthesiology and Pain Research in 1987. In 1990, Pope John Paul II honoured him for his contribution to the welfare of people worldwide (Figure 3).

The John J. Bonica distinguished lecture was inaugurated in 1984, and is presented every three years at the World Congress on Pain by a person who has made a major contribution to pain research or pain therapy (Table 1).

Acknowledgement

Portrait photograph reproduced with kind permission from the Wood Library–Museum of Anesthesiology, Park Ridge, IL, USA.

Further reading

Bonica JJ. *Principles and practice of obstetric analgesia and anesthesia*, 2nd edn. Baltimore, MD: Williams and Wilkins, 1995.

Loeser J (ed.). *Bonica's management of pain*, 3rd edn. Philadelphia, PA: Lippincott, Williams and Wilkins, 2001.

Moore DC. John J. Bonica, M.D. *Anesthesia History Association Newsletter* 1995; 13 (2): 1, 15–16. (Eulogy)

BOYLE MACHINE
BOYLE–DAVIS GAG
Henry Edmund Gaskin Boyle (1875-1941)

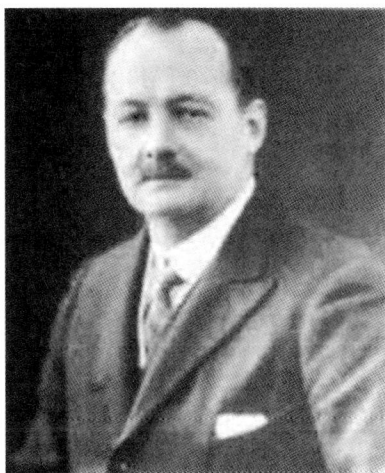

Henry 'Cocky' Boyle was born in Barbados at Porey Springs and educated at Harrison College in Bridgetown. For the remainder of his life, he made his home in England. He entered St Bartholomew's Hospital in London as a medical student in 1894 and gained his MRCS and LRCP in 1901. He worked as a casualty officer at the Bristol Royal Infirmary in Somerset and then returned to St Bartholomew's as junior resident anaesthetist. His career progressed rapidly and he was appointed visiting consultant anaesthetist to St Bartholomew's Hospital in 1903, and subsequently also to Paddington Green Children's Hospital and St Andrew's Hospital, Dollis Hill in London. Although he did not serve in France himself, his work caring for wounded soldiers as part of the Royal Army Medical Corps during the First World War in London was recognized and he was awarded the OBE for war service.

Anaesthesia at St Bartholomew's in the early years of the 20th century had developed little from the drop bottle and lint, except for a nitrous oxide and ether induction. As the patient lost consciousness, the ether was gradually turned on and the nitrous oxide discontinued. Adequate oxygenation was obtained by periodic lifting of the face piece to allow a full inspiration of room air. If the procedure lasted more than half an hour, the anaesthetist changed to open drop chloroform because prolonged ether was believed to cause pulmonary complications. The practice remained much the same until the First World War.

During the early part of the war, Boyle promoted nitrous oxide oxygen ether anaesthesia. He felt that the old 'rag and bottle' methods, good and useful as they had been, were outdated. About 1916 he persuaded the hospital to import the first Gwathmey nitrous oxide oxygen ether machine from the USA. These machines tended to develop mechanical defects, especially leakage at the gas unions. Boyle designed his own machine, using some additional ideas of Geoffrey Marshall (1887–1982). Boyle's left-handedness led to the arrangement of flow meters and vaporizers that is still used today. His early machine consisted of a somewhat clumsy and heavy wooden box with two metal crossbars from which four cylinders hung. The 'bubble-bottle' and the ether container were just above them (Figure 1). An early difficulty was the tendency for the nitrous oxide, which was not particularly pure or dry, to

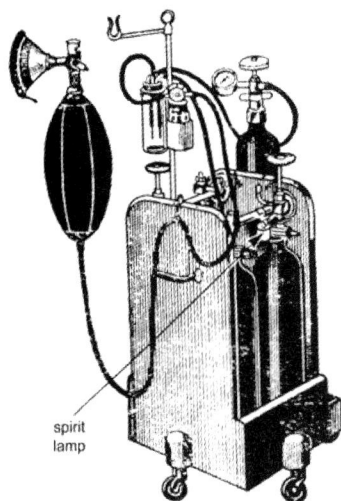

Figure 1. Boyle machine, 1917, with small spirit lamp to prevent icing in the nitrous oxide valve. (Reproduced from *Anaesthesia* 1968; 23: 103–18.)

freeze up at the reducing valve. A small metal spirit lamp was suspended so that its open flame warmed the valve – even though the ether container was only a few inches away.

The original Boyle machine was improved step by step (Figure 2, Table 1). The Boyle eponym survives in some countries, but most anaesthetic machines now carry the name of a national or multinational manufacturer and a model number. Boyle himself never received any monetary benefit from his design. The nitrous oxide oxygen ether technique quickly spread at St Bartholomew's. It was generally reserved for operations during which the anaesthetist had access to the face. One of Boyle's chief contributions to the technique was his use and promotion of endotracheal methods of delivery. At the same time he was perfecting and promoting the use of gas and oxygen in midwifery.

An important event in Boyle's life was his visit to Canada and the USA in 1921. He landed in New York where he visited James Gwathmey (1863–1944) and attended the first meeting of the Canadian Society of Anaesthetists in Niagara, Ontario. He travelled extensively in both countries and made lasting friendships with leading American and Canadian anaesthetists. Among the various ideas and appliances that he brought back was the Davis gag for dissection tonsillectomy, which he introduced to British ear, nose and throat surgeons (Figure 3). He made some slight modifications and the Boyle-Davis gag is still extensively used today.

Table 1. Evolution of the Boyle machine 1917–65

1917	Gas control by fine adjustment valve on cylinder, perforated metal tubes in 'bubble bottle' for water sight-feed meter.
1920	Chloroform bottle added.
1926	By-pass controls for regulating ether or chloroform vapour.
1930	Warm water jacket for ether bottle.
1931–33	Coxeter dry bobbin meter – gas specific glass tubes with holes. Pressure reducing regulators, Adams for oxygen, Endurance for nitrous oxide.
1937	Rotameter flow meters (not universal until after the Second World War). By-pass levers for nitrous oxide and oxygen, later only oxygen.
1939	Colour coded assemblies for each gas.
1941	Coxeter–Mushin circle absorber.
1953	Colour coded gas cylinders.
1955	Non-interchangeable pin index yokes and valves on cylinders.
1958	Bodok seal replaced washer between gas cylinder and pressure regulator.
1965	British Standard couplings from outlet of anaesthetic machine to face mask or endotracheal tube.

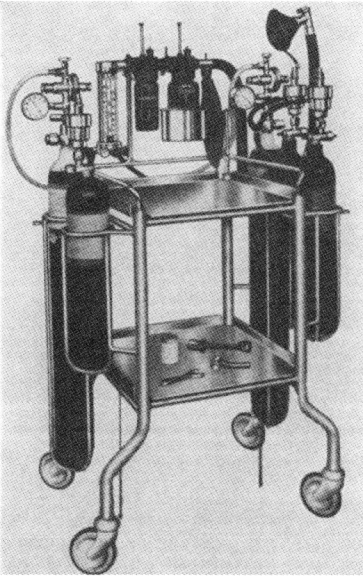

Figure 2. Boyle machine c. 1933, fitted with Coxeter bobbin meter and water bath for ether bottle vaporiser. (Reproduced from *Anaesthesia* 1968; 23: 103–18.)

Boyle was an interesting and stimulating lecturer, however, he relied on the practical instruction he gave in the operating theatres to carry on the old tradition that a 'Barts' man could always be relied upon to give a decent anaesthetic. The simple principles that he taught were well set out in an excellent and popular textbook called *Practical Anaesthetics*. Although Boyle never claimed any special scientific ability, his enthusiasm and drive did much to improve the standing of anaesthesia and anaesthetists in the first half of the 20th century.

He was a member of the original Society of Anaesthetists that was founded in London in 1893, President of the Section of Anaesthetics of the Royal Society of Medicine in 1923, a founding member of the editorial board of the *British Journal of Anaesthesia* and of the Association of Anaesthetists of Great Britain and Ireland. He was granted the Diploma in Anaesthetics without examination (but not without fee), and was one of the first pair of examiners in 1935. The Council of the Royal College of Surgeons elected him to its Fellowship without examination.

For many years Boyle's small and somewhat antiquated Saxon car was a familiar sight about the hospital and the West End of London. It hardly looked big enough to contain his heavy and bulky apparatus and his somewhat heavy and bulky self. He was a keen Mason and was at one time Master of the Rahere Lodge. A lifelong friend described him as 'a grand fellow, generous in the extreme, and one of the best of colleagues'.

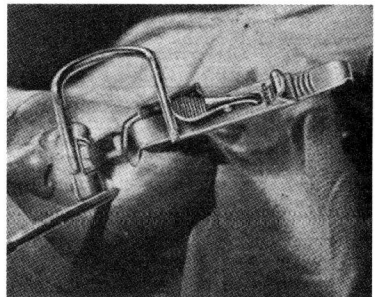

Figure 3. Boyle's 1922 version of the gag designed by Davis in America. (Reproduced from *Lancet*, 1922; 2: 1130. Elsevier Science.)

Acknowledgement

Portrait photograph reproduced with kind permission from the Wood Library–Museum of Anesthesiology, Park Ridge, IL, USA.

Further reading

Boyle HE. A combined gag and tongue retractor. *Lancet* 1922; 2: 1130.

Watt OM. The evolution of the Boyle apparatus 1917–67. *Anaesthesia* 1968; 23: 103–18.

Wilkinson DJ. Henry Edmund Gaskin Boyle (1875–1941). In: Diz JC. *Proceedings of the Fifth International Symposium on the History of Anesthesia*. Amsterdam, The Netherlands: Elsevier Science 2002.

LARYNGEAL MASK AIRWAY

Archie Brain (1942–)

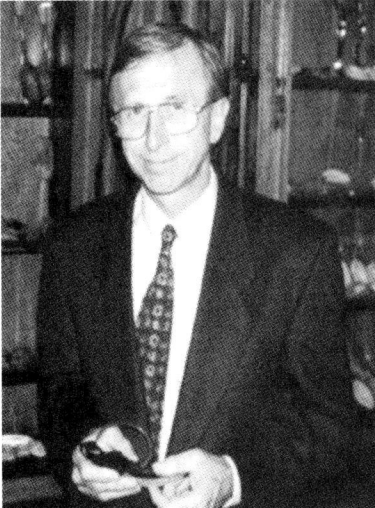

Archie Brain was born in Kobe, Japan in July 1942, son of Sir Norman and Lady Brain, British diplomats who were at that time interned there. They were allowed to leave on a Red Cross ship shortly afterwards and survived the perilous journey home to England. Brain attended the Benedictine College of Ampleforth in Yorkshire and won a scholarship to Worcester College, Oxford in 1959 to study modern languages and literature. He had a facility for languages, track athletics, spectacular absent-mindedness and winning poetry prizes, although his achievements in the sciences were notably lacking. However, after gaining his degree in 1963, he stayed on at Oxford to study basic sciences, attended the Radcliffe Infirmary as a medical student, and completed his clinical studies in 1970 at St Bartholomew's Hospital.

Brain embarked on his career in anaesthesia in Hastings, East Sussex, where the consultants were excellent and enthusiastic teachers. He obtained the Diploma in Anaesthetics within one year and in 1973, while still at registrar level, he was appointed as the sole anaesthetist in a busy five-theatre general hospital in Heemstede, The Netherlands. Brain found himself in charge of equipping and then running the whole department on his own. He stayed for four years, having been joined after 18 months by John Walker, an experienced Scottish anaesthetist. During this time he learned to speak what he describes as the 'infernally difficult' Dutch tongue and obtained the Irish Fellowship (FFARCSI).

By now married, Brain accepted a two-year contract as anaesthetist to the Seychelles Government under an Overseas Development Agency scheme, during which time his first daughter was born. He returned home in 1980 to start work at The (now Royal) London Hospital as a lecturer under Jimmy Payne. For the first time in his career, Brain found his work schedule conducive to exploring ideas that had been fermenting while he gained practical experience overseas. Within six months, he had filed 12 patent applications and started a diary of research projects.

Brain developed the concept of the laryngeal mask airway in 1980, having become disillusioned with endotracheal intubation. Face mask anaesthesia did not always provide a reliable seal or clear airway while intubation, long regarded as the gold standard for prevention of pulmonary aspiration, could lead to trauma, oesophageal or bronchial intubation and unwanted reflex responses. He wanted to make airway management less traumatic and more physiological. If the respiratory tree were seen as a tube beginning at the glottis, it seemed logical to make an end-to-end junction at this point. The space around and behind the glottis was adapted to the presence of food and liquid, and was likely to tolerate an inflated cuff with less reflex response than the trachea. He thought the new airway design was likely to overcome airway obstruction quickly and easily and to be atraumatic in unskilled hands.

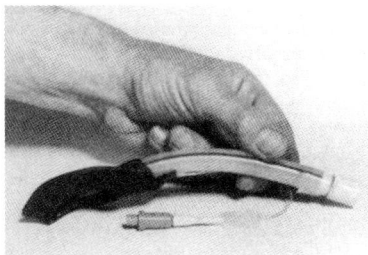

Figure 1. Prototype laryngeal mask made from Goldman nasal mask and Portex endotracheal tube. (Reproduced from *European Journal of Anaesthesiology* 1991, **Suppl 4**: 5-17.)

Plaster casts of the cadaver pharynx were roughly boat-shaped, similar to the Goldman nasal mask that Brain used for outpatient dental anaesthesia. He made his first laryngeal mask airway (LMA) prototype by joining the cuff of a Goldman nasal mask to the diagonally cut end of a 10 mm Portex endotracheal tube using acrylic adhesive. A pilot tube was inserted into a port at the narrower end of the cuff that became the proximal end of the LMA cuff, while the wider end was narrowed to fit the pharynx (Figure 1). He conducted a pilot study of three of these prototypes in 23 patients, including 16 gynaecological laparoscopies; positive pressure ventilation was used successfully in each case. He described the LMA as an alternative to the facemask or endotracheal tube, to be used with either spontaneous or positive pressure ventilation.

Payne urged him to continue his work on the LMA, even in the absence of commercial interest. Brain constructed many hundreds of prototypes while working as consultant anaesthetist at Newham General Hospital in London's East End where he had one small room that served as a laboratory. At one stage a hospital cleaner reported that he was manufacturing exotic rubber condoms. He used a variety of materials, including latex, and incorporated a posterior groove or tube in some models as an escape for regurgitated gastric fluid. He tested his models in approximately 7000 patients over the next seven years. When John Nunn from Northwick Park Hospital in Harrow, Middlesex recognized the potential of the device, serious efforts were made to manufacture it.

In February 1988, Brain demonstrated the first commercially made silicone model (Figure 2) to Colin Alexander, consultant anaesthetist in Hastings where Brain had given his first anaesthetic. Alexander and colleagues published the first description of the definitive LMA. Within 12 months of its release, more than 500 British hospitals were using the LMA, now designated the LMA-Classic.

After a year with Nunn at Northwick Park as a guest worker, in 1991 Brain joined

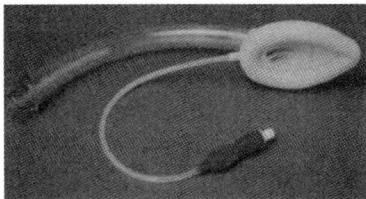

Figure 2. LMA-Classic.

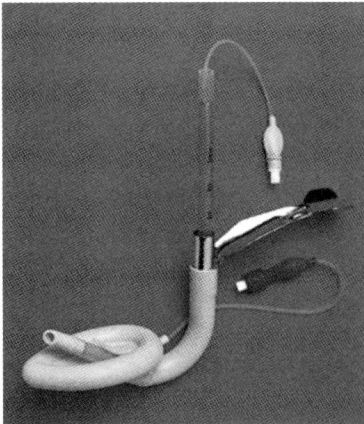

Figure 3. Intubating LMA-FasTrach.

the Royal Berkshire Hospital in Reading, Berkshire as an honorary consultant. He continued to develop new forms of laryngeal mask and became increasingly involved in teaching overseas visitors and lecturing around the world. The flexible LMA with armoured tube for head and neck surgery was released in 1993. With the help of the radiology department in Reading, magnetic resonance imaging (MRI) measurements paved the way for the development of the intubating LMA, completed in 1997 (Figure 3).

Meanwhile, Brain and a consultant colleague at the Royal Berkshire Hospital, Chandy Verghese, were testing many forms of double-tube LMA that allowed gastric drainage through one tube while an added posterior cuff allowed airway pressures up to 40 cm water. These culminated in completion of the LMA-ProSeal in 1999 (Figure 4). This device came closer to fulfilling Brain's original aim, which had always been to provide an airway device that would avoid the physiological disadvantages of the endotracheal tube and isolate the respiratory tract from the gastrointestinal tract.

Brain has received the Dudley Buxton Medal of the Royal College of Anaesthetists, and he was elected an Honorary Fellow in 2000, a very rare distinction for a British subject. The Association of Anaesthetists of Great Britain and Ireland awarded him the third Magill Gold Medal, its highest award, in 1995.

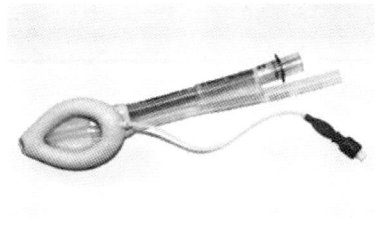

Figure 4. Double lumen LMA-ProSeal with gastric drainage tube.

Further reading

Brain AI. The development of the laryngeal mask – a brief history of the invention, early clinical studies and experimental work from which the laryngeal mask evolved. *European Journal of Anaesthesiology* 1991, **Suppl 4**: 5–17.

Brain AI. The laryngeal mask—a new concept in airway management. *British Journal of Anaesthesia* 1983; **55**: 801–5.

Brain AI, Verghese C, Strube PJ. The LMA 'ProSeal'—a laryngeal mask with an oesophageal vent. *British Journal of Anaesthesia* 2000; **84**: 650–4.

BROMAGE SCORE FOR MOTOR BLOCKADE

Philip Raikes Bromage (1920–)

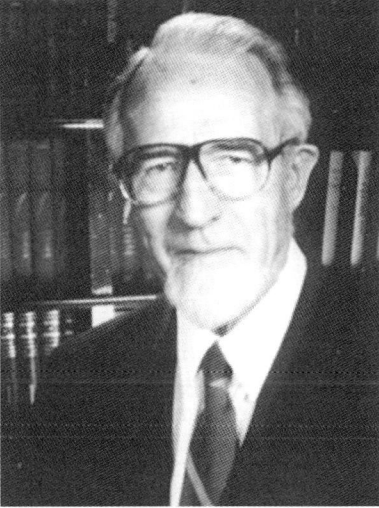

Philip Bromage was born in Richmond, London in 1920, son of Richard Raikes Bromage, an Anglican clergyman who converted to the Roman Catholic Church. His mother, Mary Hamill, came from a family of distinguished physicians on the staff of various London teaching hospitals. They were somewhat awesome figures in a world that seemed remote and unattainable to the young boy. After spending one year with relatives in South Africa, his early ambitions focused on becoming an orange farmer there. However, by his early teens, reality dawned on him. He was educated at the Benedictine College of Ampleforth in Yorkshire and, in 1938, he enrolled as a medical student at St. Thomas's Hospital in London. He graduated in medicine in 1943 and completed house officer appointments (1943–44) in ear, nose and throat surgery and orthopaedics under the great teachers George Perkins and Rowley Bristoe.

Although he was rejected for military service on medical grounds, Bromage was allowed to take the Royal Army Medical Corps short course in tropical medicine and then join the Merchant Navy (with its less rigorous selection criteria). He became a ship's surgeon on a cargo steamer converted to troop-carrying under South-East Asia command in the Burma campaign. During that time, the value of regional anaesthesia for single-handed surgery became obvious to him.

Following the end of Japanese hostilities in 1945, Bromage took an ex-service general medical post at the Municipal Hospital at Southend-on-Sea, Essex where he came under the spell of Alfred Lee. His duties included giving emergency anaesthetics at night and, being inexperienced, he ran into problems. Lee was the consultant anaesthetist, and gave Bromage some informal lessons. Lee did a large proportion of his cases under all sorts of regional anaesthesia. He was also correcting the page proofs for the first edition of *A Synopsis of Anaesthesia* – a work that has been the constant companion of British anaesthesia trainees since that time. Bromage's experience with Lee took away all thoughts of his becoming a surgeon and converted him to a career in anaesthesia. This encounter with a scholarly preceptor and a master of technique relit his enthusiasm for regional anaesthesia. Lee always insisted on disciplined documentation of technical details and clinical outcomes as basic elements of sound anaesthetic practice.

Two further registrar positions followed, one at the West Middlesex Hospital in Isleworth, Middlesex where most upper abdominal surgery was done with patients awake under a combination of bilateral intercostal and splanchnic blocks. There, with the combined essentials of anaesthesia induction rooms, efficient manpower management and swift, gentle and skilled surgery, three gastrectomies could be done routinely between lunchtime and formal afternoon tea in patients who were awake. The surgeon, always courteous, would take his patients by the hand as they left the operating room, pain-free and already starting their deep breathing and leg exercises.

The development of continuous segmental epidural analgesia created an opportunity to extend pain-free postoperative physical therapy to include ultra-early ambulation within a few hours of major abdominal or thoracic surgery (Figure 1). Two conditions had to be satisfied to make this feasible. First, proof was needed that effective bilateral analgesia was restricted to the thoracic segments, as tested by ice or pin-prick. Second, and as a prelude to safe, ultra-early ambulation, some simple bedside tests were needed to document that coordination and muscle power of the legs were adequate to prevent them buckling and causing a fall when the patient attempted to stand and walk. Thus, the technique required that adequate sensory and motor neural function be retained in spinal segments L2 to S3, supplying nerves to the joints and muscles of the legs and feet.

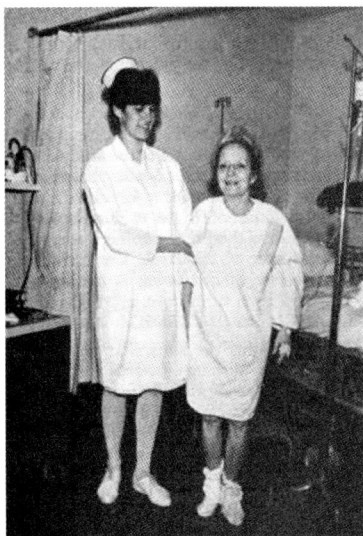

Figure 1. A 63-year-old woman walking comfortably three hours after common bile duct exploration (1967). She had a mid-thoracic epidural with 4 mL of 2% carbonated lignocaine with analgesia T4-T11. (Reproduced from *British Journal of Anaesthesia* 1967; 39: 721-9.)

As the basis for such tests, Bromage adopted four criteria (Figure 2) to score the intensity of lower limb functional impairment – this became known as the Bromage scoring system. Clearly, safe, ultra-early ambulation requires restriction of sensory blockade to the thoracic and first lumbar segments and a score of zero. Failing that, active exercises can still be done in bed and achieve scores of two or three. A block-intensity score of zero in the legs, with satisfactory anaesthetic conditions for thoracic and upper abdominal surgery without the routine use of muscle-relaxants, can be achieved. However, this requires a reversal of contemporary practice away from large-volume epidural infusions of dilute local anaesthetic and a return to the earlier regime of small volumes of surgical concentrations delivered at the appropriate segments in the mid to upper thoracic region.

Bromage held consultant posts in Portsmouth, Hampshire and Chichester, West Sussex from 1948 to 1955, during which he published the first edition of *Epidural Anaesthesia*. In 1956 he moved to Montreal where Harold Griffith had drawn worldwide attention with his work on curare 14 years earlier. Bromage believed that regional anaesthesia offered something valuable and different, especially in the days of bloody thoracoplasties under general anaesthesia. This surgical procedure provided the opportunity to study differing anaesthetic philosophies and clinical outcomes. The 'de-efferenters' used curare to block efferent nerve impulses at the neuromuscular junction and other drugs to suppress efferent autonomic impulses. Bromage and the 'de-afferenters' used local anaesthetics to protect the central nervous system by blocking afferent sensory impulses. They rejuvenated Crile's First World War concept of a protective anaesthetic shield and encouraged early pain-free ambulation after major surgery.

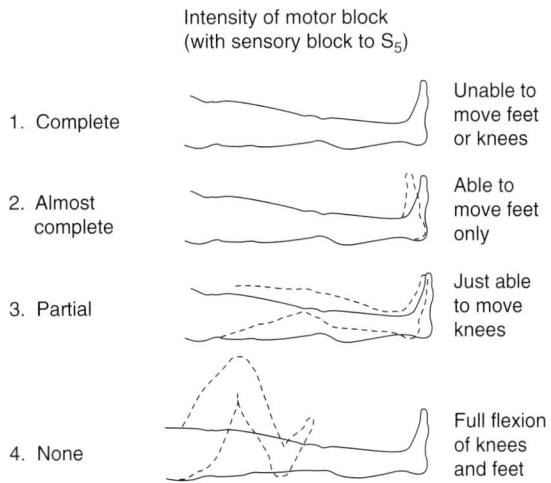

Figure 2. Assessment of intensity of motor blockade with sensory block to S5. (Reproduced from *Acta Anaesthesiologica Scandinavica 1965*, (Suppl XVI), with permission from Munksgaard International Publishers Ltd, Copenhagen, Denmark.)

Bromage was professor and chairman, McGill department of anaesthesia, Montreal during 1970–77, and post-retirement professor from 1991 to the present. He left Montreal for Durham, North Carolina in 1977, and published the second edition of *Epidural Analgesia* in 1978. He continued academic and clinical work in Denver, Colorado; Riyadh, Saudi Arabia; and Philadelphia, Pennsylvania until he retired from clinical anaesthesia in 1991.

His many honours include Doctorat Honoris Causa, Université Catholique de Louvain, Belgium (with Mother Teresa of Calcutta); the James Young Simpson Gold Medallist, Royal College of Surgeons of Edinburgh in 1982; the Gaston Labat Award of the American Society of Regional Anesthesia in 1984; Hickman Medallist, Royal Society of Medicine in 1987; the Carl Koller Medal of the European Society of Regional Anaesthesia in 1989 and the Canadian Anaesthetists' Society Gold Medal in 1995.

Acknowledgement

Portrait photograph reproduced with kind permission from McGill University Department of Anesthesia, Montreal, Canada.

Further reading

Bromage PR. A comparison of the hydrochloride and carbon dioxide salts of lidocaine and prilocaine in epidural analgesia. *Acta Anaesthesiologica Scandinavica* 1965; **Suppl XVI**: 55–69.

Bromage PR. Extradural analgesia for pain relief. *British Journal of Anaesthesia* 1967; **39**: 721–9.

Cleland JGP. Continuous peridural analgesia in surgery and early ambulation. *Northwest Medicine* 1949; **48**: 26–34.

CARLENS CATHETER

Eric Carlens (1908–1990)

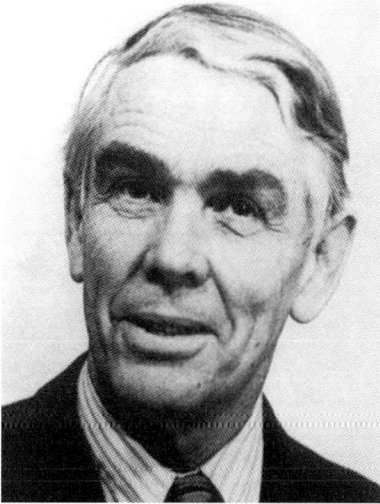

Henry Head (1861–1940), a physiologist and neurologist at The (now Royal) London Hospital in England devised the first double-lumen tube in 1889. He designed it to separate gas flows in and out of the right and left lungs during physiological experiments in a dog, and did not use it for clinical investigation in patients. He bent a fine metal cannula, to which he soldered a finer metal tube, and tied an inflatable endobronchial cuff, made of thin India rubber tubing, below the bend (Figure 1). He then attached a short piece of wide bore brass tubing to the proximal end of the cannula to lie in the trachea when the whole device was inserted through a tracheotomy. The next development came 60 years later.

Eric Carlens, who designed the Carlens double-lumen catheter, was born in Stockholm, Sweden in 1908. His father was a pharmacist and he had one sister who was a few years older than himself. When he finished school, he was diagnosed with renal tuberculosis and spent one year in a sanatorium. After that, he started his medical studies in Stockholm. Despite his earlier illness, he took part in many sports, especially rowing, where he was in the team that won the Swedish championship. He graduated in 1934 and worked in several of Stockholm's hospitals. Like many doctors at that time, he had to work without a salary for two years before he got an appointment to start his training to become an ear, nose and throat specialist at Danderyd Hospital. He defended his thesis on pneumococci in otitis media in 1943 at the Karolinska Institute.

In 1944, Carlens moved to Sabbatsberg Hospital, where he came in contact with the thoracic surgeons Clarence Crafoord (1899–1984, chief surgeon), Viking Björk and

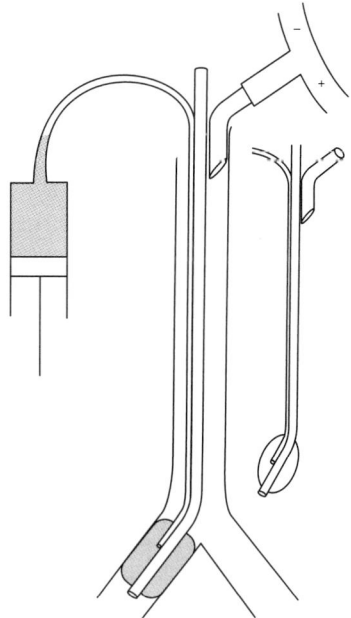

Figure 1. Head's double-lumen tube for separating right and left lung ventilation in a dog. (Reproduced from *Journal of Physiology* 1889; 10: 1–70.)

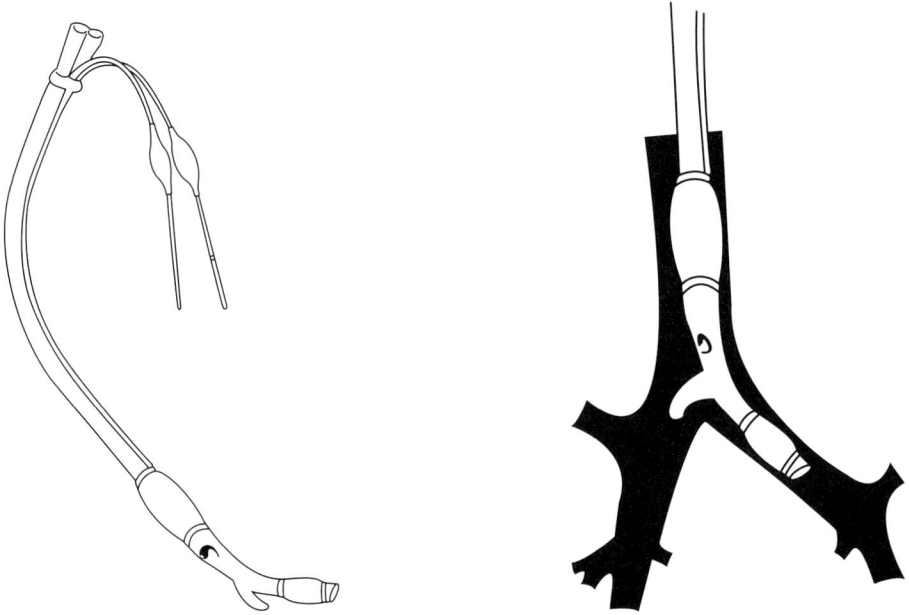

Figure 2. (Left) Carlens double-lumen tube, (right) correct position in left main bronchus. (Reproduced with permission from *General anaesthesia*, 3rd edn, London: Butterworths, 1971: 226.)

Åke Senning. Carlens and his colleagues at the department of clinical physiology became involved in the preoperative evaluation of patients, including bronchospirometry, before lung surgery. In 1948, Norris and colleagues described passing a cuffed, armoured, latex, single-lumen, 22–26 French gauge catheter into the left main bronchus under fluoroscopic control. This provided an airway to the left lung, and ventilation to the right lung was around the catheter and through the larynx. Carlens found fluoroscopy time-consuming and not always satisfactory. In 1949, he constructed a left-sided, double-lumen rubber tube with a carinal hook for use under topical anaesthesia (Figure 2). Each lumen was D-shaped in cross section, 7 mm diameter for men and 6 mm for women. The right lumen ended just above the carinal hook to provide ventilation to the right lung, and the left lumen extended as a cuffed, endobronchial tube that terminated above the orifice of the upper lobe bronchus.

Carlens inserted the catheter under topical anaesthesia. He sprayed 2% pantocaine in to the pharynx, followed by instillation to the larynx, trachea and larger bronchi, with the patient sitting facing him. He placed a curved metal stylet into the bronchial channel of the catheter and tied the carinal hook to the catheter with a moistened silk thread slipknot. He then passed the catheter through the larynx under indirect laryngoscopy (Figure 3), released the slipknot and advanced the catheter into the left main bronchus until he felt the hook on the carina. He then inflated the tracheal and bronchial cuffs. He reported the first 60 bronchospirometric examinations with no failures and no complications.

Carlens's double-lumen catheter offered advantages over a single-lumen endobronchial tube or endotracheal tube and bronchial blocker for thoracic surgery. The anaesthetist could control ventilation to each lung, including collapse of the operative lung, which enabled the development of new thoracic surgical techniques. It also provided for efficient control of secretions and prevented spread of infected material from the diseased lung to the healthy lung. The next year, Björk and Carlens

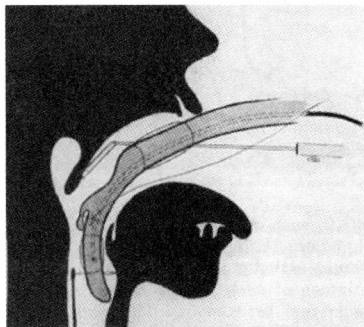

Figure 3. Carlens's insertion technique under topical anaesthesia. (Reproduced from *Anesthesiology* 1953; 14: 60–72, with permission from Lippincott Williams & Wilkins.)

used the catheter to prevent such spillover of infectious material during wedge resections for tuberculosis. In 1952, Björk, Carlens and Friberg reported its use in 500 lung resections.

In 1957, Carlens and many others moved with Crafoord to the newly formed Cardiothoracic Center at the Karolinska Hospital, situated in a new building named the Thoracic Clinics. He was appointed professor at the Karolinska Institute in 1960, and worked there until his official retirement in 1973 and for a number of years after.

In 1959 he made his second original contribution, mediastinoscopy, which he described as a method for inspection and tissue biopsy in the superior mediastinum. Taking biopsies from the superior mediastinum became a safe procedure, and major surgery could be avoided in many patients who could not be operated on due to the spread of the tumour. In 1965, mediastinoscopy also made possible the first placement, without a thoracotomy, of pacemaker electrodes on the atrium. Today computer tomography and percutaneous placement of atrial electrodes have replaced mediastinoscopy.

After his retirement Carlens continued to be active – in his own words as an 'armchair scientist' – especially in his fight against smoking. He had become a smoker in the 1940s when he was writing his thesis and inspecting his colonies of pneumococci in the laboratory. He had difficulty keeping awake and his chief advised him to start smoking: "It will keep you from falling asleep!" Carlens had already stopped smoking when the first reports of increased incidence of lung cancer in smokers appeared. When a publication appeared in 1962 from the Royal College of Surgeons in London called *Tobacco and Health*, Carlens commented sarcastically that it should rather be called 'Tobacco or Health'. He wrote articles in the local press and in medical journals to point out the enormously increased risk for smokers of developing lung cancer if they were also exposed to asbestos or radon.

Carlens was a clinician, famous for his experience and knowledge in the diseases of the oesophagus and trachea and for his skills as an endoscopist.

He looked upon himself as a coordinator for pneumologists, histologists, surgeons and epidemiologists. He was an extremely kind and sympathetic person, highly esteemed and loved by patients and co-workers at all levels. In his free time he took a great interest in art and enjoyed visiting galleries and exhibitions.

Acknowledgement

Portrait photograph from 'Thoracic and cardiovascular surgery at the Karolinska Institute', Almqvist & Wiksell International, Stockholm, 1978, with kind permission from Christian Olin (editor).

Further reading

Björk VO, Carlens E, Friberg O. Endobronchial anesthesia. Anesthesiology 1953; 14: 60–72.

Carlens E. New flexible double-lumen catheter for bronchospirometry. Journal of Thoracic Surgery 1949; 18: 742–6.

Head H. On the regulation of respiration. Journal of Physiology 1889; 10: 1–70.

JOSEPH CLOVER LECTURE

Joseph Thomas Clover (1825-1882)

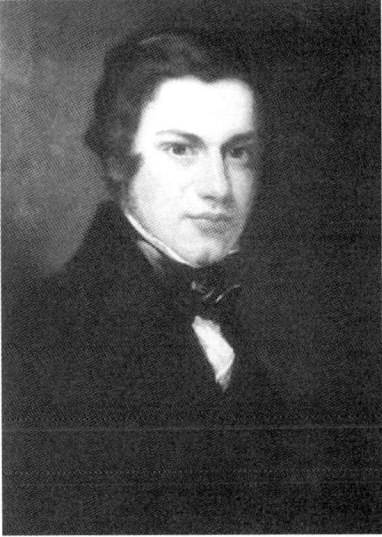

Joseph Thomas Clover was born in Aylesham, Norfolk in 1825 and was educated at the Gray Friar's Priory School in Norwich. When he was 16, he was apprenticed as a surgical dresser to a local surgeon, Charles Gibson. He entered University College Hospital (UCH) in London as a medical student in 1844, and graduated with distinction in 1846.

His personal papers for the preanaesthetic period 1841-46 contain brief notes describing 140 operative procedures. Most of these were amputations and lithotomies, although mastectomies and repairs of incarcerated hernias were regularly mentioned. There is a gap in Clover's notes for a few weeks before 21 December 1846, the day on which William Squires anaesthetized Frederick Churchill with ether at UCH for a leg amputation, and it is uncertain whether he was present.

Clover was house surgeon to James Syme (1799-1870) who, when he was moving to Edinburgh, invited Clover to be his assistant. Clover preferred to stay in London and became resident medical officer at UCH for five years, occasionally giving anaesthetics as part of his surgical duties. He passed the FRCS examination in 1850. In 1853, he entered private practice at 3, Cavendish Place where he lived for the rest of his life. He practiced for five years in general medicine, anaesthesia and urology and developed lithotrity blades to crush stones, an aspirating syringe to retrieve the fragments and a leg restraint for use during lithotomy.

Finding the life of general practice too arduous, Clover obtained appointments at UCH, Westminster Hospital and the London Dental Hospital as an anaesthetist. He became so busy that he provided over 20,000 anaesthetics in his career despite time-consuming travel by horse-drawn carriage between the hospitals and the residences of private patients. He anaesthetised socially prominent figures, including the Princess of Wales (later Queen Alexandra), Sir Robert Peel, Sir Erasmus Wilson, Florence Nightingale and the deposed Napoleon III. Unlike John Snow, Clover mentioned few details of anaesthetic administrations in his notes.

Clover realised that chloroform was safer when administered in known concentrations, and he improved on Snow's bag. Clover's bag (Figure 1) was made from waterproof silk cloth and shaped like a large pillowcase.

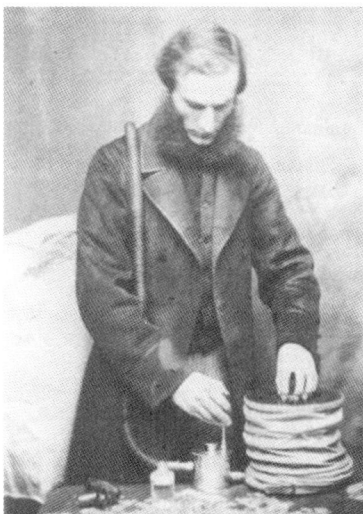

Figure 1. Clover filling the large reservoir bag with 4.5% chloroform vapour in air. (Reproduced from Barts and The London NHS Trust, London.)

The nozzle of the concertina bellows fitted into a metallic box vaporizer that contained a metallic hot water bottle. Blotting paper covered the outside of the bottle to provide a large evaporation surface area for chloroform, which was injected through a cork from a graduated glass syringe. The capacity of the concertina bellows was 1000 cubic inches (16 litres). Clover pumped that volume of air through the vaporizer as he injected 2.4 mL of chloroform, and repeated this procedure three or four times to fill the bag with 4.5% chloroform vapour. This was sufficiently strong to anaesthetize any patient within four minutes.

Rather than place the bag on the floor in the way of the surgeon, he suspended it from the back of his collar. He disconnected the large-bore flexible tube from the vaporizer and connected it to a facemask that had thin ivory inspiratory and expiratory valves supported by springs. There was an aperture in the mask to dilute the vapour or to give pure air. In 1868, he reported no deaths in 1802 administrations, although later he had one death that he attributed to his error in calculating the dilution of the chloroform. Despite the scientific ingenuity and accuracy of his bag, it was never popular.

The Royal Medical and Chirurgical Society (now the Royal Society of Medicine) established a committee in 1864 to investigate chloroform deaths. Clover was an expert assistant and conducted numerous animal experiments. Although the committee considered that his apparatus was the best available and concluded that chloroform mixtures were safe, Clover himself counselled that the pulse must be continuously observed during anaesthesia (Figure 2), and the anaesthetic discontinued temporarily should irregularities or diminished pulse volumes be noted: 'If the finger be taken from the pulse to do something else, I would give a little air'.

In 1868, T.W. Evans, an American dental surgeon practising in Paris, France, gave demonstrations of nitrous oxide anaesthesia in London. Its effectiveness and safety

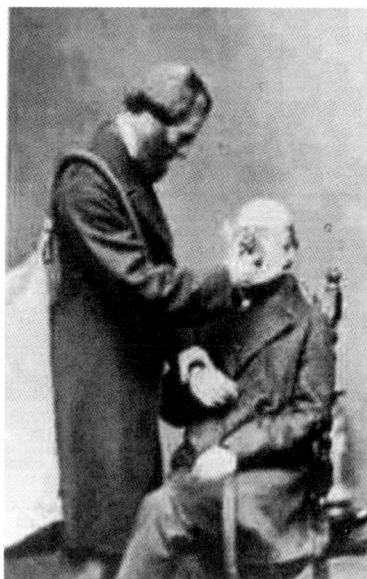

Figure 2. Clover demonstrating how he administered chloroform, with a finger on the patient's pulse. (Reproduced from Nuffield Department of Anaesthetics, Oxford.)

impressed Clover, although 'the appearance of the patients, their lividity and convulsive movements' alarmed him. Clover used his own chloroform bag and added a supplementary 200 cubic inches (3.3 L) reservoir bag near the face mask. This was opened via a stopcock after the first six or seven breaths from the main bag. He used a nasal mask to provide continuous nitrous oxide anaesthesia during dental surgery, but found that he often needed to add chloroform. Clover continued to take an interest in newer agents, especially ethidene dichloride, and in the effectiveness of different methods of artificial respiration.

In 1874, he began to introduce a series of ether inhalers for use in a nitrous oxide ether sequence and, through his success, ether came back to prominent use. He claimed the advantages were rapid response, regulated control of anaesthetic concentration and greater economic value. Many hospitals purchased these inhalers. John Nunn's reassessment of Clover's equipment nearly one century later proved that Clover's patients experienced both hypercapnia and hypoxia. However, these effects of rebreathing were minimized because Clover lifted the mask regularly to allow the patients to breathe room air. In 1877, Clover introduced his compact and robust 'portable regulating ether inhaler' (Figure 3), which was later modified by inventors, including Louis Ombrédanne (1871–1956), and used until the Second World War.

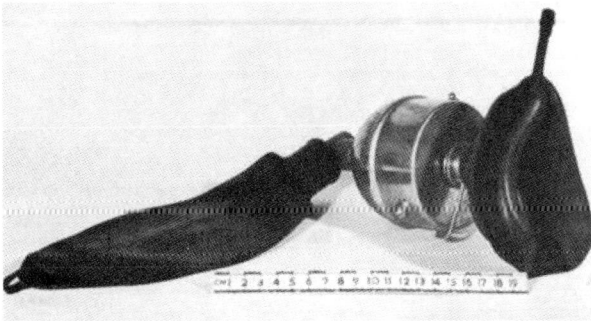

Figure 3. Clover's original portable regulating ether inhaler. (Reproduced with permission from *The development of anaesthetic apparatus*, Blackwell Scientific Publications, 1975: 17.)

Clover died of uraemia aged 57 years. He is buried near John Snow in Brompton Cemetery in London. His obituary in the *Lancet* paid him the rare but apt tribute that 'he became the companion of leading surgeons at some of their most important operations'.

In 1949, The Royal College of Surgeons established the annual Joseph Clover Lecture in recognition of his contributions as a clinician, inventor, author and leading anaesthetist in the Victorian era (Table 1). The lecture was given annually until 1958 and biennially since then, alternating with the Sir Frederick Hewitt Lecture.

Acknowledgements

Portrait photograph reproduced with kind permission from The Royal College of Anaesthetists.

Table 1. The Joseph Clover lecturers and lecture titles

Year	Lecturer	Title
1949	Archibald D. Marston	The life and achievements of Joseph Thomas Clover.
1950	John Gillies	Anaesthetic factors in the causation and prevention of excessive bleeding during surgical operations.
1951	Robert J. Minnitt	Some factors reviewed which influence the reassessment of ether as an anaesthetic agent.
1952	Robert R. Macintosh	Antecedents of early anaesthetic apparatus.
1953	Edgar A. Pask	James Brown.
1954	T. Cecil Gray	Disintegration of the nervous system.
1955	William W. Mushin	Measurement in anaesthesia.
1956	Kenneth W. Donald	The gaseous environment.
1957	Sir James R. Learmonth	A surgeon's outlook.
1958	William D.M. Paton	Mechanisms of transmission in the central nervous system.
1960	J. Alfred Lee	Joseph Clover and the contribution of surgery to anaesthesia.
1962	Geoffrey S.W. Organe	The development of intravenous anaesthesia.
1964	Emmanuel Papper	The impact of man, machines and mechanisms on the clinical practice of anaesthesia.
1966	Andrew R. Hunter	Old unhappy far off things.
1968	John F. Nunn	The evolution of atmospheric oxygen.
1970	James P. Payne	The quality of measurement.
1972	J. Gordon Robson	Science and prescience in anaesthesia.
1974	W. Derek Wylie	There, but for the grace of God...
1976	M. Keith Sykes	Anaesthesia and the lesser circulation.
1978	William W. Mapleson	From Clover to computer: towards programmed anaesthesia?
1980	D. Gordon McDowall	Anaesthesia and the brain.
1982	Peter W. Thompson	Out of this nettle...
1984	Cyril M. Conway	Trial by jury.
1986	Anthony J. Merrifield	Flight of fancy.
1988	John W. Dundee	Passing fancies or lost gems.
1990	Alastair A. Spence	*Res academica.*
1992	Cedric Prys-Roberts	Never mind the quality, feel the depth.
1994	Charles Suckling	The development of halothane.
1996	James G. Whitwam	Anaesthesia: heart of the matter or a matter of the heart.
1998	Christopher Hull	A risky business.
2000	Henry J. McQuay	Evidence matters.

Further reading

Lee JA. Joseph Thomas Clover and the contributions of surgery to anaesthesia. *Annals of the Royal College of Surgeons of England* 1960; **26**: 280–99.

Marston AD. The life and achievements of Joseph Thomas Clover. *Annals of the Royal College of Surgeons of England* 1949; **4**: 267–80.

Nunn JF. The evolution of atmospheric oxygen. *Annals of the Royal College of Surgeons of England* 1968; **43**: 200–17.

CORMACK–LEHANE
LARYNGOSCOPY GRADES

Ronald Sidney Cormack (1930–)
John Robert Lehane (1945–)

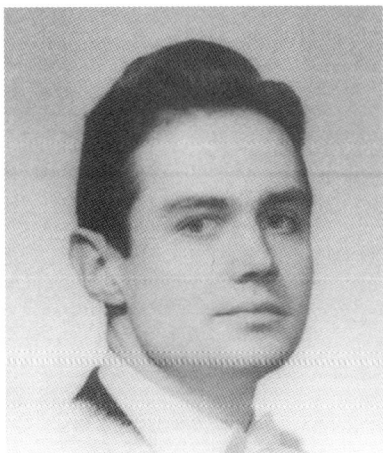

Ronald Cormack

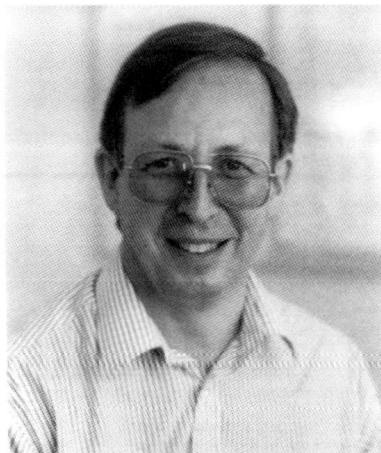

John Lehane

Ronnie Cormack's forbears were crofters in the Orkney Isles, Scotland, whose offspring migrated south. Cormack was born in 1930 in Rangoon, Burma where his father, Colonel Harry Cormack was a surgeon and the head of medical services. In the First World War his father was awarded the Military Cross for rescuing the wounded at Neuve Chappelle, France. His mother was a ward sister at Charing Cross Hospital and his wife was a staff-nurse at St Mary's Hospital in London. He graduated in medicine (BM, BCh) from Oxford in 1961.

At preparatory school he was given a child's biography of Louis Pasteur, which sparked a life-long interest in scientific research. This was reinforced at Oxford by his tutor and second cousin, D.J.C. Cunningham. Cunningham was a grandson of the famous anatomist D.J. Cunningham, whose eponymous *Textbook of Anatomy* is now in its 12th edition; and nephew of Admiral Cunningham, who master-minded the sinking of Mussolini's navy at Taranto, Italy using information from the Bletchley Park code-breakers – his weapons were archaic (Swordfish biplanes) but his information technology was state-of-the-art. Cunningham disapproved of undergraduates reading only the latest publications, arguing that the work of pioneers, even when it appeared antiquated, was often more instructive. Cormack verified this in his intubation study and in other papers covering respiratory physiology, awareness during anaesthesia, and medical statistics which were published over the following four decades.

John Lehane was born in Merseyside into a medical family. His father played a key role in work leading to the prevention of Rhesus haemolytic

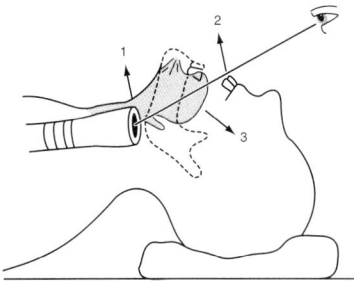

Figure 1. Difficulty arises if the relative positions of larynx (1), upper teeth (2) and tongue (3) are displaced in the direction of the arrows. Factor (3) is hard to assess from external examination.

disease and in the prevention of hepatitis B infection from transfusion. His sister, who practises in Cork, Ireland, was the anaesthetist on the team that located the first of the genes to be associated with malignant hyperthermia. John graduated in medicine from Liverpool University in 1969, passed his FFARCS in 1973 and MRCP in 1975. He moved to Northwick Park Hospital in Harrow, Middlesex in 1975 to work with John Nunn and Gareth Jones who later became professor of anaesthesia at Cambridge.

In 1972, Northwick Park Hospital opened a joint venture with the Medical Research Council (MRC), aiming to link research with everyday medicine. Cormack was appointed consultant anaesthetist, from Bristol University in Somerset where he had been a lecturer in anaesthesia. He was given overall charge of obstetric anaesthesia and worked with Lehane who supervised the epidural service. Lehane was appointed to the MRC division in 1978 and was made honorary consultant in 1980.

Cormack and Lehane studied the triennial *Reports on confidential inquiries into maternal deaths in England and Wales*. In the 1960s, pulmonary aspiration occurred when intubation was not attempted; in the 1970s intubation was routine, but aspiration still happened because of failed intubation. It is hard to think of a worse medical mishap – it focused the minds of those in responsible positions and gave rise to the laryngoscopy grades being established.

Cormack and Lehane identified two key points. Firstly, difficult intubation was well known in diseases such as ankylosing spondylitis, but textbooks at that time had no clear account of intubation in apparently normal patients. Figures 1 and 2 aimed to show why difficulty can arise, why external examination may give scant warning, and how to handle the problem. Their landmark paper in 1984 evoked immediate interest. Discussion centred mainly on whether to increase or decrease the number of grades. Over the years each anaesthetist builds up his own picture of this complex problem. However, for the beginner there is a case for keeping it simple, highlighting what separates the easy cases (Grades 1 and 2) from those which can cause failure (Grades 3 and 4). Some

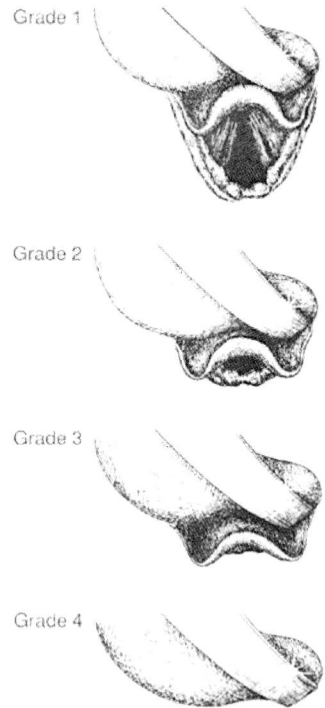

Figure 2. Typical views, assuming optimal technique. Intubation requires: Grade 1 – tube only; Grade 2 – introducer in tube, direct vision; Grade 3 – introducer in tube, blind; Grade 4 – fibreoscopy.

confusion arose over Grade 2 – if the cords cannot be seen but the arytenoids are visible, then that is still Grade 2, not 3. This decision was influenced by a letter to Cormack in 1978 from Sir Robert Macintosh who wrote; 'I can honestly say that armed with an introducer I have never failed provided I could see at least the back of an arytenoid.'

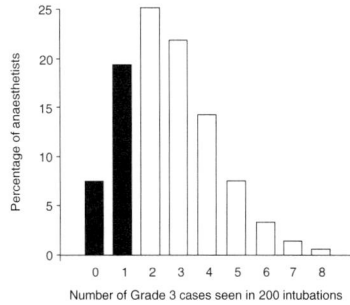

Figure 3. Predicted number of Grade 3 cases in 200 consecutive intubations if the true average is 1.3%.

If understanding the problem is 90% of the solution, then Figures 1 and 2 may be enough. However, Cormack and Lehane had a second message. If difficult intubations are not always predictable then either senior anaesthetists must do all emergency intubations or junior staff must master the art at an early stage. The simulated difficult intubation drill was designed to achieve this. Mortality related to failed intubation has fallen sharply, but is not yet zero. Cormack's statistical instinct convinced him that Poisson's distribution was crucially relevant (Figure 3). On average, 1–2% of laryngoscopies are Grade 3. It follows that some anaesthetists will meet this problem up to eight times per year, but at the other extreme, 27% will encounter it only once in a year, or not at all (the black blocks). If a serious golfer requires daily practice to keep in top form, anaesthetists need regular practice using an introducer and other intubation techniques.

The MRC withdrew from Northwick Park in the 1980s, mainly because of government cutbacks. In 1984 Lehane moved to Oxford where he is consultant anaesthetist specializing in critical care medicine and anaesthesia for ear, nose and throat surgery and trauma surgery. Cormack took early retirement to continue his research, retaining contact with MRC colleagues.

When the first microcomputers appeared in the 1970s, Cormack realized that computer simulations might solve various statistical problems for which textbook solutions were inadequate. On Fisher's exact test the standard P concept is inadequate – it was developed in relation to continuous distributions, where it works perfectly, but it is never going to make sense for quantal distributions. A slight modification of the traditional tail area idea removes the absurdities. This solution is used by clinicians who find the textbook answers unacceptable. Cormack is currently working on a beginner's textbook of statistics, which uses simulations to link the abstract idea of probability with something that can be observed. What has become complex and theoretical can be made simple and practical.

Further reading

Cormack RS. Conscious levels during anaesthesia. *British Journal of Anaesthesia* 1993; **71**: 469–71.

Cormack RS, Lehane J. Difficult intubation in obstetrics. *Anaesthesia* 1984; **39**; 1105–11.

Cormack RS, Mantel N. Doubt and certainty in statistics. *Journal of the Royal Society of Medicine* 1990; **83**: 136–7.

MALADIE DE DENBOROUGH
KING–DENBOROUGH SYNDROME

Michael Denborough (1929–)

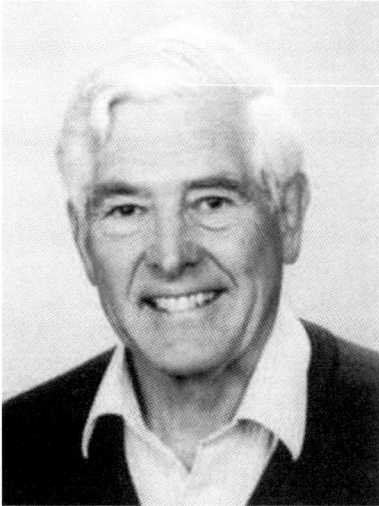

Michael Denborough was born and educated in Salisbury, Rhodesia (now Harare, Zimbabwe). He graduated in Medicine at the University of Cape Town, South Africa in 1952, obtained his DPhil from Oxford University, England in 1956, trained at the National Heart Hospital, London during 1957–58, passed the MRCP examination in 1959 and then left for Australia. Two months after taking up his appointment at the Royal Melbourne Hospital, New South Wales in 1960, he described a case of malignant hyperthermia (MH).

A 21-year-old student was run over by a car and sustained compound fractures of his right tibia and fibula. He was less concerned about his leg than by the prospect of a general anaesthetic because 10 close relatives had died during or after anaesthesia, usually for minor procedures. Ether was used in all those cases so halothane, which had recently become available, was administered cautiously. After 10 minutes he became acutely ill, his blood pressure was falling, pulse rate rising, he was cyanosed and both he and the soda lime canister felt very hot. The anaesthetic was stopped, the soda lime canister was changed, and the patient was rubbed down with ice-cold packs. He recovered and his subsequent course was uneventful. Detailed clinical examination and routine pathological and biochemical tests revealed no abnormality.

The following day, research into the deaths in the family convinced Denborough that this patient had a previously undescribed inborn error of metabolism inherited as a dominant characteristic. He described the case in the *Lancet* in the hope that others might have noted similar clinical events, but with no response. The syndrome became known as malignant hyperthermia – hyperthermia, because of the steep and rapid rise in body temperature, and malignant because the fatality rate was 70%.

One year later, the same man presented with a stone impacted in his left ureter. Every possible monitor was connected and he was given a spinal anaesthetic, which he tolerated uneventfully. The safety of local anaesthesia was reassuring because the patient came from a very large family that was prone to accidents and operations.

In 1963, Denborough learned of three anaesthetic deaths in a family in Wisconsin in the USA and further cases were published. After a child died in Ontario, Canada, Beverley Britt (an anaesthetist) along with Werner Kalow (a pharmacologist interested in MH) and Rod Gordon (professor of anaesthesia), organized inquiries throughout Canada. At the Symposium on Malignant Hyperthermia in Toronto in 1966, muscular rigidity was reported in some of the 13 cases presented. In the same year, G.M. Hall and his colleagues in London, England noticed that certain inbred pigs developed MH. Experimental work on these animals showed that the essential biochemical abnormality in MH was an elevation of calcium in muscle cells. Clinical research identified three specific human myopathies, which predispose to MH. Malignant hyperthermia is eponymously named La Maladie de Denborough in France. King was a colleague of Denborough's in Melbourne in 1973 when they described one of the three myopathies associated with MH that is now known as the King–Denborough Syndrome.

In Toronto, Kalow and Britt found that dog muscle contracted on exposure to chloroform. They studied caffeine-induced contraction in human muscle and observed that it was augmented in MH-susceptible patients. Richard Ellis and his colleagues in Leeds, England showed that it also occurred with halothane. Their specific diagnostic test, based on measuring muscle contraction *in vitro* on exposure to halothane, is used to identify MH susceptibility and for genetic counselling.

In November 1969, a second case occurred at the Royal Melbourne Hospital. A 51-year-old man had sustained a compound fracture of the right leg in a motor accident. He had no family history of anaesthetic problems and had been administered ether uneventfully for an appendicectomy when he was 21. When he was given halothane and succinylcholine (suxamethonium), he became acutely ill, his right arm became rigid and he died 24 hours later. His serum creatine kinase rose to 20,500 IU per litre just before he died. Clearly, the anaesthetic drugs had induced severe rhabdomyolysis in a susceptible individual and this implied an underlying muscle disease. The propositus in the original Melbourne family was contacted and his serum creatine kinase was found to be very high. His father and a paternal aunt also had raised serum creatine kinase and clear evidence of a clinical myopathy. His sister's serum creatine kinase was also raised but his brother's was normal.

Denborough moved to the Australian National University in Canberra, New South Wales in 1974. In 1976, Bill Bowman, from the University of Strathclyde, Scotland suggested to Denborough that, if elevated myoplasmic calcium was the essential cause of MH, a new drug called dantrolene that specifically lowered myoplasmic calcium should be an effective antidote and treatment. Its effectiveness was confirmed in halothane and caffeine-induced contractions in pig muscle *in vitro*, and subsequently also *in vivo* in pigs (Figure 1) and humans. Dantrolene proved to be a life-saving treatment and it was required to be immediately available wherever general

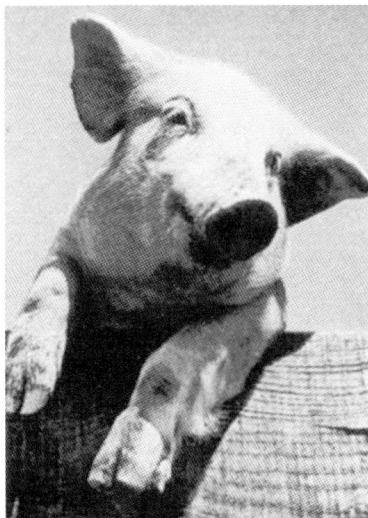

Figure 1. The pig that Denborough used in his malignant hyperthermia experiments.

anaesthesia is used. Its early use in the treatment of MH has reduced the fatality rate from 70% to 5%.

Muscle membrane disorders that predispose to MH may also predispose to other clinical presentations. A surgeon in Wagga Wagga, two hours from Canberra, telephoned Denborough for advice on a moribund young army officer trainee who was bleeding from the bowel as a result of severe heatstroke sustained in a route march in very hot conditions. The surgeon said that it looked like MH. Denborough sent him a vial of the experimental dantrolene by army motorcycle for intravenous infusion and within an hour the patient improved dramatically. Muscle biopsy showed that he was MH-susceptible and an inquiry revealed that he was related to a previously investigated MH family. Many patients with severe heatstroke have since been shown by biopsy to be susceptible to MH.

Denborough is also a political activist. He initiated a scientific protest against a French atmospheric nuclear test in 1970, convened a symposium on Australia and Nuclear War in 1983, and founded the Nuclear Disarmament Party in 1984.

His honours include the Eric Susman Prize for Medical Research, Royal Australasian College of Physicians in 1972; Gold Medal, Fifth International Congress on Neuromuscular Diseases, Marseille in 1982; and Honorary Fellowship, Australian and New Zealand College of Anaesthetists in 1993. He became Emeritus Professor in 1995 and a Member of the Order of Australia in 1999.

Further reading

Denborough M. Malignant hyperthermia. *Lancet* 1998; **352**: 1131–36.
Denborough MA, Lovell RRH. Anaesthetic deaths in a family. *Lancet* 1960; **2**: 45.
King JO, Denborough MA. Anaesthetic-induced malignant hyperpyrexia in children. *The Journal of Pediatrics*1973; **83**: 37–40.

DRIPPS, ECKENHOFF AND VANDAM'S 'INTRODUCTION TO ANESTHESIA'

The forerunner of Dripps, Eckenhoff and Vandam's *Introduction to Anesthesia* first appeared as a privately printed, spiral bound pamphlet in the department of anesthesiology of the University of Pennsylvania in Philadelphia. The first hardcover edition of *Introduction to Anesthesia* was published by W.B. Saunders in 1954. Later editions were multi-authored by members of the University of Pennsylvania and have been translated into several foreign languages. The comprehensive ninth edition was published in 1996.

Robert Dunning Dripps (1911–1973)

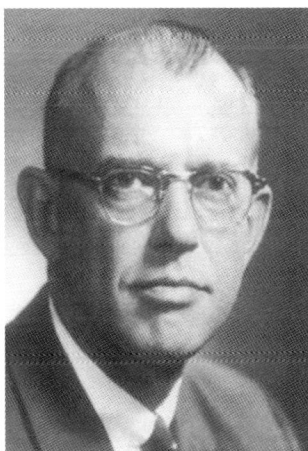

Robert Dripps was born in Philadelphia in 1911, the son of a lawyer and grandson of a Presbyterian minister. He attended Germantown Academy and Princeton University, New Jersey and the University of Pennsylvania School of Medicine where he graduated MD in 1936. He helped to support himself as a special correspondent, reporting sporting events for the *New York Times*. He was also among the first reporters on the scene in the Lindbergh kidnapping case. He interned at the University of Pennsylvania Hospital and was an instructor in pharmacology from 1938 to 1940. After training in anaesthesia under Ralph Waters in Madison, Wisconsin, he returned to the University of Pennsylvania Hospital in 1942 where he was associate professor of surgery until his retirement in 1972.

He regarded every anaesthetic as a pharmacological study and taught his trainees to do likewise. Seventeen of his residents and fellows became departmental chairmen at American universities, and six in overseas universities that included the National University at Seoul in South Korea, and Pahlavi University in Iran. He was also a spiritual man and a humanitarian, serving with the Medical Mission to Greece and Italy in 1948, and much later with Project Hope in Ceylon (now Sri Lanka) and Tunisia.

He collaborated in research with Julius Comroe and many others from 1939 to 1973 and contributed to leading textbooks, including Goodman and Gilman's *Pharmacological Basis of Therapeutics*. He was president of the Pennsylvania State Society of Anesthesiologists, the Association of University Anesthetists, the Halsted Society (the first anaesthetist so honoured) and the American Board of Anesthesiology. He was chairman of committees of the National Institutes of Health, the World Health Organization and the National Academy of Sciences National Research Council. He received the Distinguished Service Award of the American Society of Anesthesiologists in 1965. He was elected to Fellowship of the Faculties of Anaesthetists of the Royal Colleges of Surgeons of England and Ireland. The University of Pennsylvania established the Robert Dunning Dripps Professorship and the Robert Dunning Dripps Memorial Fund in the early 1970s and the Robert Dunning Dripps Library of Anesthesia in 1980.

James Edward Eckenhoff (1915–1996)

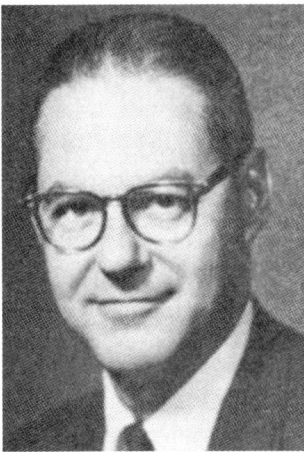

James Eckenhoff was born on the eastern shore of Maryland in 1915. He supported himself through Transylvania College in Lexington, Kentucky and the University of Kentucky, and graduated MD from the University of Pennsylvania School of Medicine in 1941. Following internship in Kentucky, he served as a battalion surgeon and later as an anaesthetist in the 107th Evacuation Hospital in the European theatre of operations during the Second World War.

He returned to the University of Pennsylvania in 1945 as a Harrison Fellow in Anesthesiology in the pharmacology department. The department of anesthesiology, under Dripps, was closely allied with the pharmacology department. Eckenhoff's research led to the first coherent account of the relationship between coronary arterial blood flow and systemic blood pressure, cardiac output, cardiac work and oxygen consumption, and the effects of certain drugs.

This laboratory experience added to his natural talents as a teacher and physician when he returned to clinical work in 1947, and he soon became a professor. He was the first to use nalorphine hydrochloride in the treatment of neonatal asphyxia, and he was also the first to use hyaluronidase with local anaesthetic agents. He spent a period with the World Health Organization (WHO) Anaesthesia Teaching Centre in Copenhagen, Denmark and on his return to Philadelphia in 1952 he promoted the Danish treatment of barbiturate poisoning by supportive, physiological measures instead of using analeptic drugs. In 1966, Eckenhoff moved from Philadelphia to be chairman of the department of anesthesiology at Northwestern University in Chicago, Illinois and was dean of the Medical School from 1970 until his retirement in 1983.

Eckenhoff was editor of *Anesthesiology* during 1958–62, Hunterian Professor of the Royal College of Surgeons of England in 1965, and chairman of the board of the ASA Wood Library–Museum of Anesthesiology from

1967 to 1970. He received the Distinguished Service Award of the American Society of Anesthesiologists in 1980. The Eckenhoff Lectureship at the University of Pennsylvania, Philadelphia, and the Eckenhoff Library Fund at Northwestern University Medical School, Chicago are named in his honour.

Leroy David Vandam (1914–)

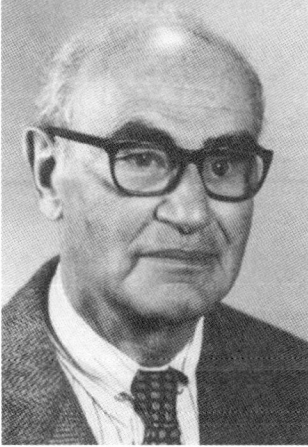

Leroy Vandam was born in New York City in 1914. He attended Townsend Harris Hall, an experimental preparatory school, where he won several art prizes and a short-term scholarship for study at the Metropolitan Museum of Art. He graduated MD from New York University Bellevue Medical School. During medical school he wondered whether to become a full-time artist, but decided against it.

He took one year of surgical pathology at Beth Israel Hospital in Boston, Massachusetts before becoming a surgical resident. Towards the end of his residency, he suddenly developed a scotoma in his left eye. Despite this, he served for several months in the Fourth Auxiliary Surgical Group (a mobile surgical unit) in 1943, but received an honourable medical discharge when he suffered repeated retinal haemorrhages in both eyes. He resumed his work in 1945 as a Fellow in Surgery at The Johns Hopkins Hospital in Baltimore, Maryland until a massive intraocular haemorrhage with severe pain necessitated a retrobulbar block and ultimately enucleation of the eye.

Vandam became interested in anaesthesia during treatment at the Wilmer Eye Institute in Baltimore when Austin Lamont, one of the first two medically qualified anaesthetists at The Johns Hopkins Hospital, interviewed him. Aged 33, he started his anaesthesia residency under Dripps at the University of Pennsylvania in 1947. Three years later, in response to Foster Kennedy's 1950 paper on grave neurological complications of spinal anaesthesia, Dripps and Vandam prospectively studied 10,098 spinal anaesthetics at their hospital. They found only minor problems that were attributable to lumbar puncture or prior neurological conditions.

Vandam spent three months as instructor at the WHO Centre of Anaesthesia in Copenhagen in 1953, and moved to Boston in 1954 as director of the Division of Anesthesia at Peter Bent Brigham Hospital and Clinical Professor of Anesthesia at Harvard Medical School. He was on the Committee of the National Halothane Study in 1963. His publications covered a broad field, but especially the physiology of circulation and circulatory behaviour during anaesthesia, and he was editor of *Anesthesiology* during 1962–70. He received the Distinguished Service Award of the American Society of Anesthesiologists in 1977.

Acknowledgement

Portrait photograph of Dripps reproduced from *Anesthesia and Analgesia* 1963; **42**: 332–3 with permission from Lippincott Williams & Wilkins; Portrait photograph of Eckenhoff reproduced from *Anesthesia and Analgesia* 1963; **42**: 607–8 with permission from Lippincott Williams & Wilkins; Portrait photograph of Vandam reproduced with kind permission from the Wood Library–Museum of Anesthesiology, Park Ridge, IL, USA.

Further reading

DRIPPS:

Anonymous. We salute … Robert D. Dripps, M.D. *Anesthesia and Analgesia* 1963; **42**: 332–3.

Wollman H. Robert Dunning Dripps 1911–73. *Anesthesiology* 1974; **40**, 114–15.

ECKENHOFF:

Anonymous. We salute … James E. Eckenhoff, M.D. *Anesthesia and Analgesia* 1963; **42**: 607–8.

Ellison N. James E. Eckenhoff, M.D., 1915–1996. *ASA Newsletter* 1997; **61 (Suppl 1)**: 31.

VANDAM:

Anonymous. We salute … Leroy D. Vandam, M. D. *Anesthesia and Analgesia* 1960; **39**: 28.

Dripps RD, Vandam LD. Long-term follow-up of patients who received 10,098 spinal anesthetics. Failure to discover major neurological sequelae. *Journal of the American Medical Association* 1954; **156**: 1486–91.

Vandam LD. On the Craggy Path to Anesthesiology. In: Fink BR, McGoldrick KE (Eds) *Careers in Anesthesiology, Volume IV*. Park Ridge, IL: Wood Library–Museum of Anesthesiology 2000: 162–81.

Minimal alveolar concentration (MAC)

Edmond I Eger II (1930–)

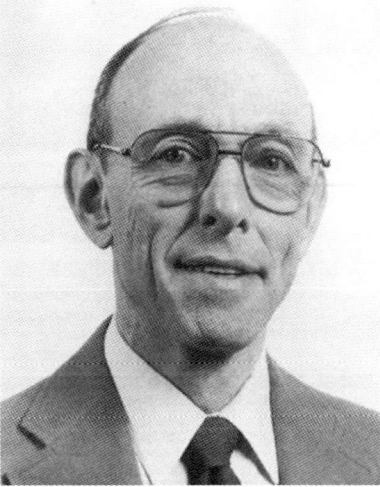

Ted Eger was born in Chicago, Illinois in 1930. There were three 'Eds' in the house and his mother said it was too complicated. If she called for Ed, three would come running – so one became Ted. He graduated from the University of Illinois in 1951, received his MD degree from Northwestern University Medical School, Chicago in 1955, and interned at St Luke's Hospital in Chicago. Following his residency in anaesthesia with Stuart Cullen (1907–79) at the State University of Iowa hospitals and Veterans Administration Hospital in Iowa City, he was appointed chief of the anesthesia and operative section at the US Army Hospital in Fort Leavenworth, Kansas from 1958 to 1960.

Eger joined the University of California, San Francisco in 1960, where he began his illustrious career as a researcher. He was also an interesting and inspiring teacher. Over the next eight years, he rose to the rank of professor. The clarity of his writing and his lecturing ability enabled him to make the complex, theoretical aspects of uptake and distribution of volatile agents both understandable and clinically useful. In the 1960s, long before the days of anaesthetic agent monitors, he taught us why and how we use anaesthetics in the operating room.

Eger developed the concept of minimum alveolar concentration (MAC) for gaseous and volatile anaesthetic agents as a practical measure of anaesthetic depth, and as a means of comparing their potencies. Along with Giles Merkel, he published a study in 1963, which compared the effects of halothane and halopropane on physiological parameters in dogs. In order to do this, they needed an index of comparison that they defined as 'the minimal anesthetic concentration in the alveolus required to keep a dog from responding by gross movement to a painful stimulus'. The stimuli included tail clamping or varying electrical currents applied to sensitive mucous membranes. They studied each of six dogs on four occasions at minimal intervals of two weeks. Only one agent was used in each study so that each dog served as its own control. No single physiological parameter could be used to measure progressive depth of anaesthesia, whereas MAC 1.0 was remarkably constant. To their delight, MAC was reproducible for

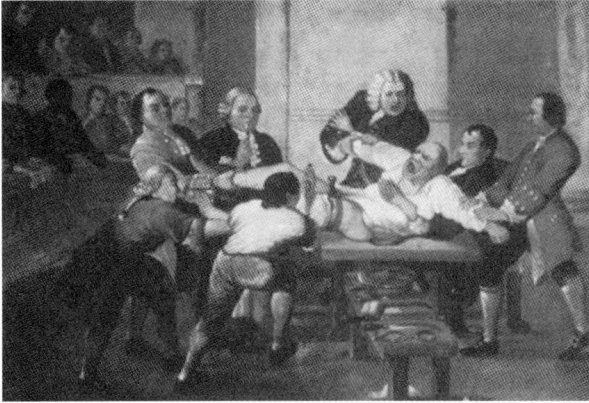

Figure 1. Amputation scene in 1776. (Reproduced with kind permission from the Royal College of Surgeons of England.)

both agents during either spontaneous or controlled ventilation, and was not critically dependent on the type or intensity of the noxious stimulus.

Eger's definition of MAC is reminiscent of John Snow's succinct comment more than 100 years earlier that; 'Ether contributes other benefits besides . . . preventing pain. It keeps patients still, who otherwise would not be.' Figure 1 depicts an amputation scene in 1776, in which MAC was zero and the patient was moving vigorously. In the first 100 years of anaesthesia, before the introduction of muscle relaxants and accurately calibrated vaporizers, lying still was the defining criterion of adequate anaesthesia. It applied equally to all inhaled anaesthetics, whereas other physical signs such as Guedel's eye signs, sympathetic activity and respiratory changes varied from one agent to another.

Eger's later studies in humans showed that although the effect of modifying factors such as age, premedication, opioids and comorbid conditions are known, they are relatively small. He established equipotent doses of clinically used inhalational anaesthetics. This permitted, for the first time, precision in studies of their comparative pharmacology in humans. He defined MAC as the 'minimal alveolar concentration of anesthetic at 1 atmosphere that produces immobility in 50 per cent of those patients or animals exposed to a noxious stimulus'. Because the noxious stimulus in humans is the surgical skin incision, only one observation can be made in each patient. The alveolar concentration is held constant for 15 minutes at one of several predetermined levels, the levels chosen being above or below the estimated MAC value. The percentage of patients who move at each concentration is plotted, and the concentration (MAC) that prevents 50% of patients from moving is estimated from a visual line of best fit (Figure 2).

Calibrated vaporizers outside the circuit indicate the concentration coming from the

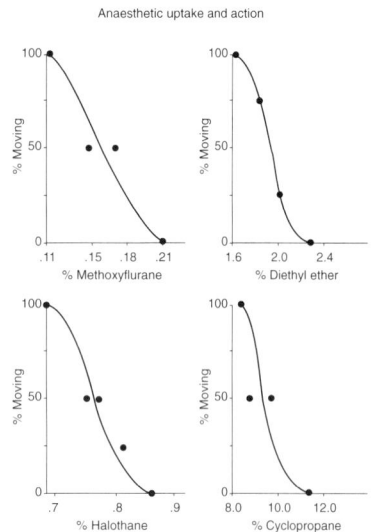

Figure 2. Visual line of best fit for MAC values.

machine, not the concentration in the patient's alveoli or brain. They do not account for rates of uptake and distribution of different agents according to their solubility, or of the influence of fresh gas flow, minute volume ventilation or cardiac output. Eger focused attention on the fact that MAC equals the partial pressure of anaesthetic at the anaesthetic site of action. This assumes that, given sufficient time for equilibration, partial pressures in arterial blood and at the site of action are equal. Eger used this concept for all early human pharmacological studies of enflurane, isoflurane, desflurane and sevoflurane.

His bibliography of nearly 500 publications reads like the index of a textbook: anaesthetic systems, uptake, elimination, MAC, theories of anaesthesia, factors which affect anaesthetic requirement, mechanism of action, metabolism, toxicity, and cardiorespiratory effects of anaesthesia. Eger compiled his research into a book, *Anesthetic Uptake and Action*. His real interests are in pharmacokinetics and mechanisms of inhaled anaesthetic action, and MAC was a means to an end.

Few individuals made a greater impact on clinical anaesthesia in the latter part of the 20th century than Ted Eger. He is a kind and generous man who has freely given his time, his energy and his counsel. He has enthused young physicians to the fun and usefulness of research. He has helped trainees to pursue their own research interests, to solve problems, and to mature into independent investigators. Many of his research trainees have chosen full-time academic careers.

He has four children and nine grandchildren of whom he is inordinately proud. He is married to Dr Lynn Spitler and loves poetry and walking in the mountains.

Eger's honours and awards include the ASA Award for Excellence in Research in 1989; Distinguished Service Award of the American Society of Anesthesiologists in 1991; and Honorary Fellowship of the Faculty of Anaesthetists of the Royal College of Surgeons in Ireland.

Acknowledgement

Portrait photograph reproduced with kind permission from the Wood Library–Museum of Anesthesiology, Park Ridge, IL, USA.

Further reading

Anonymous. We salute . . . Edmond I Eger II, M. D. *Anesthesia and Analgesia* 1976; 55: 604–5.

Eger EI. *Anesthetic uptake and action*. Baltimore, MD: Williams and Wilkins, 1974.

Eger EI, Saidman LJ, Brandstater B. Minimum alveolar anesthetic concentration: a standard of anesthetic potency. *Anesthesiology* 1965; 26: 756–63.

EPSTEIN MACINTOSH OXFORD (EMO) VAPORIZER

Hans G. Epstein (1909–)

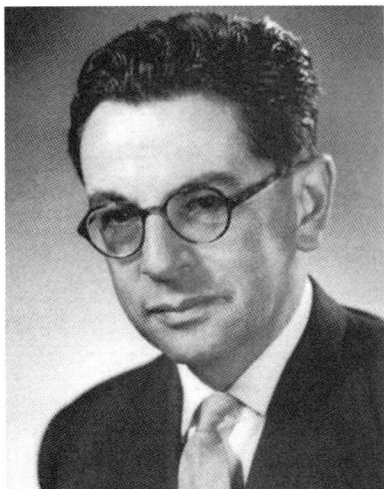

Hans Epstein was born in Berlin, Germany in 1909. He was educated at schools in Switzerland and Bavaria, passed Staatexamen and obtained his PhD in physics in Berlin in 1934. He left Germany before the outbreak of the Second World War and found temporary employment in England as personal assistant to Lord Cherwell, director of the Clarendon Laboratory in Oxford where K. Mendelssohn PhD, a fellow refugee, had a permanent post.

Oxford vaporizer (1941)

Robert Macintosh, Nuffield Professor of Anaesthetics at Oxford, was grateful for his experience with an improvised Flagg can during the Spanish Civil War. It convinced him that war conditions required easily portable anaesthetic machines that did not depend on heavy cylinders of compressed gases. Richard Salt, technician in charge of the Nuffield department workshop, had been Macintosh's handyman and chauffeur at his former private anaesthetic practice in Mayfair, London. He constructed a slightly modified Flagg can that Macintosh designed but they had no means of testing it.

Early in 1940, Macintosh accepted the suggestion from Mendelssohn, whose advice he had sought for the prototype drawover design of the Oxford vaporizer, of appointing Epstein as a research assistant in Oxford. About that time, Lord Cherwell told Epstein that he would have to leave Clarendon because he was German, and offered him a choice of working in the department of physiology or pharmacology. Epstein chose pharmacology and became a member of the Nuffield Department of Anaesthetics until his retirement in 1976. Epstein improvised his 'home-made' optical analysers and was able to analyse the vaporizer.

During 1940, several basic prototype models of the Oxford vaporizer were constructed. The first model (Figure 1) used the latent heat of crystallization of calcium chloride, itself heated by hot water, to maintain a constant temperature and thus a constant vapour pressure of ether in the vaporizing chamber. This ensured accuracy of vaporizer settings. Between 1940 and 1943, Epstein assembled various designs of optical analysers and respiratory simulators in the laboratory of the department of pharmacology.

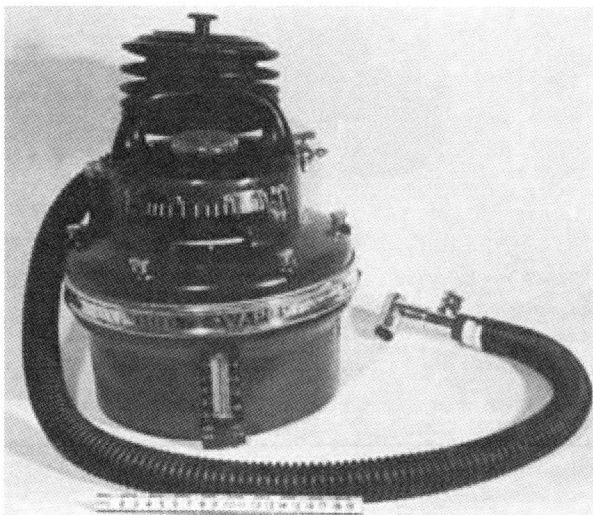

Figure 1. Oxford vaporizer. (Reproduced with kind permission from the Association of Anaesthetists of Great Britain and Ireland.)

He analysed all experimentally made inhalers and vaporizers, including the plenum devices for which Mendelssohn, Pask and Salt had opted. Mass production became a reality when Lord Nuffield supplied experienced production engineers and ample facilities in his nearby Morris Motors factory. By the end of 1942, production was in full swing. Most of the first 1000 vaporizers presented by Lord Nuffield were checked in Epstein's laboratory with improved analytical equipment.

When these Oxford vaporizers were delivered to the army, medical officers of other units soon showed interest. Popularity gradually spread throughout various branches of the Allied Medical Services, but a strangely bureaucratic obstacle arose for airborne troops. Although they transported and parachuted large amounts of ammunition, regulations forbade them to carry flammable liquids including ether.

Epstein Suffolk Oxford (ESO) inhaler (1942)

The importance of the weight of an anaesthetic device that was to be carried in a knapsack by the parachutist led to the development of the ESO inhaler. The chemist S.F. Suffolk had already joined Epstein for testing and improving the Oxford vaporizer when the lightweight drawover inhaler for chloroform was proposed. Instead of keeping the temperature constant (thermostat principle), the ESO inhaler used a simple manually operated thermocompensator and a liquid-filled, thin-walled metal bellows as a thermocontroller. It incorporated a modified Oxford inflating bellows and was firmly attached to a plate for easy insertion into the wadded aluminium case, which contained basic accessories and could withstand being dropped by parachute.

Epstein Macintosh Trilene (Emotril) inhaler (1949)

Home births accounted for almost one-half of all British births at the end of the Second World War, but there was a steady move to hospital deliveries in the post-war years. Epstein developed the Emotril inhaler (Figure 2) to provide safer and more convenient midwife-supervised self-administered analgesia than Minnit's nitrous oxygen and air machine. The inhalers met

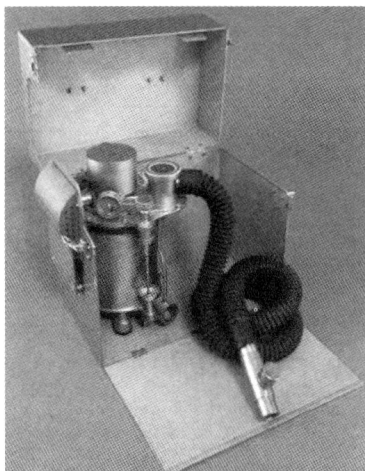

Figure 2. Epstein Macintosh trilene (Emotril) inhaler. (Reproduced with kind permission from the Association of Anaesthetists of Great Britain and Ireland.)

stringent criteria and were suitable for use during either a home or hospital birth. The delivered concentration had to be within 20% of the 'normal' 0.5% and 'weak' 0.35% settings, in a temperature range of 13–35°C, minute volume 7–20 litres per minute and respiratory rate of 12–30 breaths per minute, even if the inhaler was shaken before use or transported upside down. In 1950, the Medical Research Council (MRC) and the Central Midwives Board accepted the results of an extensive bedside clinical trial of the Emotril in parturient mothers by E.H. Seward, research anaesthetist at the Nuffield department. In 1954, after further multicentre trials supervised by the MRC committee on analgesia, the Ministry of Health approved its use by midwives.

Epstein Macintosh Oxford (EMO) inhaler (1956)

The Nuffield department began development of the EMO drawover ether vaporizer (Figure 3) in the early 1950s, as a successor to the Oxford vaporizer. Technical staff of the Pentland Company, which later amalgamated with Longworth of Abingdon to become Penlon, cooperated from 1952 to 1956 before the first commercial model went into production. Use of intravenous induction agents and muscle relaxants avoided the need for prolonged delivery of high ether concentrations. By making the outer surface of the inhaler sufficiently large with good thermal conductivity and incorporating ample heat capacity, heat inflow from the environment could fully compensate for any temperature drop for up to 6% ether at expected respiratory minute volumes. Nevertheless, large evaporation areas were incorporated to enable delivery of higher concentrations, although with less accuracy. In contrast to the Oxford vaporizer, no special heat source was required and the main container was no longer an insulator, but was made from a good heat-conducting aluminium alloy.

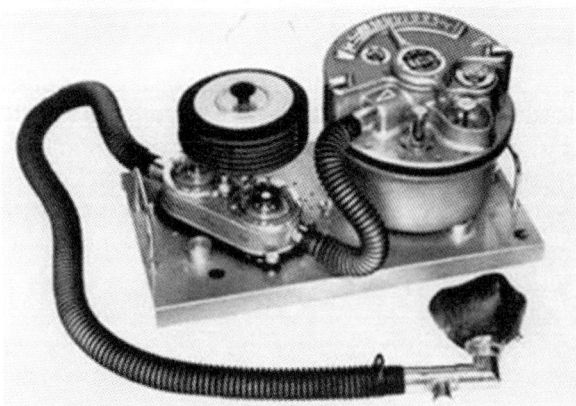

Figure 3. Epstein Macintosh Oxford (EMO) inhaler. (Reproduced with kind permission from the Association of Anaesthetists of Great Britain and Ireland.)

Oxford miniature vaporizer (OMV) (1966)

The OMV was introduced in 1966 for halothane and other agents (Figure 4). It was to be used in series with the EMO to provide a smoother inhalation induction before switching over to ether.

Some features are common to all these eponymous devices. Foremost was the attainment of a low resistance at all concentration settings or temperatures so that spontaneous inspiration would not be impeded. The imposition of a low resistance in drawover vaporizers led to many design difficulties compared with plenum apparatus that has a positive pressure gas supply. The story of the EMO illustrates Macintosh's approach to improving anaesthesia, not only in Britain but also around the world. Its reliability, simplicity, portability and use of room air as the carrier gas commended it for use in developing countries. Compared with plenum systems, the safety of the EMO and OMV increases in proportion to remoteness from centres of advanced learning and availability of oxygen cylinders.

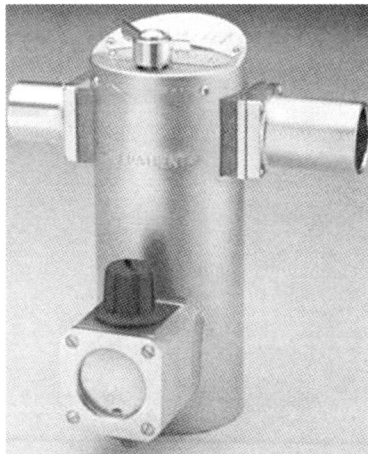

Figure 4. Oxford miniature vaporizer (OMV). (Reproduced from Penlon.)

Further reading

Epstein HG, Macintosh RR. An anaesthetic inhaler with automatic thermocompensation. *Anaesthesia* 1956; 11: 83–8.

Epstein HG, Macintosh RR. Analgesia inhaler for trichlorethylene. *British Medical Journal* 1949; 2: 1092–4.

Epstein HG, Macintosh RR, Mendelssohn K. The Oxford vaporiser No. 1. *Lancet* 1941; 2: 62–4.

Esmarch bandage

Johan Friedrich von Esmarch (1823–1908)

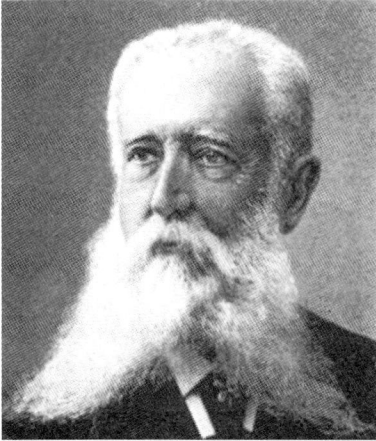

Friedrich von Esmarch was born in 1823 in Tönning in a part of Denmark inhabited by people of German language and culture. It is now Schleswig–Holstein in Germany, just south of the Danish border. Esmarch was the son of a country doctor and accompanied his father on his rounds. He showed a special interest in surgery when he was a medical student at the universities of Kiel and Göttingen in Germany. He graduated in 1848 and became assistant to the surgeon, Bernhard von Langenbeck (1810–87), after whom the tissue retractor is named. In the same year, war broke out between Denmark and Germany and Esmarch at once joined the German forces as a military surgeon (Figure 1).

He was soon taken as a prisoner of war, but he was exchanged for a Danish doctor and returned to Kiel. Langenbeck had moved to Berlin, so Esmarch visited surgical clinics in Germany, Austria, Hungary, France and Britain during 1848 with a view to an academic career in surgery. Once more, on returning to Kiel, he not only became assistant to Georg Stromeyer, Professor of Surgery at the Christian Albert University, but also became his son-in-law. When Stromeyer was promoted to the Chair of Surgery in Hanover in 1854, Esmarch hoped to succeed him in Kiel, but the ruling Danes delayed his appointment for three years. His further experience of military surgery in the war of 1866 against Austria resulted in his classic book, *On Resection in Gunshot Injuries,* and in the Franco–Prussian war of 1870–71 he served in an administrative capacity as surgeon general to the German Army.

Anaesthetists know Esmarch's name because

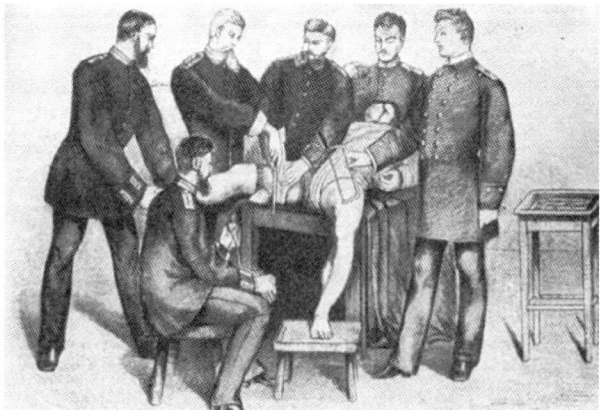

Figure 1. Esmarch as a military surgeon, performing an amputation under anaesthesia. (Reproduced with permission from *Notable names in medicine and surgery,* H.K. Lewis & Co, 1959: 99.)

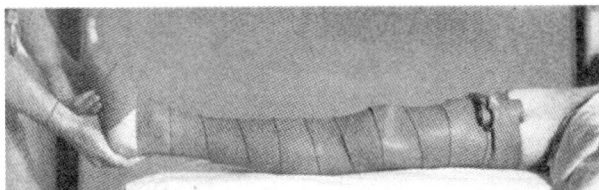

of the rubber bandage (Figure 2) that is used to permit orthopaedic surgery and other operations on the extremities to be carried out through a bloodless field. He described the bandage in 1873 at the German Surgical Congress. Bier's technique of intravenous regional analgesia would not have been possible without the Esmarch bandage to exsanguinate the limb and act as a tourniquet to limit the spread of procaine.

Esmarch's other contributions to anaesthesia were his simple wire frame mask for open drop ether anaesthesia in 1877, and his more elaborate set of equipment for open drop chloroform anaesthesia, for use in military surgery. The latter was available in a leather compendium (Figure 3) which contained tongue forceps, a mouth gag, a mask and a calibrated dropper bottle. The basket-shaped wire mask was designed to fit the contour of the face around the mouth and nose. One end was curved to form a handle, and a knitted or woven fabric was stretched over the frame to allow free passage of air. A curved dropper tube passed through the cork of the calibrated bottle and reached nearly to the bottom while a shorter tube admitted air into the bottle.

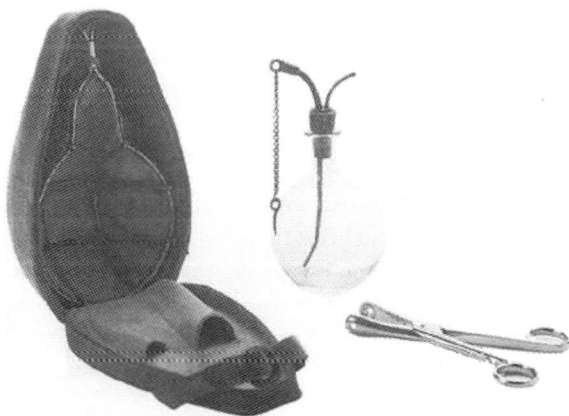

Figure 3. Esmarch chloroform anaesthesia set 1880. (Reproduced with permission from *Anaesthetic equipment in the history of German anaesthesia*, Verlag DrägerDruck, 1997: 24.)

Esmarch's manoeuvre was his widely known technique for managing acute airway obstruction during anaesthesia; 'In asphyxia, open the mouth at once, and press the lower jaw forwards with both hands by placing the forefinger behind the ascending ramus, so that the lower teeth project in front of the upper . . . If this cannot be accomplished because of convulsive contraction of the muscles, separate the teeth with a dilator, seize the end of the tongue with the fingers, or with the tongue forceps, and draw it out of the mouth as far as possible.'

Esmarch was an early and ardent supporter of the antiseptic system for surgery and the treatment of wounds. He visited Joseph Lister to see the system in practice. During a visit to London for the International Medical Exhibition in 1881, he became familiar with the St John's Ambulance

Association, a charity devoted to providing first aid to the injured. He introduced first aid into Germany as the Samaritan Association and was a strong advocate that it should be performed by laymen in the early treatment of trauma. He promoted the idea that soldiers on active war service should carry their own first aid kit and be trained in its use.

Esmarch's first wife died in 1870. In 1872 he married the Princess Henrietta of Schleswig–Holstein, who was the aunt of the Empress Augusta of Germany (1858–1921). He thus became uncle of the Kaiser William II (1859–1941), the 'Kaiser Bill' of the First World War. A Samaritan cross, the family crest, and a bloodless arm on his coat of arms marked the surgical accomplishments for which his name is remembered.

Acknowledgement

Portrait photograph reproduced with kind permission from *Notable names in medicine and surgery,* H.K. Lewis & Co, 1959: 98.

Further reading

Esmarch JFA von. Ueber Kunstliche Blutleere bei Operationem. *Sammlung Klinischer Vortrage* 1873; **58**: 373–84. (Translated by Whitley G.: Esmarch F. On the artificial emptying of blood-vessels in operation. In: *Clinical lectures on subjects connected with medicine, surgery, and obstetrics.* London: New Sydenham Society 1876: 84–96.)

Lee JA. Some foundations on which we have built. *Regional Anesthesia* 1985; **10**: 99–109.

Schulte am Esch J, Goerig M (Eds). *Anaesthetic Equipment in the History of German Anaesthesia.* Lübeck: Dräger, 1997: 24.

FINK EFFECT – DIFFUSION ANOXIA

Bernard Raymond Fink (1914–2000)

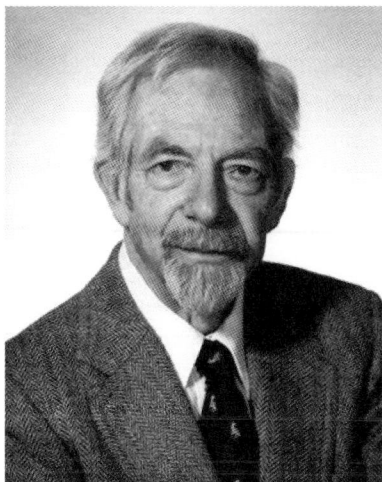

Ray Fink was born in London, England in 1914. He grew up in Antwerp, Belgium and entered the University of London aged 16 years. He completed his BSc in 1934 and graduated in medicine (MB, BS) in 1938. He interned at Randfontein Hospital in Randfontein, South Africa and served as Captain in the South African Medical Corps during the Second World War, tending soldiers from Africa and Europe. After one year of postgraduate medicine at University College Hospital in London, he returned to Randfontein and became medical superintendent of Moroka Methodist Mission Hospital during 1947–49. He denounced apartheid and preached against the use of Nazi-linked human experimental data by some of his colleagues. In 1950, he and his wife decided not to raise their family in an apartheid South Africa and immigrated to the USA.

Fink completed his anaesthesia residency at Beth Israel Hospital in New York City in 1952 when he was already 38 years old. He spent the next 12 years on the staff of Presbyterian Hospital, New York City practising clinical anaesthesia, and at Columbia University where he conducted landmark research. He made his mark within months of joining the faculty by inventing the 'Fink non-rebreathing valve' for use in children. It allowed single-handed assisted respiration at a time when other non-rebreathing valves required both hands, one to occlude the expiratory orifice of the valve and the other to squeeze the reservoir bag. Although the Fink valve was later superseded, it was innovative and useful at that time. He subsequently developed the vallecular extension airway by adding a Macintosh blade tip to a Waters airway, which worked particularly well in edentulous patients when mask anaesthesia was common.

Fink began his 1955 paper on diffusion anoxia, known to some anaesthetists as the Fink effect, in his elegantly simple style; 'Some patients become cyanotic during recovery from general anesthesia despite apparently good ventilation. The cyanosis appears more definitely and more frequently in patients who have been anaesthetised with nitrous oxide–oxygen mixtures." Other authors had made a similar observation, but had offered no explanation for its occurrence. Fink applied his knowledge of physics and pharmacology. From a comparison of the physical properties

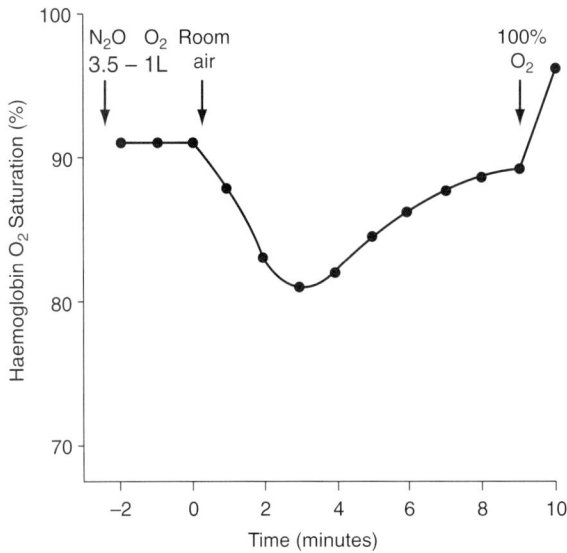

Figure 1. Arterial oxygen saturation during recovery from nitrous oxide-oxygen anaesthesia. (Reproduced from *Anesthesiology* 1955; 16: 511–99, with permission from Lippincott Williams & Wilkins.)

of anaesthetic gases and vapours, it was apparent that nitrous oxide was present in considerable volume in the blood. He calculated that a woman weighing 57 kg, after equilibration with 75% nitrous oxide, would have more than 28 litres of nitrous oxide dissolved in her blood. At the end of the case, when a patient began to breathe room air, nitrous oxide would diffuse out of the blood and into the lungs. This would mix with the room air drawn into the alveoli during inspiration and reduce the alveolar partial pressures of oxygen and nitrogen to below normal. He measured oxygen saturation for 10 minutes after surgery in eight healthy patients who breathed 75% nitrous oxide during minor gynaecological operations. Arterial oxygen saturation fell an average of 7.9% (Figure 1) on room air, while expiratory volume exceeded inspiratory volume by 3.3–6.9 litres in the first 10 minutes. The diffusion anoxia from nitrous oxide, which was at its maximum in the first few minutes, could be avoided by giving 100% oxygen for several minutes by mask and then by nasal catheter.

Fink began his studies on the larynx at Columbia University in the mid-1950s. He conducted original investigations into the anatomical and physiological mechanisms of laryngeal opening and closing, phonation and other laryngeal functions. Laryngologists recognize his contributions to understanding normal laryngeal function, and to explaining the surgical limits that are compatible with retention of laryngeal function. His observations of the folding mechanism of the epiglottis during swallowing are models of simplicity and elegance. In 1964, during this work, he moved to the University of Washington in Seattle as Director of Anesthesia Research. His first book on the larynx, *The Human Larynx: a Functional Study*, was published in 1975. The second, *Laryngeal Biomechanics* in 1978, with anatomical artist Robert Demarest (Figure 2), won the 1978 and 1979 book award from the Anesthesia Foundation.

During the last two decades of his life, Fink directed much of his formidable intellect to historical aspects of anaesthesia. His brilliant 1984 Lewis Wright Memorial Lecture, *Leaves and Needles: The Introduction of Surgical*

Local Anesthesia, won international renown. He was Editor-in-Chief of the *Proceedings of the Third International Symposium on the History of Anesthesia* that was held in Atlanta, Georgia in 1992, and was president of the Anesthesia History Association. He served as a trustee of the ASA Wood Library–Museum of Anesthesiology in Park Ridge, Illinois and was

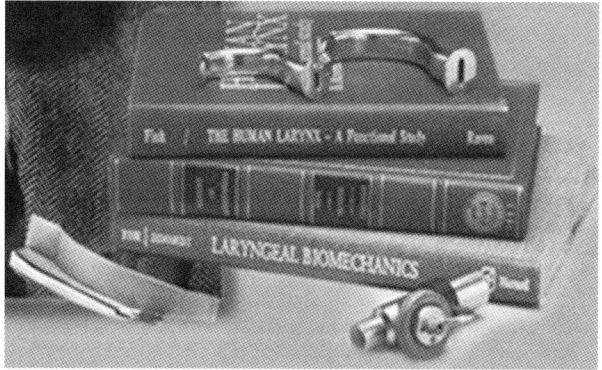

Figure 2. Fink's books and items of equipment. (Reproduced with kind permission from the Wood Library–Museum of Anesthesiology, Park Ridge IL, USA.)

chairman of its publications committee. In the mid-1990s, he launched the *Careers in Anesthesiology* series that documents the lives of anaesthetists of the latter half of the 20th century who had distinguished or interesting careers. Most of the contributions are autobiographical although some, like Fink's, have been completed posthumously.

He could speak and write in seven languages. He was as comfortable reciting poetry, discussing philosophy, or translating the works of Claude Bernard (1813–78) and Nikolai Pirogoff (1810–81) as he was discussing molecular mechanics or pharmacokinetics. He was the consummate intellectual and so much more; he was totally principled, graceful, benevolent, courtly and gentle. He had rare qualities that touched our hearts and minds. He blended science with service, history, philosophy and humanism. He compelled not only respect, but also deep affection, from all who knew him.

Fink received awards and honours and gave many eponymous lectures in the USA and abroad. He was elected to Fellowship of the Faculty of Anaesthetists of the Royal College of Surgeons of England in 1980, received the ASA Award for Excellence in Research in 1987 and the Distinguished Service Award of the American Society of Anesthesiologists in 1993.

Acknowledgement

Portrait photograph reproduced with kind permission from the Wood Library–Museum of Anesthesiology, Park Ridge, IL, USA.

Further reading

Epstein RM. ASA Award: B. Raymond Fink. *Anesthesiology* 1987; **67**: 456–8.
Fink BR. Diffusion anoxia. *Anesthesiology* 1955; **16**: 511–19.
McGoldrick KE. In Memoriam: B. Raymond Fink, M.D. (1914–2000) *Bulletin of Anesthesia History* 2001; **19(1)**: 3.

FLAGG CAN

Paluel Joseph Flagg (1886-1970)

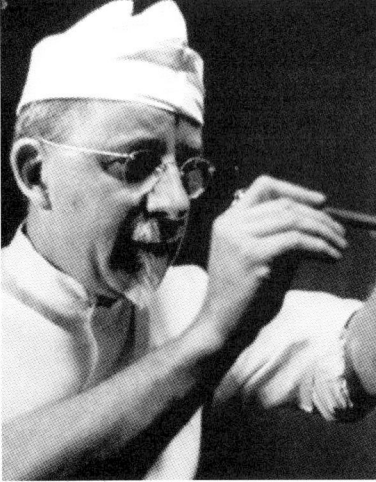

Paluel Flagg was born in 1886. He graduated in the first medical school class from Fordham University in Bronx, New York in 1909, and interned at St. Joseph's Hospital and the Lying-in Hospital in Providence, Rhode Island. He published his first article on ether in 1911 and in 1913 he decided to devote himself exclusively to anaesthesia. He worked in New York City during the First World War as a member of the Roosevelt Hospital reserve unit. In 1916, he completed the first edition of his book *The Art of Anaesthesia* that ran to a seventh edition in 1944 and was Anesthetist-in-Charge at St Vincent's Hospital in New York City from 1916 to 1934.

Flagg described his simple ether vaporizer, the Flagg can, in 1916 in the first edition of *The Art of Anaesthesia*. The earliest design consisted merely of an ether can with a perforated lid. He induced anaesthesia using the open drop method on a towel cone. He passed a catheter or small rectal tube into one of the nostrils, fitted this into a piece of rubber tubing, and attached the tubing to an ether can (Figure 1). He then poured a small amount of ether onto lint or a sponge in the can. Great care was needed in keeping the can upright to prevent liquid ether from finding its way into the catheter. Later modifications included a side draw tube and a gauze covering over the top of the can onto which the ether was dropped (Figure 2). Flagg demonstrated its effectiveness when Robert Macintosh visited him in the 1930s. In 1936, Macintosh went to Spain to provide anaesthesia for maxillofacial surgery cases during the Civil War, only to find no Boyle's machine and no cylinders of

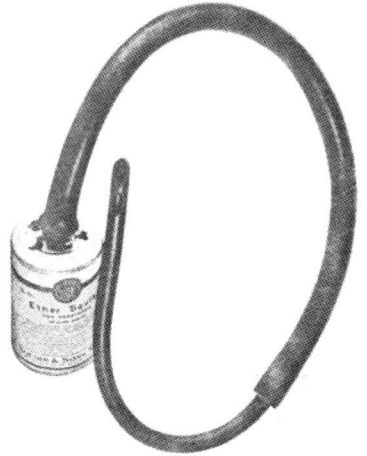

Figure 1. Flagg can with nasopharyngeal airway. (Reproduced with pemission from *The Art of Anaesthesia*, 2nd edn, Lippincott Williams & Wilkins, 1916.)

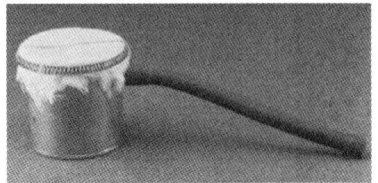

Figure 2. Gauze-covered Flagg can with side draw tube. (Reproduced with permission from *The Art of Anaesthesia*, 6th edn, Lippincott Williams & Wilkins, 1939.)

oxygen or nitrous oxide. His earlier amusement at the Flagg can turned to gratitude as he improvized one from an empty tin of golden syrup and found it worked well. This experience led to the development of the more precise wartime Oxford ether vaporizer.

Samuel Meltzer (1851–1922), John Auer (1875–1948) and Charles Elzberg (1871–1948) introduced endotracheal anaesthesia in 1910, but their methods required extra equipment. In the 1920s, Eastman Sheehan, a New York plastic surgeon who had worked with Ivan Magill in London, England told Flagg of Magill's two-tube method. This method required a special holder for the endotracheal insufflation catheter and separate expiration tube. Flagg realized that if the glottis tolerated this holder, he could use a single wide-bore tube and eliminate all other apparatus. He invented Flagg endotracheal tubes that remained unchanged for 20 years. The Flagg laryngoscope (Figure 3) was one of the earliest to have batteries in its handle.

In the early 1930s, he was struck by the obvious respiratory obstruction from amniotic fluid in a newborn baby. Unable to find any information in the medical literature, he contacted a pathologist at the New

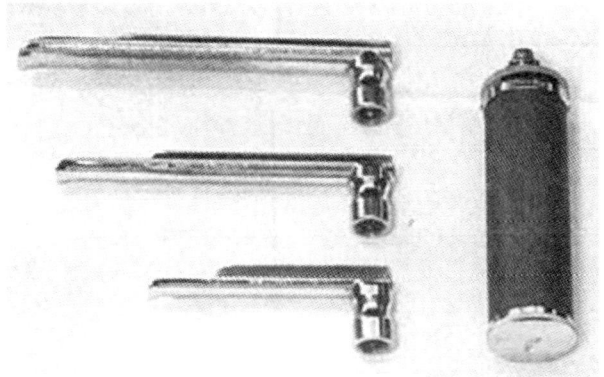

Figure 3. Flagg laryngoscope. (Reproduced with permission from *Clinical anesthesia*, W.B. Saunders Company, 1942: 285.)

York Lying-in Hospital, made measurements on cadaver infants, and constructed the infant insufflation tube that was consequently used in many clinics. Successful management of asphyxia in the newborn suggested to Flagg that similar treatment might be used in asphyxia from drowning in seawater, carbon monoxide poisoning, electrocution, foreign body obstruction or during anaesthesia. He determined the magnitude of the problem from the vital statistics of New York City, and published a provocative paper, *Asphyxial death, a professional disgrace*, in 1933. Along with other prominent doctors, Flagg led the movement to form the Society for the Prevention of Asphyxial Death (SPAD), and became its president. The American Medical Association (AMA) and two New York medical societies approved SPAD in less than one year, and the surgeons general of the armed forces and US Public Health Service sat on its advisory board throughout its 23 years. He included the results of a survey of asphyxia neonatorum in American and Canadian medical schools in his second book, *The Art of Resuscitation*, in 1944.

Flagg believed that anaesthesia societies were in a blind alley whose horizons were limited by the requirements of the surgeon. He advocated that well-trained technicians should work under the supervision of a physician-administrator to provide anaesthesia, resuscitation and inhalation therapy services. Organized anaesthesia was trying to eliminate these groups, and expressed little interest in resuscitation outside the operating theatre. In December 1936, the AMA appointed a committee on resuscitation with Flagg as chairman. The AMA House of Delegates accepted its 1937 report and recommendations, but allocated no funds for implementation. Flagg carried out some of the major recommendations at his own expense.

Flagg spent more than 40 years teaching doctors and paramedics respiratory and cardiac resuscitation. When mouth-to-mouth resuscitation and closed-chest cardiac massage became used routinely in the early 1960s, he reminded people that the brain dies of hypoxia long before the heart and re-emphasized the vital importance of proper oxygenation by preaching; 'Intubate first, then massage'.

Early in Flagg's career, an irascible surgical colleague employed the routine 'blame the anaesthetist' technique for a bad outcome. Flagg met this with a stony silence. That night, he wrote to the surgeon that there were three ways to react to his behaviour. He could tell him to go to hell and they would break permanently, he could take it and be a mutt, or he could say; 'Let's sit down and talk it over'. The following day the surgeon telephoned Flagg and invited him to lunch, which was the beginning of a lifelong friendship. Flagg's spirit of independence, and unwillingness to be beholden to anyone was responsible for many of his difficulties and much of his success. He was appalled by the flimsy assumptions, unproven hypotheses and theories that were taught as facts. He believed that a safe, established routine should have priority over a continuous introduction of new agents, and that progress in anaesthesia is determined by reducing morbidity and mortality.

Acknowledgement

Portrait photograph reproduced with kind permission from the Wood Library–Museum of Anesthesiology, Park Ridge, IL, USA.

Further reading

Flagg PJ. *The Art of Anaesthesia*. Philadelphia, PA: Lippincott, 1916.

Macintosh R. Saved by the Flagg. In: Atkinson RS, Boulton TB (Eds) *The History of Anaesthesia*. London: Royal Society of Medicine Press, 1989: 8–9.

THE FOREGGER COMPANY

Richard von Foregger (1872–1960)

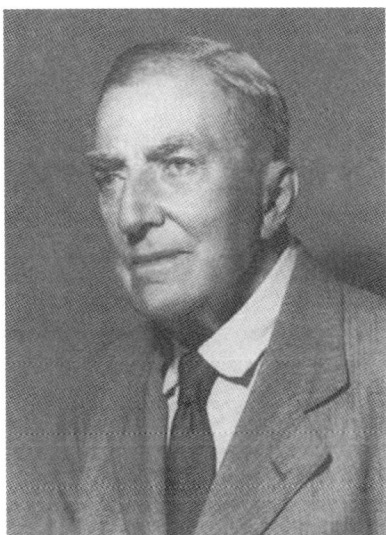

Richard von Foregger was born in Vienna, Austria in 1872, the son of a socially prominent Viennese family. His father was a lawyer and a member of the Austrian Senate. He learned Russian from his mother who was born in Odessa, Ukraine, and he was fluent in German, French and English. He studied at the University of Munich, Germany where he participated in fencing and acquired a large scar across the bridge of the nose in a duelling match. He went on to the Universities of Stuttgart, Germany and Bern, Switzerland where he received his PhD in chemistry in 1896. He immigrated to America in 1898 and worked for the General Electric Company until 1905. He then worked for the Roessler and Hasslacher Chemical Company in New York City until 1914.

Foregger had a special interest in the alkaline earth peroxides and superoxides. On 24 February 1902, the *Niagara Falls Gazette* reported that Foregger had spent six hours in a sealed six feet by three feet box with an oxygen generator, although there was only enough air for 20 minutes (Figure 1). In 1906, at the New York King's County Pharmaceutical Society, he demonstrated his small portable oxygen generator that produced pure oxygen and absorbed carbon dioxide when water was added to fused sodium peroxide. He and co-worker George Brindley calculated that 18 kg of sodium peroxide would keep nine men alive in a submarine for 14 hours. Later he modified the oxygen generator to become an oxygen–ether apparatus.

In 1914 he set up The Foregger Company in New York City for the manufacture of the oxygen generator and anaesthetic equipment. His office overlooked the New York Public Library and adjacent Bryant Park, and his workshop was in a barn at Roslyn, Long Island. He corresponded with manufacturers, surgeons, anaesthetists, nurse anaesthetists, hospital

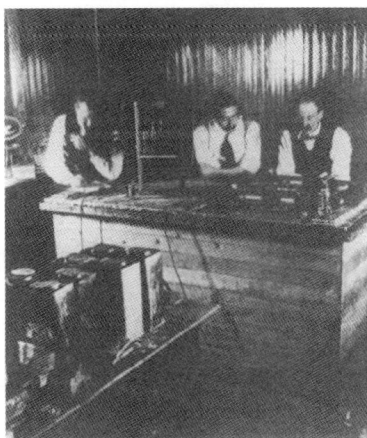

Figure 1. Richard Foregger (centre) behind the airtight box used in experiments at the Niagara Electrochemical Company (Reproduced from *Anesthesiology* 1996; 84: 190–200, with permission from Lippincott Williams & Wilkins.)

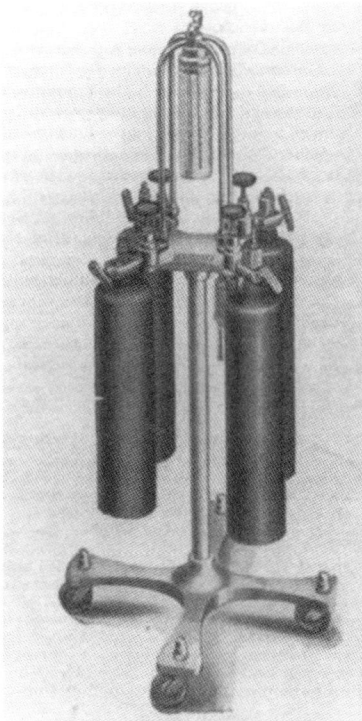

Figure 2. Gwathmey apparatus 1926. (Reproduced from *Anesthesiology* 1996; **84**: 190–200, with permission from Lippincott Williams & Wilkins.)

superintendents, Foregger salesmen, dealers and representatives. He enjoyed being at medical meetings to discuss new ideas or improvements in equipment, either at his display booth or at the hotel in the evening. Anaesthetists brought their ideas and designs to him, and he developed, manufactured and patented the equipment but he had no commercial relationship with any of them. Many anaesthetists were proud to see equipment named after them in Foregger's influential catalogue that he personally prepared every two years.

Foregger first met the New York anaesthetist James Gwathmey in 1907 and built the Gwathmey anaesthetic apparatus (Figure 2) from 1914 onwards. It had control valves for oxygen and nitrous oxide but no reducing valves. Each gas passed into a tube calibrated with a succession of openings and then through water into a glass mixing chamber.

In 1923, Ralph Waters was in private practice at Sioux City, Iowa. He gave Foregger the design of his to-and-fro carbon dioxide absorber for use in closed-circuit anaesthesia (Figure 3). This required fine adjustment for oxygen delivery so, in 1924, Foregger designed a water sight flowmeter. The principle was well known but its application for anaesthetic gases was new. Yandell Henderson and Howard Haggard, professors of applied physiology at Yale University in New Haven, Connecticut recalibrated and tested the first flowmeters. In early 1927, Foregger constructed a carbon dioxide absorber with unidirectional valves for anaesthesia apparatus. The apothecary system of ounces and gallons was used in medicine and engineering in the 1920s. Foregger vigorously promoted the metric system through his company's catalogue, and used it on his anaesthetic equipment. His success in this field was a major accomplishment.

Two German surgeons, Helmut Schmidt (1895–1979) of Hamburg and Hans Killian (1892–1982) of Freiburg, visited several American centres in 1928 and met Foregger at the 7th Annual Congress of Anesthetists in Minneapolis, Minnesota. They asked Foregger

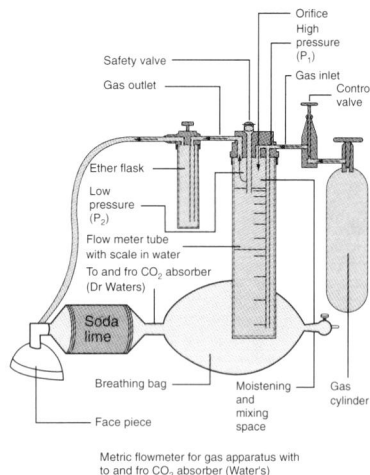

Figure 3. Diagram of carbon dioxide absorption circuit and flowmeter with metric scale. (Reproduced from *Anesthesiology* 1996; **84**: 190–200, with permission from Lippincott Williams & Wilkins.)

why the to-and-fro closed absorption system was used in America, and not the circle system that was used in Germany. Foregger soon introduced a circle system with very sensitive flutter valves to direct the gas stream. He acknowledged that DrägerWerk of Lübeck in Germany had long experience in building self-contained oxygen breathing apparatus for mine rescue work, and had preceded him with their circle absorber system for anaesthesia. At the 1929 Congress, Brian Sword (1889–1956) reported its use in 1200 cases.

In 1940, a Foregger military model anaesthetic apparatus tipped over and damaged the water flowmeter. Waters suggested changing to the rotameter, but Foregger resisted. The rotameter had been used in Germany in 1910 and again in 1923, and in England since 1937. Foregger eventually put the rotameter on his machines in 1950 and by 1958 it had almost replaced the obsolete water flowmeter.

He manufactured the original Guedel–Waters inflatable cuffs for endotracheal tubes and Waters's metal oropharyngeal airway. During the 1940s he worked with Arthur Guedel to construct anatomically correct oropharyngeal airways made of rubber and later of plastic. His development of laryngoscopes involved working with Arthur Guedel, Ralph Waters, Robert Miller and Robert Macintosh. His 1959 catalogue showed 20 different shaped laryngoscope blades in several sizes. He produced many devices that Paluel Flagg of New York City designed for anaesthesia and resuscitation. The Copper Kettle vaporizer that Lucien Morris invented in 1952 was one of the last major appliances that he developed and manufactured.

The last 14 years of his private life were surrounded by turmoil, which interfered with his business life. His physical condition began to deteriorate, and later he developed a paranoid psychosis. He died at the age of 87. The Foregger Company was subsequently acquired by other firms and was eventually liquidated.

Acknowledgement

Portrait photograph reproduced from *Anesthesiology* 1996; **84**: 190–200, with permission from Lippincott Williams & Wilkins.

Further reading

Cope DK. James Tayloe Gwathmey: Seeds of a developing specialty. *Anesthesia and Analgesia* 1993; **76**: 642–7.

Foregger R. Richard von Foregger, Ph.D., 1872–1960. *Anesthesiology* 1996; **84**: 190–200.

von Foregger R. New pharmaceutical sources of oxygen. *American Druggist and Pharmaceutical Record* 1906; **48**: 155–7.

GOLDMAN VAPORIZER
GOLDMAN NASAL MASK

Victor Goldman (1903–1994)

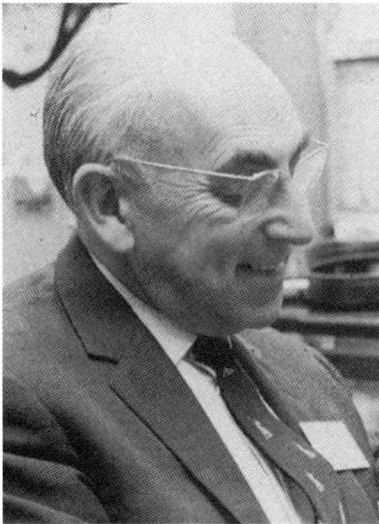

Victor Goldman was born in Birmingham, England in 1903. He was educated at King Edward's School, Birmingham and took his medical training in Birmingham where he was awarded the Gold Medal in surgery and graduated in medicine in 1927. He was resident anaesthetist at the Royal Free Hospital in London during 1935–39 and obtained the Diploma in Anaesthetics in 1936.

During the Second World War he was a senior specialist anaesthetist to the Ministry of Pensions from October 1939 to December 1940, and advisor in anaesthetics to the Northwest Army India Command from January 1941 until his discharge in November 1945. He then took up anaesthetic appointments in London at the Eastman Dental Clinic; the Royal Free Hospital; Queen Mary's Hospital, Stratford; Sutton and Cheam Hospital and Battersea General Hospital.

Goldman made many contributions to anaesthesia through his writing and inventions. In the 1930s he published articles on the new agents Evipan (hexobarbitone) and Vinesthene (divinyl ether) in dental anaesthesia, which was a special field of interest throughout his career. He described 'an improved electric laryngoscope' in 1936, five years before Robert Macintosh of Oxford and Robert Miller of San Antonio, Texas introduced theirs. The first edition of his book, *Aids to Anaesthesia*, was published in London in 1941. He wrote journal articles in the 1940s on giving anaesthetics in tropical climates, regional anaesthesia and the place of the anaesthetist in the surgical team.

He designed a Vinesthene inhaler for guillotine tonsillectomies and dental extractions in children. The contents of a 3 mL or 5 mL ampoule were shaken into the inhaler. The Vinesthene was vaporized by the child's to-and-fro breathing into the bag or by oxygen fed into the bag. Anaesthesia lasted for one minute after which it lightened owing to redistribution of the Vinesthene. In 1936, he designed a drip-feed vaporizer that required an average of two drops of Vinesthene per breath to supplement nitrous oxide and oxygen anaesthesia.

Several anaesthetists besides Goldman designed nasal masks so that inhalation anaesthesia in the dental chair could continue while the dentist

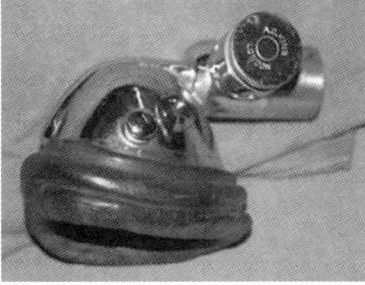

Figure 1. Goldman nasal mask. (Reproduced with kind permission from the Association of Anaesthetists of Great Britain and Ireland.)

worked in the patient's mouth. One prototype, made by the Cyprane Company in Keighley, Yorkshire, England, incorporated a whistle that reassured the dentist that the patient was breathing freely. Its absence warned of airway obstruction. Goldman's design (Figure 1) had studs for attachment of a head harness to free the anaesthetist's hands.

Goldman welcomed the introduction of halothane in 1956, and promoted its use in dental anaesthesia. In 1959, he made his first simple, low cost halothane vaporizer that could not deliver more than 2% halothane. He constructed this vaporizer from a glass bowl that was fitted below the mechanical fuel pump to trap sediment in British army vehicles. He used it to supplement nitrous oxide for short operations in children. However, as its popularity spread, anaesthetists soon found it less satisfactory for long operations. It had no temperature compensating mechanism, and output fell as the halothane cooled. Goldman produced a more efficient mark II vaporizer (Figure 2) by modifying the size and shape of the opening in the ports and limiting movement of the inner sleeve. He added volume markings on the glass, and introduced 'click stops' for the concentration-regulating lever. In 1966, he measured delivered halothane concentration during a one and a half hour operation. Output still fell, but he could partially circumvent this by regularly topping up with halothane at room temperature.

In 1960, Goldman visited the USA and Canada, where he had many friends and colleagues. He visited clinics and hospitals in New York City, New York; Madison, Wisconsin; the Mayo Clinic in Rochester, Minnesota and the Ether Dome in Boston, Massachusetts. He attended the Second World Congress of Anaesthesiologists in Toronto, Ontario and afterwards visited clinics in Toledo and Cleveland, Ohio.

Richard Bodman, at St Paul's Hospital, London, created a simple closed circuit (Figure 3) that used a Waters soda lime canister, mark II Goldman vaporizer, a T-piece and unidirectional valves. He found this safe and satisfactory for closed-circuit halothane and oxygen with spontaneous respiration. He set the vaporiser setting at '2' for induction in adults and reduced it to '1' after three minutes. The inspired concentration fell exponentially to a little over 1% as a steady state developed. The improved safety of this in-circuit vaporizer, compared with the ether bottle when it is first turned on, was due to its inability to deliver a

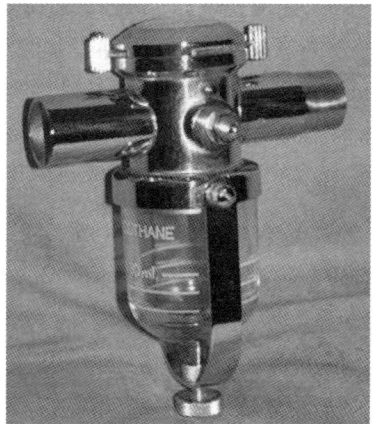

Figure 2. Goldman halothane vaporizer mark II. (Reproduced with kind permission from the Association of Anaesthetists of Great Britain and Ireland.)

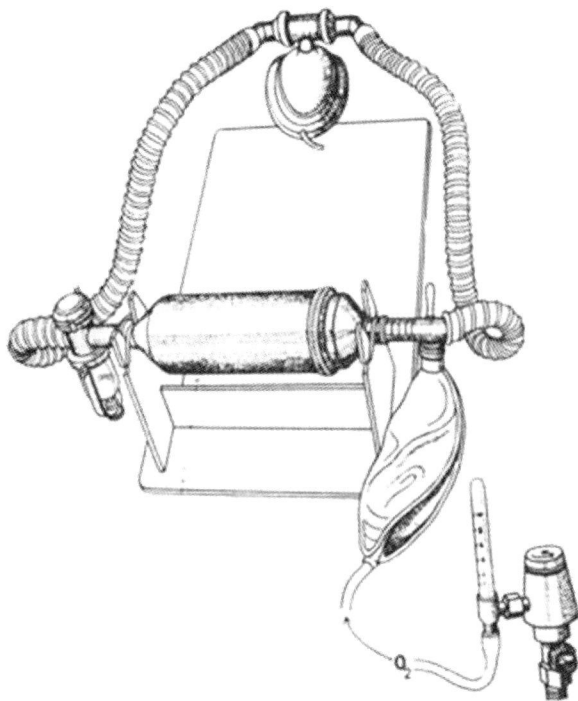

Figure 3. Goldman vaporizer in closed circuit. (Reproduced from *Anaesthesia* 1967; 22: 476–86.)

dangerously high halothane concentration.

Goldman devoted much of his career to the improvement and safety of outpatient dental anaesthesia. In 1958, he reviewed death rates from the 1920s to 1950s from anaesthesia in dentists' surgeries. The surgery was often a large room in the dentist's own house. Patients were commonly anaesthetized sitting up in the dental chair without tracheal intubation. Most cases only lasted a few minutes and Goldman believed that, with a throat pack in place and a clear airway, this was safer than the morbidity from intubation if the supine position were adopted. The death rate with intravenous barbiturates was higher than with inhalation anaesthetics, and he warned strongly against their general use in the dental surgery. He knew he was recognized as an authority on dental anaesthesia, and his firmly opinionated attitude did not endear him to some other eminent anaesthetists.

Goldman was a member of many anaesthesia societies, including the Association of Anaesthetists of Great Britain and Ireland, the Section of Anaesthetics of the Royal Society of Medicine, The International Congress of Anaesthetists and the American Society of Anesthesiologists.

Acknowledgement

Portrait photograph reproduced with kind permission from the Eastman Dental Hospital, London, UK.

Further reading

Bodman RI, Gerson G, Smith K. A simple closed circuit for halothane anaesthesia. *Anaesthesia* 1967; 22: 476–86.

Goldman V. Deaths under anaesthesia in the dental surgery. *British Dental Journal* 1958; 105: 160–3.

Goldman V. The Goldman halothane vaporiser mark II. *Anaesthesia* 1962; 17: 537–9.

GORDH NEEDLE

Torsten Gordh (1907–)

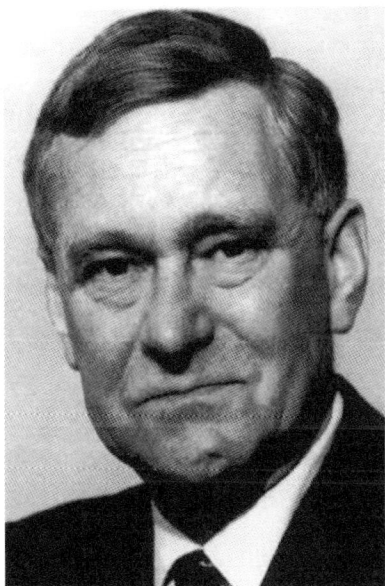

Torsten Gordh was born in Sweden in 1907 and was the eldest of six children. His father was a land surveyor and his mother was the daughter of a clergyman. His application to train as a surveyor was rejected so he decided to upgrade his mathematics. He did not understand the first lecture at the University of Uppsala, Sweden and decided to study medicine instead. He spent seven and a half years at the medical school of the Karolinska Institute in Stockholm where he graduated in 1935.

Gordh wanted to be a surgeon and worked for a year and a half at a well-respected hospital in Örebro before becoming a junior surgical resident with Gustaf Söderlund – Professor at the University Clinic of the Serafimer Hospital in Stockholm. Like all the surgical residents at that time, Gordh spent his first six months as a 'dripper'. This meant dripping ether on a mask for all patients, even though he had no anaesthesia training.

Swedish doctors who travelled to Great Britain and the USA admired the quiet and peaceful anaesthetics they saw there and wanted the same in Sweden. Söderlund suggested to Gordh that he should study anaesthesia. Gordh's answer was; 'I'll think about it'. Some months later, a plastic surgeon who had trained in England mentioned that Michael Nosworthy (1902–80), senior consultant anaesthetist at St Thomas' Hospital in London was in town and that Gordh should meet him. They met for six hours and Nosworthy presented the whole story of the rapidly developing specialty of anaesthesia. Gordh was convinced that anaesthesia was applied physiology and pharmacology at its best, that its advancement was necessary for good surgery, and that he would pursue it.

Nosworthy then arranged for Gordh to become a resident with Ralph Waters at the University of Wisconsin in Madison. Gordh left for the USA in October 1938 to be a resident with free board, lodging and laundry and was paid 25 dollars each month. What struck him most was that a doctor provided close supervision of every patient under anaesthesia and recorded pulse, blood pressure and respiration every five minutes. He appreciated the importance of Waters' basic precepts of patient safety and comfort, teaching and research, and he followed them throughout his career. Through errors he also learned how easy it was to overdose and kill a dog in the laboratory.

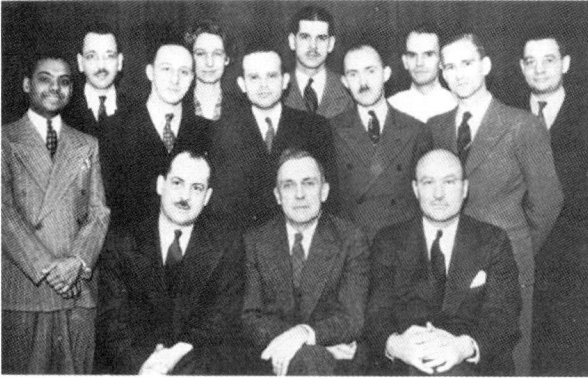

Figure 1. 'Aqua alumni' 1939. (Left to right) Back row: William Cassels, Virginia Apgar, Harvey Slocum, Allen Conroy, Ivan Taylor. Middle row: Barney Sircar, Digby Leigh, Hubert Hathaway, William Neff, Torsten Gordh. Seated: Emery Rovenstine, Ralph Waters, Maurice Seevers. (Reproduced with kind permission from the University of Wisconsin, Madison.)

Gordh spent 15 months in Madison (Figure 1) and one month travelling to other centres of interest. He arrived home in Sweden on 8 April 1940, one day before the German occupation of Norway and Denmark. After one week with his family, he started work as an anaesthetist at the newly opened Karolinska Hospital University Clinic.

Gordh always acknowledged that Thore Olovson (1904–87), a surgeon at St Görans Hospital, Stockholm in the late 1930s, and Helge Meyer, an engineer at the instrument firm of Stille–Werner (now Stille Surgical AB) in Stockholm, constructed the original intravenous needle with wings at the head end and a rubber membrane inserted in a detachable ring (Figures 2 and 3). It was fixed in position with adhesive tape over the wings and could remain patent for several days. Olovson designed it so that four-hourly heparin injections could be made through the rubber diaphragm to treat postoperative thrombosis without disturbing the patient. The needle was taken apart for sterilization and the diaphragm could be replaced at any time.

When Gordh returned from Madison, Meyer showed him the Olovson needle. Gordh said it was 'like a gift from heaven'. He found it so useful that in 1945 he described it in *Anesthesiology*, quoting Olovson's original paper. Intravenous anaesthesia previously required anaesthetists to fix both the syringe and its needle on the forearm with tape. Even special syringe holders were devised to address the problem. Gordh used the Olovson needle for intravenous anaesthesia and later added an inlet at the end for an intravenous drip and blood transfusion. Many anaesthetists visited the Karolinska Hospital after the war; they saw Gordh using the technique and referred to it as the 'Gordh needle'. It was the forerunner of disposable plastic intravenous cannulae that became available in the 1960s. When Olovson died, Gordh wrote that anaesthetists, nurses and patients from all over the world could send Olovson a grateful thought.

In 1943, the chemists Nils Loefgren and Holger Erdtman at the Department of Organic Chemistry, University of Stockholm, synthe-

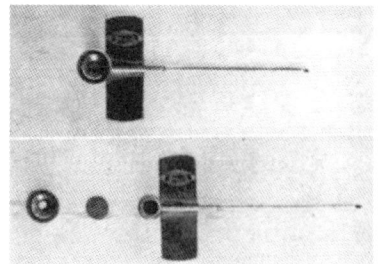

Figure 2. At the base of the needle there is a ring screw at a right angle to the shaft. Inside the ring is a rubber diaphragm 1.5 mm thick. A metal wing for adhesive fixation to the skin is placed at the base. (Reproduced from *Anesthesiology* 1945; 6: 258–60, with permission from Lippincott Williams & Wilkins.)

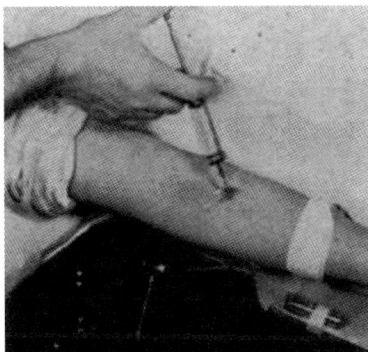

Figure 3. Injection through the diaphragm of the Gordh indwelling needle. (Reproduced from *Anesthesiology* 1945; **6**: 258–60, with permission from Lippincott Williams & Wilkins.)

sized a series of 16 basic anilides that were different in chemical structure from the cocaine and procaine groups of local anaesthetics. Early in 1943, the chemist Bengt Lundquist, tested the compounds on himself – on his tongue, finger blocks and even spinals. He told Loefgren that LL30 was the best. The pharmaceutical company, Astra, bought the patent application and worldwide marketing and distribution rights for Xylocain (lignocaine, lidocaine) in November 1943. Gordh began clinical trials in 1944. He presented his findings at the Swedish Anaesthesia Club in 1947 and published his landmark paper on Xylocain for infiltration analgesia, conduction anaesthesia, spinal blocks and surface analgesia in *Anaesthesia* in 1949.

Gordh was the first medically trained anaesthetist in Sweden and the father of Scandinavian anaesthesia. The decade from 1945 to 1955 saw anaesthesia being recognized as an important branch of medicine in Sweden. The Anaesthesia Club became the Swedish Society of Anaesthesiologists and *Acta Anaesthesiologica Scandinavica* began publication. The next decade saw the development of subspecialization and intensive care, and the establishment of the first Swedish Chair in Anaesthesia at the Karolinska Institute in 1963. Gordh was the first chairman from 1964 to 1974.

Gordh was one of the five initial members of the Interim Committee that, in 1955, led to the formation of the World Federation of Societies of Anaesthesiologists, and he became a member of its executive committee. When he retired from the Karolinska Institute in 1974, his friends, colleagues and firms raised money to establish the Torsten Gordh Lecture Fund. His honours include the Gaston Labat Award of the American Society of Regional Anesthesia in 1979; the Ralph M. Waters Award and Lecture, Midwest Anesthesia Conference in 1982; and the Carl Koller Medal of the European Society of Regional Anaesthesia in 1986.

Gordh has many talents – he could have been a professional magician with his quick movements, impish eyes and conjuring repertoire.

Acknowledgement

Portrait photograph reproduced with kind permission from the Wood Library–Museum of Anesthesiology, Park Ridge, IL, USA.

Further reading

Anonymous. We salute ... Torsten Gordh, M.D. *Anesthesia and Analgesia.* 1964; **43**: 199–200.

Gordh T. A new, simple and practical needle for intravenous anesthesia. *Anesthesiology* 1945; **6**: 258–60.

Gordh T. Xylocain – a new local analgesic. *Anaesthesia* 1949; **4**: 4–9, 21.

The Liverpool technique

Thomas Cecil Gray (1913–)

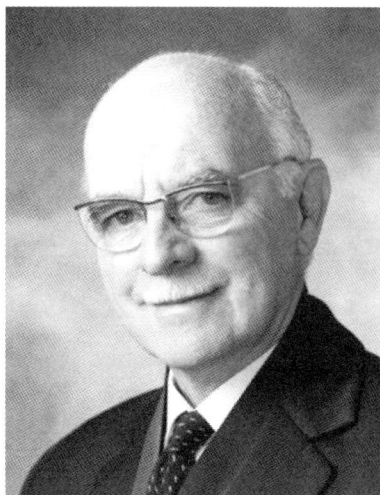

Cecil Gray was born in Liverpool, Merseyside in 1913. His father, Thomas, also Liverpool-born and of Irish stock, was proprietor of the ancient Liverpool 'Clock Inn'; his mother, Ethel, came from the village of Bollington, near Macclesfield in Cheshire. Gray developed childhood asthma and was sent to a preparatory boarding school run by nuns in the milder climate of Bath, Somerset. He continued his education at the Benedictine College of Ampleforth in Yorkshire. Seeing perfection in the life of the monks, on leaving school he decided to try his vocation. After two months in the monastery, it was clear to all except Gray that he did not have one. He returned home to the disappointment of his mother and the joy of his father!

He applied to read medicine at Liverpool University, and graduated with a Bachelor of medicine and a Bachelor of surgery in June 1937, with distinction in anatomy. He went straight into general practice in Liverpool as assistant to an excellent family doctor and teacher. In January 1939, he bought a single-handed practice in Wallasey, Merseyside. Greatly helped by his wife, he quickly built it up to provide a good living. When the Second World War erupted, he was found unfit for military service because of his asthma.

Gray became interested in anaesthesia when he anaesthetized his own private patients who needed surgery. He engaged a part-time assistant in his practice to enable him to attend a hospital on two afternoons a week to study for the Diploma in Anaesthetics, which he passed in November 1941. He sold his practice and became a full-time anaesthetist.

Gray felt fit for army service and, with uxorial approval, volunteered for another medical in November 1942. He was found fit and served in North Africa as anaesthetist to a mobile neurosurgical unit. In 1944, he became critically ill with bronchopneumonia. He was saved by four-hourly intramuscular injections of trial samples of crystalline penicillin. He returned to England on a hospital ship, was discharged, and resumed his hospital duties in Liverpool. In 1945, he was appointed as a part-time university demonstrator in anaesthesia.

He resumed a friendship with John Halton (1903–68), an innovative anaesthetist who was then working with Hugh Morriston Davies, a distinguished surgeon who was establishing a thoracic surgical unit in Mersey-side. Halton joined the US Air Force Officers' Mess at the Burtonwood Bomber Base outside Liverpool where he heard about the use of curare in anaesthesia by Harold Griffith in Montreal, Quebec. Halton persuaded one of his American friends to bring some over for him.

The curare arrived in the form of Intocostrin (Squibb). Halton shared it with Gray, and a trial using it in conjunction with cyclopropane anaesthesia was agreed. When the supply of Intocostrin was exhausted, Gray reminded Halton of the curarine used in physiology classes to explore neuromuscular transmission. Curarine (Burroughs–Wellcome) was a crystalline alkaloid, d-tubocurarine chloride, first isolated in 1935 from crude curare by Harold King in London's Wellcome Laboratory. Gray obtained a box full of ampoules of curarine, each containing 100 mg of crystalline powder. When total sterility was ascertained, Halton and Gray started clinical trials by tipping one ampoule into 500 mL of normal saline and using it as an intravenous infusion, changing the infusion to plain saline when the desired effect was achieved. The dose required was soon determined and Burroughs–Wellcome supplied ampoules containing 15 mg of tubocurarine in 1 mL of saline.

The striking results were first reported to a meeting of the Liverpool Medical Institution in January 1946. Results in 1049 further cases were reported to the Section of Anaesthetics of the Royal Society of Medicine, London, under the title *A Milestone in Anaesthesia? (d-tubocurarine chloride)* on 1 March 1946. Gray upended current thinking in 1947 when he wrote in his MD thesis, 'The aim should be to use very light anaesthesia and to provide good operating conditions with the relaxant drug.' This principle guided his future teaching and research.

Pulmonary hyperventilation, resulting in a degree of hypocarbia, became a feature in intubated, curarized patients. It was found to reduce the amount of both anaesthetic and relaxant required. Hyperventilation (hypocarbia) was added to the triad of 'narcosis, analgesia (reflex depression) and muscle relaxation' necessary for anaesthesia, thus making it a pyramid. This approach to anaesthesia, with reversal of the relaxant using neostigmine and atropine, became known as the 'Liverpool technique'. It calls for meticulous technique, especially when nitrous oxide is used as the sole anaesthetic, as was Gray's practice. He avoided what he called the 'smelly agents', referring especially to ether and halothane.

An original contribution of Gray's department was the 'day-release course' for junior anaesthetists preparing for anaesthesia examinations, which attracted students from the UK, Europe, the Far East, Australia, Africa and India. Gray had a brilliant team of co-workers in Liverpool, including Jackson Rees, an outstanding pioneer in the modernization of paediatric anaesthesia. Others were appointed to professorial chairs in Liverpool, Manchester, Belfast, Birmingham, Pecs (Hungary), Cape Town, Sydney, Hyderabad (India) and Boston.

Gray was appointed full-time reader in anaesthesia and head of department in 1947 and in 1959 he was awarded a personal chair with the title of professor. He was editor of the *British Journal of Anaesthesia* from 1948 to 1963. He was a founder member of the Board of the Faculty of Anaesthetists of the Royal College of Surgeons, its vice-dean from 1952 to 1954 and dean from 1964 to 1967. In 1970 he was appointed dean of faculty of medicine in Liverpool. His many awards include the CBE; Knight Commander of the Order of St Gregory from Pope John Paul II; Hickman Medallist of the Royal Society of Medicine in 1972; he was elected to Honorary Membership in 1977 and awarded the John Snow Silver Medal in 1982 of the Association of Anaesthetists of Great Britain and Ireland.

Gray retired in 1976 to be with his wife who died of cancer in 1978. Their son David, an anaesthetist, was born in 1939 and daughter Beverley was born in 1942. He married again in 1979 and he and his American wife have a son, James, born in 1981. Although retired for over 20 years, Gray is still kept busy with worldwide correspondence, medical meetings and writing.

Further reading

Gray TC. A reassessment of the signs and levels of anaesthesia. *Irish Journal of Medical Sciences.* 6th Series 1960: 499–508.

Gray TC, Halton J. A milestone in anaesthesia? (d-tubocurarine chloride). *Proceedings of the Royal Society of Medicine* 1946; **39**: 400–10.

King H. Curare alkaloids. I. tubocurarine. *Journal of the Chemical Society* 1935; **57**: 1381–9.

HAROLD GRIFFITH SYMPOSIUM

Harold Randall Griffith (1894–1985)

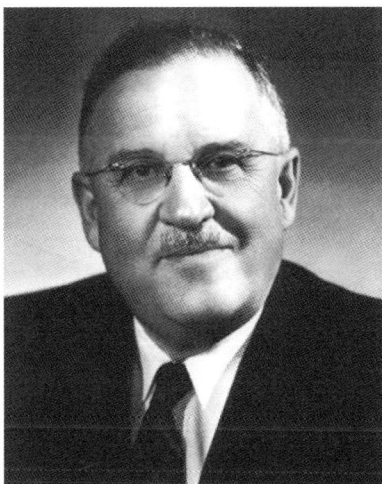

Harold Griffith was born in Montreal, Quebec in 1894. His father, a physician, had also trained in homoeopathic medicine and was one of the founders of the Montreal Homoeopathic Hospital that opened in 1894. It was renamed Queen Elizabeth Hospital in 1951 and closed in the 1990s. Griffith attended school in Montreal, won a scholarship to McGill University, Montreal and completed his BA degree and one year of medicine before the outbreak of the First World War. He volunteered for army service in 1914, served for three years in the 6th Field Ambulance of the Canadian Expeditionary Force, and was awarded the Military Medal for gallantry at the battle of Vimy Ridge. He transferred to the British Navy as a Probationary Surgeon Sub-Lieutenant until the end of the war.

Griffith returned to Montreal in the autumn of 1918. He resumed his medical studies, graduating in medicine and surgery from McGill University in 1922 and gaining a Doctorate of Homoeopathic Medicine from Hahnemann Medical College in Philadelphia, Pennsylvania in 1923. He became interested in anaesthesia early in his medical training. His first paper was based on the 400 anaesthetics he had given as a medical student and was published in 1922.

He became Chief of Anaesthesia at the Montreal Homoeopathic Hospital in 1923, and held the post until 1959. His father was medical director there and his younger brother Jim was the chief of surgery. Although he had no formal training in anaesthesia, he soon began to write papers on ethylene and endotracheal anaesthesia. This brought him to the attention of Frank McMechan (1879–1939) of Cleveland, Ohio and founder of the International Anesthesia Research Society; Ralph Waters of Madison, Wisconsin and Wesley Bourne of Montreal. They recruited him to help in the advancement of anaesthesia as a specialty.

Griffith taught himself to intubate the trachea early in his career after losing a patient to hypoxia from intense laryngospasm in 1925. At that time, there was no manufacturer of endotracheal tubes so he ordered extralarge urinary catheters (up to size 34 French gauge) specially made by a manufacturer in Paris, France. In 1933, Waters drew Griffith's attention to cyclopropane and closed-circuit anaesthesia. Griffith adopted the new agent enthusiastically, using assisted or controlled ventilation when necessary. His status as a clinician, researcher and teacher grew rapidly.

Griffith first used curare in anaesthesia on 23 January 1942. In an interview more than 30 years later he described how this came about:

> 'Like everyone else, I knew that there was a need for better muscular relaxation during certain surgical procedures so I pricked up my ears when, in 1940, Dr Lewis Wright told me of his idea that curare might provide that relaxation. He told me of the work of Dr A.E. Bennett, of Nebraska, who had been using the new preparation, Intocostrin to soften the convulsions of patients undergoing shock therapy for psychiatric disease. Because curare had a fabulous reputation as a poison, I was only mildly interested, but I kept thinking of the possibilities.
>
> I met Dr Wright again in 1941, and asked him how he was getting along with his idea. He said he still thought that curare might be of value to the anaesthetist but he hadn't been able to get anyone to try it in the Operating Room. I argued to myself that if it did not kill Dr Bennett's patients it could hardly do any serious harm to ours, because the major danger would be respiratory paralysis and even at that time anaesthetists were accustomed to maintaining controlled respiration over long periods so I asked Dr Wright to send me some Intocostrin.
>
> On January 23, 1942 at the Homoeopathic Hospital in Montréal (now the Queen Elizabeth Hospital) my resident, Dr Enid Johnson, and I administered the first dose to a young man undergoing appendectomy...'

He had acted courageously and responsibly, knowing that he could intubate the trachea and provide controlled ventilation if necessary. Griffith observed rapid relaxation of the abdominal muscles, he was able to reduce the concentration of cyclopropane and did not need to assist ventilation. When he and Johnson had given Intocostrin to 24 more patients, they concluded that the drug could be used safely and successfully and published their results in July 1942. Reaction was swift; those who did not try the drug were often scathing in their condemnation. They implied that Griffith had acted irresponsibly in using the poison but he was eventually vindicated.

Griffith was a Wing Commander in the Royal Canadian Air Force during the Second World War, and thus served in all three armed services. He developed a rapid training programme for physicians who would be going overseas to administer anaesthetics. This gave him the experience to organize the McGill University training programme in anaesthesia. He joined Wesley Bourne, the newly appointed first professor and chairman, at McGill University in 1946 and succeeded him from 1951 to 1956.

Griffith became the first president of the Canadian Anaesthetists' Society during 1943–46, and president of the International Anaesthesia Research Society in 1948. From 1951 to 1955 he was involved in what he considered to be his greatest contribution to anaesthesia, the organization of the World Federation of Societies of Anaesthesiologists. He was elected president at its first meeting in The Netherlands in 1955, and permanent founder president at the second World Congress in Toronto, Ontario in 1960. His name is now enshrined in the Harold Griffith Symposium, which is a feature of each World Congress and is given by one or more distinguished speakers.

Harold Griffith was Hickman Medallist of the Royal Society of Medicine in 1956; he received the Distinguished Service Award of the American Society of Anesthesiologists in 1959; and was appointed an Officer of the Order of Canada in 1974. Canada post issued a 40-cent stamp of Harold Griffith on 15 March 1991, one of a group of four famous Canadian physicians (Figure 1). There is now an endowed Harold R. Griffith research chair in anaesthesia at McGill University to honour this man who dedicated his life to the practice of anaesthesia. Many senior anaesthetists still remember him affectionately as 'Uncle Harold'.

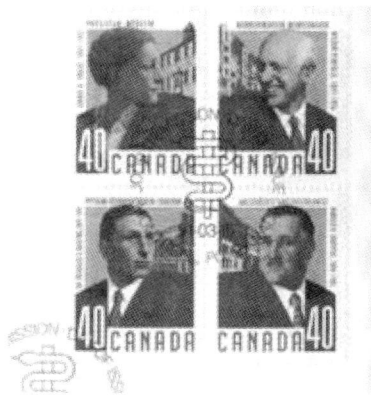

Figure 1. Commemorative stamps issued by Canada Post on March 15, 1991 to honour four Canadian physicians: Jennie Trout (1841–1921), Wilder Penfield (1891–1976), Sir Frederick Banting (1891–1941) and Harold Griffith.

Acknowledgement

Portrait photograph reproduced with kind permission from McGill University Department of Anesthesia, Montreal, Canada.

Further reading

Bodman RI, Gillies DM. *Harold Griffith: the evolution of modern anaesthesia.* Toronto, Ontario: Hannah Institute and Dundurn Press, 1992.

Griffith HR, Johnson GE. The use of curare in general anesthesia. *Anesthesiology* 1942; 3: 418–20.

Maltby JR, Shephard DAE (Eds). Harold Griffith – his life and legacy. *Canadian Journal of Anaesthesia* 1992; **39 (Suppl 1)**: 1–145.

GUEDEL ORAL AIRWAY
GUEDEL SIGNS OF ETHER ANAESTHESIA

Arthur E. Guedel (1883–1956)

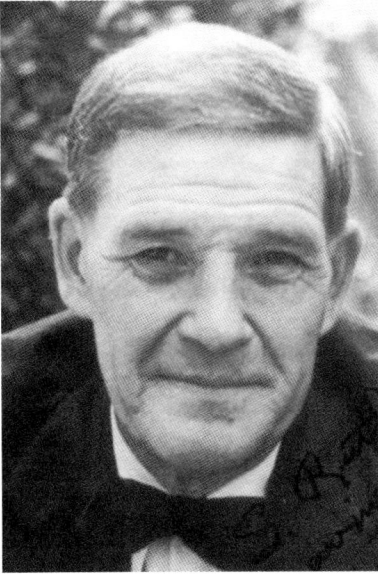

Arthur Guedel was born in Cambridge City, Indiana in 1883 and attended grade school in Indianapolis, Indiana. He lost three fingers from his right hand when he was 13, but he went on to become an accomplished pianist, organist and composer. His family could not afford to send him to high school. He continued his education under the guidance of a high school teacher and was admitted to the Medical College of Indiana in Indianapolis in 1903. He graduated in 1908 and interned for six months at the City Hospital in Indianapolis where he was required to administer ether and chloroform. He became interested in anaesthesia and when he opened his first general practice in 1909, he supplemented his income by providing anaesthetic services to hospitals and dental offices.

Guedel served as an anaesthetist in the American Expeditionary Forces in France in the First World War. He and his colleagues performed heroically but, even by working non-stop for 72 hours after a battle, they could not attend to the thousands of wounded men needing surgery. He developed a training school for orderlies and nurses to learn how to administer anaesthesia, and then made short visits to each local hospital every day or two by motorcycle to instruct and supervise them. He created a wall chart that showed the stages and physical signs of ether anaesthesia to enable the trainees to assess depth of anaesthesia (Figure 1). This classification of stages of anaesthesia was used throughout the world for more than 50 years. After the war, he spent a year in Minneapolis, Minnesota and then returned to the private practice of anaesthesia in Indianapolis.

Guedel and Ralph Waters became acquainted at meetings of the Anaesthesia Travel Club, the American Society of Anesthesiologists, and other anaesthesia societies. Although they never lived in the same city, they discussed ideas through regular correspondence and visits. Guedel created the first inflatable cuffs for endotracheal tubes from the fingers of rubber gloves in the basement laboratory of his home. From 1926 to 1928 he experimented on the composition of cuff and tube – whether the cuff should be above, below or at the vocal cords; how far the tube should

	Respiration		Ocular movements	Pupils no premedication	Eye reflexes	Secretion of tears	Laryngeal and pharyngeal reflexes	Respiratory response to skin incision	Muscular tone
	Intercostal	Diaphragm							
Stage 1			Voluntary control			Normal			Normal
Stage 2					Eyelash / Lid		Swallowing Retching Vomiting		Tense Struggling
Stage 3 (Plane I)									
Stage 3 (Plane II)					Conjunctival / Corneal		Glottic		
Stage 3 (Plane III)					Pupillary light reflex				
Stage 3 (Plane IV)									
Stage 4									

Figure 1. Guedel's signs of ether anaesthesia. (Reproduced with permission from *A synopsis of anesthesia*, 2nd edn, John Wright & Sons, 1950: 41.)

extend beyond the cuff; and inflation techniques and pressures. Waters joined him in the final stages of this enterprise.

Guedel demonstrated the safety of his technique by filling an intubated patient's mouth with water, but a second demonstration failed. He wrote to Waters in April 1928; 'If you try it, be sure to aspirate all the water before you remove the catheter [tube]. I left it to an intern and he didn't. Result, annoying laryngospasm ...' In the same letter he proposed the 'dunked dog' demonstration (Figure 2). This featured his own dog, Airway, who was anaesthetized, intubated and immersed in an aquarium at the beginning of a lecture. After the demonstration was complete, the dog was retrieved from the water, allowed to awaken, shake himself and exit to the applause of the audience. His assignment completed, Airway enjoyed an honourable retirement with the Waters family in Madison, Wisconsin.

Guedel moved to Pasadena, California for health reasons in 1928 to be clinical professor of anesthesia at the University of Southern California and staff anaesthetist at the Cedars of Lebanon Hospital in Los Angeles. In the same year Chauncey Leake (1896–1978), an eminent pharmacologist, moved from the University of Wisconsin, Madison to the University of California Health Center in San Francisco. Leake had begun a study with Waters on carbon dioxide anaesthesia and confirmed the findings of Henry Hill Hickman. Leake enlisted Guedel's expert assistance to study the anaesthetic effects of divinyl ether in dogs. They showed that it was safe and effective, but were prevented from proceeding to clinical trials in patients by a stiffly conservative professor of neurosurgery. They collaborated on other research, including inhalation of 30–70% carbon dioxide (which produced transitory improvement in catatonic schizophrenia) and the early use of thiopental.

Metal pharyngeal airways could be traumatic to the patient's lips, teeth or pharynx, so in 1933,

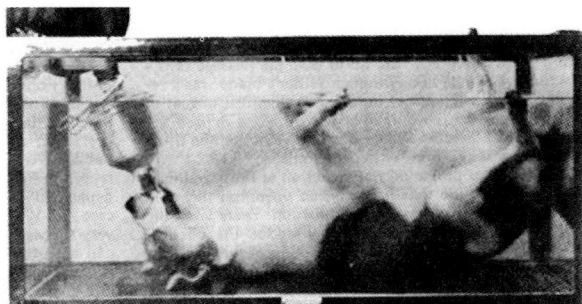

Figure 2. The 'dunked dog' demonstration. (Reproduced from *Clinical anesthesia* 4th edn, 2001: 17, with permission from Lippincott Williams & Wilkins.)

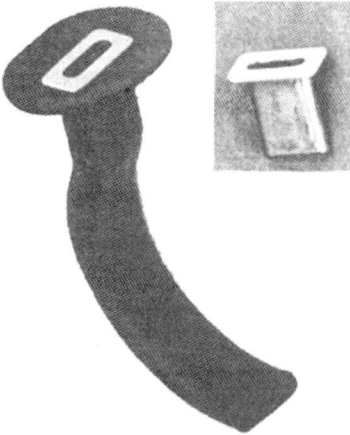

Figure 3. Guedel oral airway. (Reproduced from *Journal of the American Medical Association* 1933; **100**: 1862.)

Guedel designed one in moulded rubber (Figure 3) with a metal insert to prevent occlusion by biting. His design has stood the test of time for nearly 70 years.

Guedel's research background, combined with his clinical experience during peace and war, was the basis for *Inhalation Anesthesia, a Fundamental Guide* which was published in 1937. He presented a wealth of information in a readable fashion, interspersed with illustrative case reports and mistakes to teach important principles. It was essential for teachers and students in medical school, but it also provided valuable practical guidance for general practitioners and specialist anaesthetists. He produced a second edition in 1951.

Guedel pushed himself hard and often suffered from insomnia. In one particularly hectic period, he took barbiturates to get to sleep and developed a dependence on them. Then he began taking amphetamines to be alert in the mornings. He was soon taking larger doses of both drugs, one to ensure sleep and one to wake up. When he realized that he was caught in a vicious circle, he had the strength of character to stop taking either and overcame both addictions. He was disturbed by what he had been through, and made efforts to warn other physicians of this great risk.

However, angina, arthritis, and emphysema crippled him and he retired from clinical practice in 1941. He and his wife continued to provide hospitality in their home to visiting colleagues. His workshop became a meeting place for anaesthetists and residents in training. In his last years, he required supplemental oxygen but he continued to visit laboratories and hospitals, asking questions and offering helpful suggestions.

In 1941, Guedel was the first Hickman Medallist of the Royal Society of Medicine from outside the British Isles. He also received the Distinguished Service Award of the American Society of Anesthesiologists in 1950. The Arthur E. Guedel Memorial Anesthesia Center in San Francisco opened in 1964. It has a fine library of current and historical writings and is a fitting tribute to the high esteem in which he was held.

Acknowledgement

Portrait photograph reproduced with kind permission from the Wood Library–Museum of Anesthesiology, Park Ridge, IL, USA.

Further reading

Guedel AE. A nontraumatic pharyngeal airway. *Journal of the American Medical Association* 1933; **100**: 1862.

Guedel AE, Waters RM. A new intratracheal catheter. *Anesthesia and Analgesia* 1928; **7**: 238–9.

Waters R. Eminent anaesthetists, No. 7 Arthur E. Guedel. *British Journal of Anaesthesia* 1952; **24**: 292–9.

FREDERIC HEWITT LECTURE

Sir Frederic William Hewitt (1857–1916)

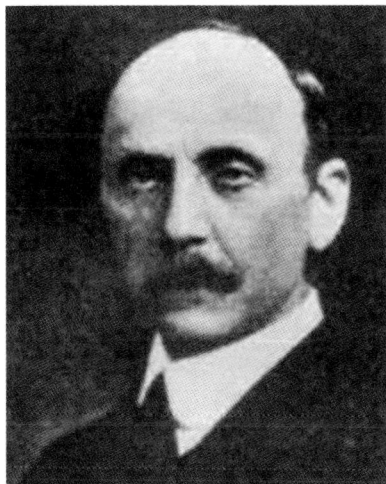

Frederic Hewitt followed John Snow and Joseph Clover as the foremost British anaesthetist. His father was an agricultural chemist whose home was in Badbury in Wiltshire. Frederic was born in London, the eldest of six children, and was educated at Merchant Taylors' School in London. He spent two years at the Royal School of Mines in South Kensington, London and went up to Christ's College, Cambridge in 1876. He graduated in medicine from St George's Hospital Medical School, London with MRCS in 1882 and MB, BChir in 1883. He was popular with a lively sense of humour and the hospital gazette published several of his humorous poems. He obtained his Cambridge MD in 1886.

His eyesight gave him trouble at Cambridge and, as it later got worse and was unlikely to improve, he decided to pursue anaesthesia as a career. Such a decision was practical in the 1880s when general anaesthesia was given by holding a mask over the patient's face and feeling his or her pulse. Hewitt was appointed anaesthetist to Charing Cross Hospital in 1884, the National Dental Hospital in 1885 and The (now Royal) London Hospital in 1886. Surgeons regarded him as a practical and very safe anaesthetist. He was well known for his coolness and determination in difficult situations.

Hewitt described a new method of administering nitrous oxide gas for short dental procedures in the *Lancet* in 1885. Patients inspired about half the contents of a nine-litre Cattlin bag (which contained 100% nitrous oxide) to the point of anaesthesia and hypoxia. The mask was then withdrawn and simple extractions completed immediately as the patient breathed room air.

He was aware that Edmund Andrews in Chicago, Illinois in 1869, and S. Klikowitsch in St Petersburg, Russia in 1881, had used 20–25% oxygen in nitrous oxide. Freedom from cyanosis and other signs of hypoxia convinced Hewitt that nitrous oxide, unlike nitrogen, did not act by causing anoxia. In 1889, he described his apparatus for administering nitrous oxide and oxygen mixtures via a tube to a reservoir bag and via a regulating stopcock to the mask (Figures 1 and 2). He used 13% oxygen for dental work and short minor operations. His apparatus was bulky and required considerable skill in its use, so it never achieved widespread popularity.

Nitrous oxide, oxygen and ether or chloroform only became popular at the end of Hewitt's life when the first Gwathmey apparatus with sight-feed

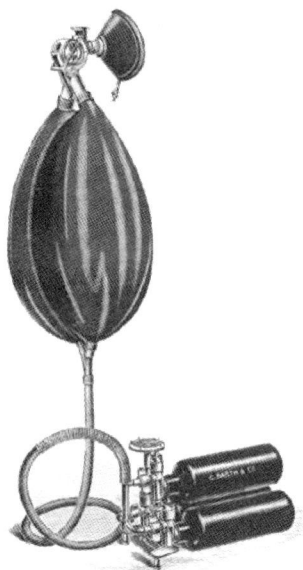

Figure 1. Hewitt's nitrous oxide oxygen apparatus. (Reproduced with permission from *The administration of nitrous oxide and oxygen for dental operations*, 4th edn, Claudius Ash, Sons & Co, 1911: 25.)

flowmeters became available. Abdominal operations were still performed under ether or chloroform anaesthesia. Hewitt modified Junker's chloroform inhaler in 1892 to prevent it from spilling liquid chloroform into the patient's mouth and improved the design of dental mouth-props. His first book *Anaesthetics and their Administration* was published in 1893 and *The Administration of Nitrous Oxide and Oxygen for Dental Operations* followed in 1897. Both books ran to five editions.

Hewitt was appointed anaesthetist to King Edward VII in 1901. Three days before the King's scheduled coronation, Sir Frederick Treves, surgeon to the King, warned Hewitt that his services might be needed for an operation on the King. When Hewitt entered Buckingham Palace the following day, the King's physicians were present but Hewitt insisted on examining the King himself. He found that the King's chest expansion was poor and that he could not lie flat with comfort. Hewitt had to anaesthetize him partly propped up. He used a mixture of two parts chloroform and three parts ether on a Skinner's (open) mask for induction of anaesthesia and ether for maintenance. An appendix abscess was drained and the operation was completed in 40 minutes. The King quickly recovered from the anaesthetic. The doctors then went downstairs to a very good luncheon. Hewitt recorded that; 'The champagne, as one might have expected, was very good.' After his appointment as anaesthetist to the King in 1901, Hewitt became very busy in private practice and had to give up many of his hospital appointments.

Hewitt drew attention to the frequency and danger of respiratory obstruction above the larynx during anaesthesia. He described the first oral airway in 1908 (Figure 3). It had a circular metal ring with a deep groove to fit between the teeth and a bevelled rubber tube not more than 8 cm long with an internal diameter of 12 mm. It was intended for use only when respiration was obstructed and was inserted with the bevel upwards to face the laryngeal orifice.

In 1893, Frederick Silk (1858–1943), anaesthetist to Guy's Hospital, founded the Society of Anaesthetists in London, of which Hewitt was a founder member. In 1901, the Society

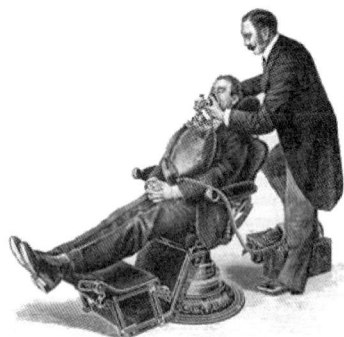

Figure 2. Nitrous oxide oxygen administration in the dental chair. (Reproduced with permission from *The administration of nitrous oxide and oxygen for dental operations*, 4th edn, Claudius Ash, Sons & Co, 1911: 25.)

asked the General Medical Council (GMC) to consider including anaesthetics in the medical curriculum. The council's educational committee replied that, although proper instruction was desirable, it should not be

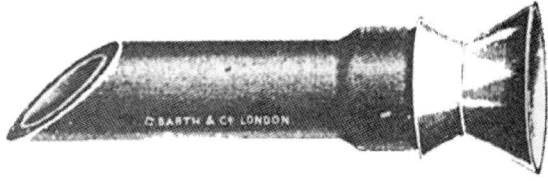

Figure 3. Hewitt oral airway. (Reproduced with permission from *Lancet* 1908; 1: 490–1, Elsevier Science.)

compulsory. Hewitt wrote letters and lectured on this topic and on deaths under anaesthesia, particularly dental anaesthesia. In 1903, he wrote to the *Lancet*, recommending that large hospitals should have an anaesthetic department with a director, additional anaesthetists and resident anaesthetists. In 1908, Hewitt read a paper on the prevention of deaths under anaesthesia. He persuaded the Medico-Legal Society to request that the

Table 1. Frederic Hewitt lecturers and lecture titles

Year	Lecturer	Title
1950	George Edwards	Frederic William Hewitt (1857–1916).
1951	Ralph M. Tovell	New horizons in anaesthesiology.
1952	Charles F. Hadfield	Random reminiscences of fifty years.
1953	Frankis T. Evans	Freedoms of anaesthesia.
1954	Hugh J.V. Morton	Education and recreation during routine work.
1955	M.H. Armstrong Davison	*Ut non percipiatur dolor.*
1956	Ronald F. Woolmer	Artistry and science in anaesthesia.
1957	Michael D. Nosworthy	Pseudo-science and modern anaesthesia.
1959	C. Langton Hewer	Forty years on.
1961	Robert P.W. Shackleton	In my end is my beginning.
1963	Archibald H. Galley	The debt of anaesthesia to pharmacy.
1965	Sir Ivan Magill	An appraisal of progress in anaesthetics.
1967	G. Jackson Rees	The influence of clinical practice on research in anaesthesia.
1969	James D. Robertson	Anaesthetics and their administration.
1971	Cyril F. Scurr	Evolution and revolution in anaesthetic training.
1973	Brian A. Sellick	The contribution of surgery to anaesthesia.
1975	A. Crampton Smith	The business of anaesthesia.
1977	Douglas D.C. Howat	Anaesthesia as a career.
1979	James Parkhouse	The journey and the arrival.
1981	Edgar A. Cooper	Dead in time and space.
1983	John E. Riding	Still more to learn.
1985	John E. Utting	Nemesis and anaesthesia.
1987	D. Bruce Scott	The need to know.
1989	Donald Campbell	Mere dispensers of drugs.
1991	Rt. Rev. David Jenkins	Death as a fact of life.
1993	Michael Halsey	The debt of science to anaesthesia.
1995	Pierre Foëx	Anaesthesia: heart of the matter or a matter of the heart.
1997	Anthony Angel	Fact, fiction and fantasy in anaesthetic research.
1999	David J. Hatch	The quality agenda.
2001	Rev. Dr. John Searle	Dead or alive – principled pragmatism at the end of life.

GMC insist on instruction in anaesthetics in medical schools and to ask the Privy Council to consider legislation. In 1909 the GMC complied. The draft of the Bill was eventually accepted by parliament but passage was post-poned because of other business in 1912, then by the outbreak of war in 1914, and the Bill was never passed.

Hewitt was made a member of the Royal Victorian Order (fourth class) in 1902 for personal service to the King, and in the same year was appointed physician–anaesthetist to St George's Hospital. He was in great demand as a lecturer and attended many meetings. He did more than anyone else in his time to advance the status of the anaesthetist and the specialty of anaesthesia. In 1911 he became the first anaesthetist to be honoured with a knighthood in recognition of his services to medicine.

The Faculty of Anaesthetists of the Royal College of Surgeons, now the Royal College of Anaesthetists, inaugurated the Frederic Hewitt Lecture in 1950 (Table 1). It was given annually until 1957 and now alternates bienni-ally with the Joseph Clover Lecture.

Acknowledgement

Portrait photograph reproduced from the Royal College of Physicians.

Further reading

Edwards G. Frederic William Hewitt (1857–1916). *Annals of the Royal College of Surgeons of England* 1951: **8**: 233–45.

Hewitt FW. An artificial 'air-way' for use during anaesthetisation. *Lancet* 1908; **1**: 490–1.

Howat DDC. Sir Frederic William Hewitt MVO MD. Part I: early life and work on nitrous oxide. *Journal of Medical Biography* 1999; **7**: 5–10. Part II: The Anaes-thetic Bill and professional and private life. *Journal of Medical Biography* 1999; **7**: 63–8.

HICKMAN MEDAL

Henry Hill Hickman (1800–1830)

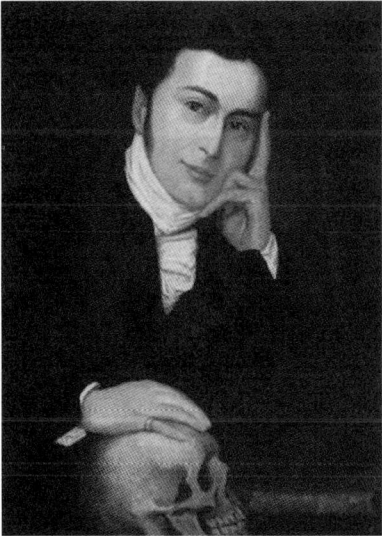

Henry Hill Hickman was a member of a well-known Shropshire family that settled in Bromfield, near Ludlow in Shropshire. He was born there in 1800, the seventh of 13 children. He studied in Edinburgh, Scotland where he was a member of the Royal Medical Society, and matriculated in 1819. He did not graduate in medicine from Edinburgh, but he was admitted as a Member of the Royal College of Surgeons (MRCS), London in 1820 and set up practice in Ludlow in 1821.

Several chemists in the late 18th and early 19th centuries contributed to the rapid increase in knowledge of the chemistry of gases. They exploited the gases for treatment of diseases, but never as an adjuvant for surgery. It was Hickman who had the idea that inhalation of gases could produce anaesthesia and also Hickman who proved it. He recognized that gases introduced into the lungs entered the bloodstream and might therefore provide sleep during surgery. He tested his hypothesis in small animals by administering carbon dioxide to produce temporary, reversible 'suspended animation'. Although his protocols do not supply all the details of the experiments, it is clear that he was investigating true anaesthesia because he used asphyxia in some experiments and carbon dioxide in others.

His first experiment involved partial asphyxiation of a puppy under a bell jar (Figure 1) by excluding atmospheric air for 17 minutes until respiration ceased. He cut off one of its ears without causing pain, respiration soon returned and the ear healed perfectly in three days. Four days later, he exposed the same puppy to carbon dioxide and painlessly cut off the other ear, which healed in four days. Two weeks after that he repeated the asphyxiation and cut off the puppy's tail. He made a painless incision over the loin muscles and tied a ligature through it. The wound

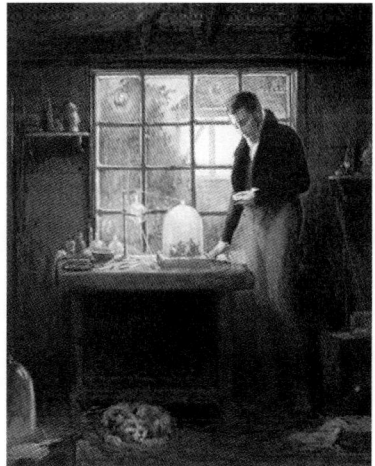

Figure 1. Hickman performing experiments on suspended animation. (Reproduced with kind permission from The Wellcome Library, London, UK.)

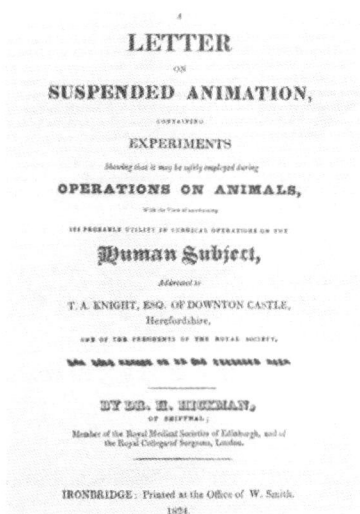

LETTER
ON
SUSPENDED ANIMATION,
CONTAINING
EXPERIMENTS
Showing that it may be safely employed during
OPERATIONS ON ANIMALS,
With the View of ascertaining
ITS PROBABLE UTILITY IN SURGICAL OPERATIONS ON THE
Human Subject,
Adressed to
T. A. KNIGHT, ESQ. OF DOWNTON CASTLE,
Herefordshire,
ONE OF THE PRESIDENTS OF THE ROYAL SOCIETY,
&c. &c. &c.

BY DR. H. HICKMAN,
OF SHIFFNAL,
Member of the Royal Medical Societies of Edinburgh, and of
the Royal College of Surgeons, London.

IRONBRIDGE : Printed at the Office of W. Smith.
1824.

Figure 2. Title page of Hickman's pamphlet. (Reproduced from *Henry Hill Hickman, MRCS (1800–1830) and anaesthesia 1981*: 4, Leeds University Printing Service.)

became inflamed and suppurated, but healed completely in 12 days.

His next experiment was to place a mouse under a bell jar that he filled with carbon dioxide. Respiration ceased in three minutes. He cut off all four legs painlessly at the first joint and revived the mouse by plunging it into a basin of cold water. The stumps healed and he set the mouse free after two weeks. He also gave carbon dioxide to an adult dog, a rabbit and a kitten. He cut off their ears without causing pain, noted the time for the wounds to heal and the time to complete recovery.

Hickman was confident of the accuracy of his experiments but he needed confirmation of his experiments in human patients. He sought help from colleagues, but apparently they did not recognize the value of his work, or even consider it worthy of examination. He therefore wrote a letter on 21 February 1824 to Mr. T.A. Knight of Downton Castle near Ludlow who was a Fellow of the Royal Society and a friend of Sir Humphry Davy (1778–1829), President of the Royal Society.

> Dear Sir,
> ...There is not an individual who does not shudder at the idea of an operation, however skilful the surgeon or urgent the case, knowing the great pain that the patient must endure, and I have frequently lamented, when performing my own duties as a Surgeon that something has not been thought of whereby the fears may be tranquillised and suffering relieved.... I have been induced to make experiments on Animals, endeavouring to ascertain the practicability of such treatment on the human subject, and by particular attention to each individual experiment, I have witnessed results which show that it may be applied to the animal world, and ultimately I think will be found used with perfect safety and success in Surgical operations.... I have no hesitation in saying that suspended animation may be continued a sufficient time for any surgical operation providing the Surgeon acts with skill and promptitude.... From a number of others I have selected the experiments now sent; each is correctly noted in as few words as possible, which I think will prove a vast object.
>
> With great respect,
> I am, Dear Sir,
> Your Obedient Servant,
> (Signed) H. H. Hickman.

There is no evidence that the Royal Society ever formally received his ideas. His second communication was a fresh version of an open letter to T.A. Knight, in the form of a small pamphlet in August 1824 (Figure 2), but there was no response. Even Davy, who was approached directly by Knight, showed no interest. In April 1828 Hickman visited Paris and addressed a letter to King Charles X of France. The letter described his theory and sought permission to demonstrate his discovery to a meeting of the Royal Academy of Medicine. His letter was brought before a meeting of the Academy on 21 October 1828 but was met with derision and contempt except from the Paris surgeon Baron Larrey (1766–1842) who offered himself for a demonstration. The demonstration never took place and the matter was dropped. Hickman returned to England and settled in Tenbury Wells, near Ludlow. He died two years later at the age of 30.

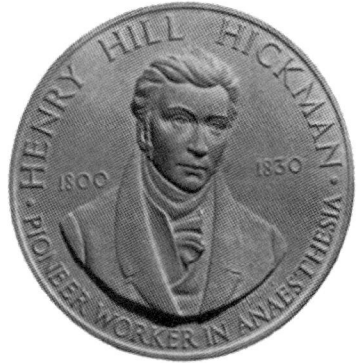

Figure 3. Henry Hill Hickman Medal.

Hickman was belatedly honoured in 1930 on the centenary of his death. The Wellcome Historical Medical Museum in London arranged a fine exhibition and reception that Henry S. Wellcome (1853–1936) and other dignitaries attended. In 1931, the Royal Society of Medicine received £200 to establish a bronze medal to commemorate the work of Henry Hill Hickman in anaesthesia. The Hickman Medal (Figure 3) has been awarded every three years since 1935, on the recommendation of the council of the Section of

Table 1. Hickman Medallists

1935	Wesley Bourne	McGill University, Montreal, Canada
1938	Ivan W. Magill	Westminster Hospital, London
1941	Arthur E. Guedel	Los Angeles, California, USA
1944	Ralph M. Waters	University of Wisconsin, Madison, USA
1947	Robert R. Macintosh	Nuffield Department of Anaesthetics, Oxford
1950	Robert J. Minnitt	Royal Infirmary, Liverpool
1953	John Gillies	Royal Infirmary, Edinburgh
1956	Harold R. Griffith	McGill University, Montreal, Canada
1959	Michael D. Nosworthy	St Thomas's Hospital, London
1962	Ronald Woolmer	BOC Research Department, Royal College of Surgeons
1965	C. Langton Hewer	St Bartholomew's Hospital, London
1968	James Raventos	Imperial Chemical Industries, Manchester
1972	T. Cecil Gray	University of Liverpool
1975	J. Alfred Lee	Southend-on-Sea Hospital, Southend-on-Sea
1978	William W. Mushin	University of Wales, Cardiff
1981	Andrew R. Hunter	University of Manchester
1984	W. Derek Wylie	St Thomas's Hospital, London
1987	Philip R. Bromage	King Khalid University Hospital, Riyadh, Saudi Arabia
1990	G. Jackson Rees	Alder Hey Hospital, Liverpool
1993	Brian A. Sellick	Middlesex Hospital, London (retired)
1996	John F. Nunn	Northwick Park Hospital, Harrow
1999	William W. Mapleson	University of Wales, Cardiff

Anaesthetics (Table 1). It is awarded for original work of outstanding merit in anaesthesia or directly related subjects, and is open to any person of any nationality, not necessarily in the medical profession. There is also a Hickman professor of anaesthesia in Birmingham and an anaesthetists' Hickman Society in England.

Acknowledgement

Portrait photograph reproduced with kind permission from The Wellcome Library, London, UK.

Further reading

Anonymous. Souvenir Henry Hill Hickman Centenary Exhibition 1830–1930, at the Wellcome Historical Medical Museum.

Atkinson RS. Henry Hill Hickman revisited. *The History of Anaesthesia Society Proceedings* 1996; 19: 22–4.

C.J.S.T. [Wellcome Historical Medical Exhibition Research]. Henry Hill Hickman. A forgotten pioneer of anaesthesia. *British Medical Journal* 1912; 1: 843–5.

HINGSON–EDWARDS CAUDAL NEEDLE

Robert Andrew Hingson (1913–1996)

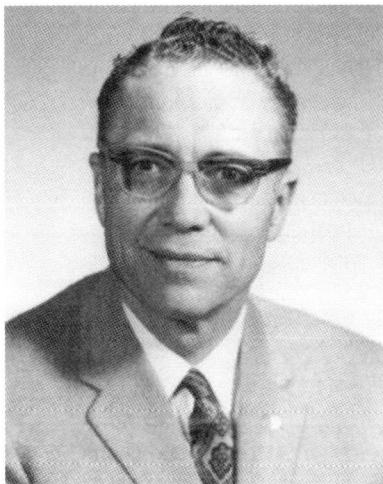

Robert Hingson was born in Anniston, Alabama in 1913. A former slave helped to raise him, and she made him sensitive to the plight of Afro-Americans in the south. He gained his Bachelor of arts from the University of Alabama in 1935 and Doctorate of medicine from Emory University in Atlanta, Georgia in 1938. He delivered 82 babies as a junior medical student. Many of the mothers had no anaesthesia and provided full sound effects for the 'help me Jesus' stage of labour. This experience helped to determine his interest in pain relief, especially in obstetrics. He interned at the US Marine Hospital on Staten Island, New York, and joined the US Coast Guard Service as a public health officer. He then spent a two-year anaesthesia fellowship at the Mayo Clinic in Rochester, Minnesota under John Lundy (1894–1973), who was an advocate of regional anaesthesia.

Hingson returned to the Staten Island hospital in 1941 as chief of anaesthesia, by which time it was an obstetric hospital. He and an obstetrician, Waldo B. Edwards, knew that a single lumbar epidural injection of piperocaine produced analgesia when the cervix was fully dilated, but they wanted to provide pain relief throughout prolonged or difficult labour. They adapted the continuous spinal technique of William Lemmon, a surgeon in Philadelphia, to provide continuous caudal analgesia. They designed the 19-gauge Hingson–Edwards caudal malleable stainless steel needle (Figure 1) to pass through the sacral hiatus. The needle hub was connected by rubber tubing through a three-way tap to a 5 mL syringe and 135 mL reservoir bottle containing 1.5% piperocaine (Figure 2). They could induce analgesia in the patient's room and continue it during transfer to the delivery room and until the baby was delivered. They had no complications in their first report of 33 cases.

Hingson suggested the use of continuous caudal block for battlefront and other trauma surgery. His technique was later extended to the upper abdomen. The editor of

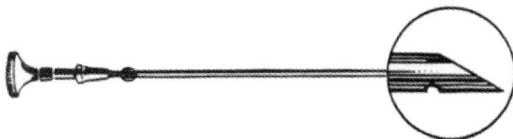

Figure 1. Hingson–Edwards caudal needle. This malleable needle was easily bent and could be straightened for reuse. (Reproduced from *Anesthesia and Analgesia* 1966; 45: 520–6.)

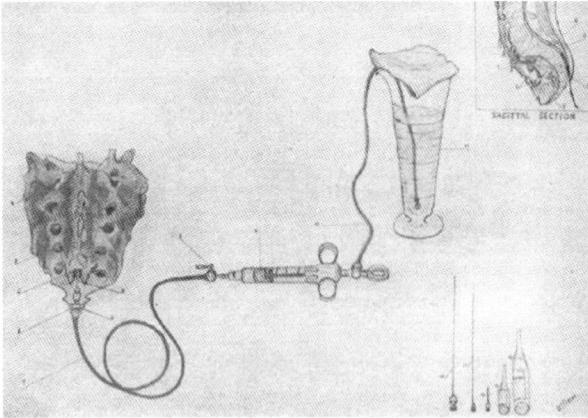

Figure 2. Hingson's method of continuous caudal analgesia. (Reproduced from American *Journal of Surgery* 1942; 57: 459–64.)

the Journal of the American Medical Association came to Staten Island to watch the 29-year-old Hingson at work and encouraged him to publish his findings. Hingson did so and soon received invitations to speak at medical schools and meetings.

Over the next few years, Hingson held clinics in obstetric analgesia throughout Europe and Canada as well as in the USA. He moved to the Philadelphia Lying-In Hospital in 1943, where he established an obstetric caudal analgesia service and published his first book, *Control of Pain in Childbirth*, in 1944 with Clifford Lull. He established a third obstetric caudal analgesia service at the University of Tennessee in Memphis where he was professor of anesthesiology from 1945 to 1948.

Next, he moved to The Johns Hopkins University in Baltimore, Maryland as associate professor of anesthesia in the department of obstetrics. Charles Flowers, a young obstetrician, had similar interests and was soon administering regional analgesia. When caudal analgesia was difficult for anatomical reasons, they found that continuous lumbar epidural with a ureteral catheter worked well. They published their results in 1949, nearly a decade before other American and Canadian centres introduced the technique. Hingson also visited Sweden in 1949 and introduced the new local anaesthetic lignocaine (lidocaine) into the USA.

Hingson retired from the Public Health Service in 1951 to be chairman of the Department of Anesthesiology at Case Western Reserve University in Cleveland, Ohio. During his 17-year tenure, he developed a department of medically qualified anaesthetists as he phased out the first American department of nurse anesthesia, founded by Agatha Hodgins in 1915.

During his time at Staten Island in 1941–43, Hingson looked after a merchant seaman who had experienced a high-pressure trauma that had forced diesel oil into his hand without a visible surface wound. Hingson used the phenomenon to develop a technique of injection. He and an engineer designed the Hypospray – a small jet injector whose high pressure forced fluid into the subcutaneous tissue without a break in the epidermis. It was hand-held, delivered a precise, preset volume from an ampoule, and pain was minimal. It was used initially for administering local anaesthetics, ephedrine, insulin and penicillin. Later, he and a few departmental colleagues in Cleveland inoculated 12,000 post office union members against influenza on one Saturday.

Production-line immunization began in 1956 when Hingson and his team inoculated children with the Salk polio vaccine in Cleveland, Ohio. Eventually more than 300,000 patients were immunized via jet injection, primarily against polio and influenza. For Hingson, the most important benefit of the Hypospray was that it did not frighten children undergoing vaccination nearly as much as a syringe and needle.

In 1958, in association with the Baptist World Alliance, Hingson and his team inoculated approximately 90,000 people throughout Asia and Africa against typhoid, cholera and polio. The vaccines and transportation were gifts from pharmaceutical firms. In 1962, he led a team that immunized 1,000,000 people against smallpox during a major epidemic in Liberia, West Africa, using donated injector guns and vaccines. This feat demonstrated to the World Health Organization what was possible and they eradicated small-pox worldwide using similar equipment. These large-scale medical missions were the impetus for his establishing the Brother's Brother Foundation. In 1969, he moved to the University of Pittsburgh, Pennsylvania with permission to take two months off each year for foreign inoculation tours. He left academic anaesthesia in 1973 to devote his time to the Brother's Brother Foundation. Today, along with medical and agricultural supplies, the Foundation receives yearly donations of educational materials to be distributed to schools and medical institutions. Its intraocular lens programme distributes and implants lenses to restore vision to cataract sufferers.

Hingson received the Gaston Labat Award of the American Society of Regional Anesthesia in 1991. Nearly every country in which he served awarded him its highest humanitarian honour. He was nominated for a Nobel Peace Prize, and in 1987 he received the President's Volunteer Action Award from President Ronald Reagan.

Acknowledgement

Portrait photograph reproduced with kind permission from the Wood Library–Museum of Anesthesiology, Park Ridge, IL, USA.

Further reading

Edwards WB, Hingson RA. Continuous caudal anesthesia in obstetrics. *American Journal of Surgery* 1942; **57**: 459–64.
Hingson RA, Hughes JG. Clinical studies with jet injection. A new method of drug administration. *Anesthesia and Analgesia* 1947; **26**: 221–30.
Rosenberg H, Axelrod JK. Robert Andrew Hingson: his unique contributions to world health as well as to anesthesiology. *The American Journal of Anesthesiology* 1998; **25**: 90–3.

THE GEOFFREY KAYE MUSEUM
OF ANAESTHETIC HISTORY

Geoffrey Kaye (1903-1986)

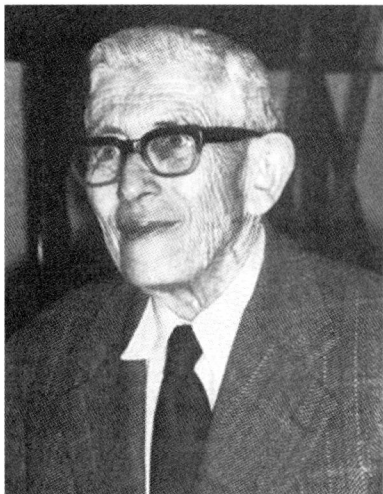

Geoffrey Kaye was born in 1903 in Melbourne, Victoria, Australia. He was educated in England at Peterborough Lodge Preparatory School and Gresham's School in Holt, Norfolk. These years gave him a formal style and approach that set him apart from his more casual Australian colleagues. He graduated in medicine from the University of Melbourne Medical School in 1926, and by 1927 had decided to specialize in anaesthesia. Being unmarried and having a private income of one thousand pounds a year from his father, gave him the privilege to choose the unremunerative field of anaesthesia. Most early Australian doctors, like those in other countries, had to make a living and could only afford to be part-time anaesthetists. Kaye became Australia's second full-time specialist anaesthetist after Rupert Hornabrook, who was appointed to the Royal Melbourne Hospital in 1909.

In 1929 another Melbourne anaesthetist, Frederick Green, was appointed vice-president of the Section of Anaesthetics for the Australasian Medical Congress in Sydney. He had heard of Kaye, the resident staff anaesthetist at the Alfred Hospital in Melbourne, who had shown dedication and enthusiasm. Kaye was an honorary research worker at the Baker Institute of Research and planned to take a research position at St Thomas's Hospital in London, England in 1930. Green became ill and could not do the work for his promised paper on anaesthetic mortality and thought he might not be able to attend the Congress. Kaye was interested in the topic, did the statistical work for Green and, at the age of 26, presented the paper. He discussed the pathological findings of 107 deaths under anaesthesia that the Melbourne coroner had investigated during 1919-29. Francis McMechan from the USA, who had founded the American Society of Anesthetists in 1912, was in the audience and 'could not help but congratulate Dr. Kaye on his paper'. McMechan arranged for Kaye to visit the USA and Canada where he met leading anaesthetists in Philadelphia, Louisville, Toledo, Madison, Rochester, Buffalo and Montreal. He attended postgraduate courses and anaesthetic meetings, and became a life-long friend and correspondent of Ralph Waters.

Kaye returned to Australia in 1931 and was determined to found a society of anaesthetists. His meticulous observance of formalities was helpful during the foundation and early days of the Australian Society of Anaesthetists. He corresponded with anaesthetists in every state and arranged a foundation meeting in Hobart, Tasmania, on 19 January 1934. He was not quite 31 years old. The Society's first Annual General Meeting was held in Melbourne in 1935, and the second in Adelaide, South Australia in 1937. He kept members interested, informed and stimulated by regular memoranda and newsletters until the outbreak of the Second World War. He lived to participate in its 50th anniversary celebrations.

During his visit to the USA, Kaye developed an intense interest in anaesthetic apparatus that led to his foundation of an anaesthetic museum in 1937. This is now The Geoffrey Kaye Museum of Anaesthetic History that is housed at Ulimaroa – the home of the Australian and New Zealand College of Anaesthetists in Melbourne (Figure 1). He founded it only three years after the Australian Society and it holds many items that Kaye collected during his working life and his retirement (Figures 2 and 3). Duplicates of early items are sectioned to display their inner workings. These include cylinder valves, flow-meters, pressure reducing valves and many anaesthetic machines. The museum has moved from an upstairs room of the College to a large area of the foyer where more display cabinets have been added and a display of a 'period' operating room is planned.

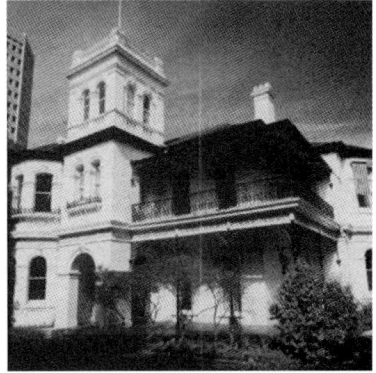

Figure 1. Ulimaroa, home of the Australian and New Zealand College of Anaesthetists in Melbourne. (Reproduced with kind permission from the Geoffrey Kaye Museum.)

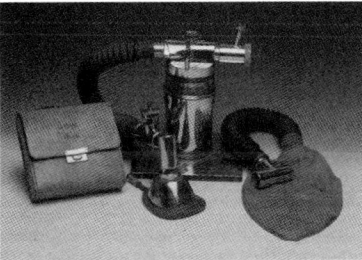

Figure 2. Kaye's version of the Marrett portable drawover ether apparatus. (Reproduced with kind permission from the Geoffrey Kaye Museum.)

At the outbreak of the Second World War, Kaye enrolled in the Australian Army Medical Corps. Later, when serving in the Middle East, he was appointed its first advisor in anaesthetics. His unpublished war diary reveals his persistent efforts to provide modern anaesthesia under the difficult campaign conditions. During periods of inactivity, he organized a 'Hole and Corner University' in a tent with volunteer teachers. Its curriculum offered such diverse subjects as surveying, theory of flight, nature study and elementary Japanese language. The army later incorporated it into its official Education Corps programme, staffing it with full-time tutors.

In 1932, Kaye edited the Baker Institute's first monograph, *Practical Anaesthesia,* compiled by

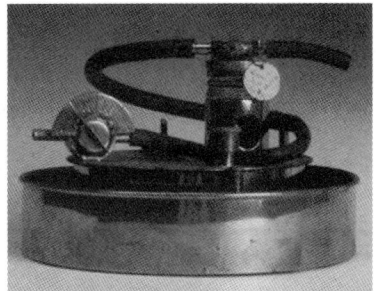

Figure 3. Blow over ether army vaporizer. (Reproduced with kind permission from the Geoffrey Kaye Museum.)

the anaesthetists of the Alfred Hospital. He wrote *Anaesthetic Methods* with Robert Orton and Douglas Renton, which was published in 1946. His publications appeared in many anaesthesia and experimental science journals, both in Australia and in other countries. Those in the Society's *Newsletter* provide a historical record of changes in techniques and apparatus. His non-medical articles covered *Religious Beliefs of Ancient Egypt* (1923), *Petra* (1944), *Old English Glass* (1960), *Antique English Silver* (1961), *Chinese Monochromes of the 18th Century* (1962), serious and light verse, and tales and essays such as *Pipes of Yesteryear* and *Aldstadt-in-Forest*

Geoffrey Kaye was a physician, scientist, researcher, organizer and an inveterate correspondent. He was an idealist in his earlier years. He believed that a national society should be a purely scientific body, with its own research laboratories, standards laboratory, lecture halls for congresses and a comprehensive library and museum. The Society developed into a strong and meaningful body but his ideals were impossible to achieve given the geography of Australia and its political changes. In 1957, he withdrew from anaesthetic practice, the Society and the Faculty of Anaesthetists. He confined his activities to university teaching, research in his private laboratory, pursuits in his machine workshop and becoming a computer expert.

The Australian Society of Anaesthetists honoured him with Life Membership in 1964. He received the Faculty of Anaesthetists of the Royal Australasian College of Surgeons's highest accolade, the Orton Award in 1974 and was elected to Honorary Fellowship of the Faculty in 1978. By the time he died in 1986, he was revered by Australian anaesthetists as an almost legendary figure.

Acknowledgement

Portrait photograph reproduced with kind permission from the Geoffrey Kaye Museum.

Further reading

Penn HP. The Geoffrey Kaye Anaesthetic Museum. *Anaesthesia and Intensive Care* 1972; 1: 106–8.

Wilson G. Geoffrey Kaye, MD (Melb.), MBBS, FFARACS (Hon.), FFARCS, DA (RCP&S) 1903–1986. *Anaesthesia and Intensive Care* 1987; 15: 107–9.

Wilson G. *One grand chain: the history of anaesthesia in Australia 1846–1962, Volume I 1846–1934.* Melbourne, NSW: Australian and New Zealand College of Anaesthetists, 1995.

THE CHARLES KING COLLECTION OF ANAESTHETIC EQUIPMENT

Charles King (1888–1966)

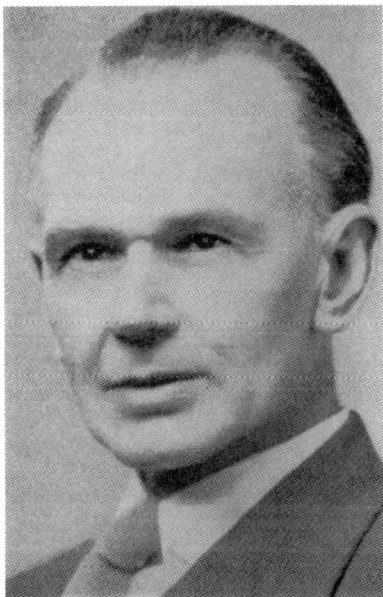

Charles King was born in Islington, London in 1888. He attended the local primary school, and then Owens, a private school near the Angel, Islington. He left school at the age of 14 to be apprenticed to a local engineering firm. When he completed his apprenticeship, he joined a medical supply company as a salesman.

King had joined a City of London Territorial Unit while he was an apprentice and at the outbreak of the First World War he was immediately called up. He fought in each major battle on the French Front from 1914 to 1918, and was wounded three times. When he returned home at the end of the war, his old job no longer existed. He set up his own business from home, selling medical supplies to hospitals and local doctors with whom he had contact before the war. However, he felt he needed to be in London's West End to be nearer to the private nursing homes and fashionable medical premises of Harley Street. He borrowed £100 from an uncle to purchase the lease of 34 Devonshire Street (Figure 1) and sold general medical supplies, instrument cabinets, sterilizers, operating tables, and especially ear, nose and throat equipment and instruments.

He began to specialize in anaesthetic apparatus in the early 1920s, when F.P. de Caux, an anaesthetist at the North Middlesex Hospital, London, returned from the USA with a McKesson demand-flow

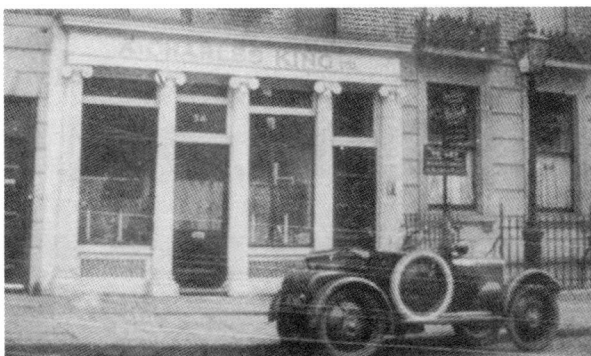

Figure 1. Premises of A. Charles King at 34 Devonshire Street. His 1922 Rover car in the foreground had an 8hp, two-cylinder, air-cooled engine and a top speed of 30–35 mph. (Image courtesy of Margaret King.)

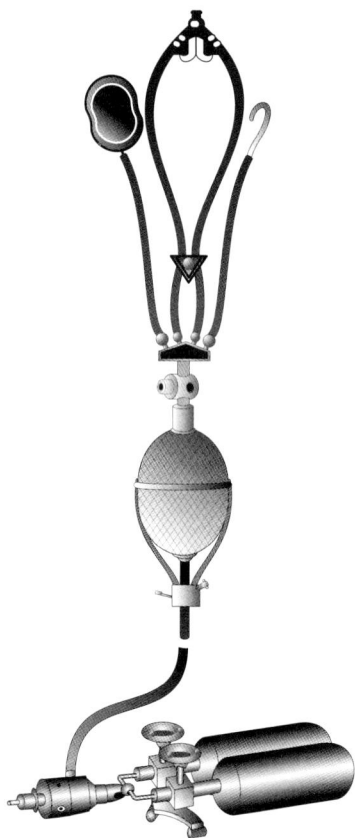

Figure 2. de Caux-McKesson dental apparatus.

nitrous oxide–oxygen apparatus. King obtained the British franchise and was soon selling as many as he could import. He also produced a modified version that he sold as the de Caux–McKesson dental apparatus (Figure 2). He provided anaesthetists with nitrous oxide and oxygen cylinders, as well as a rapidly widening selection of anaesthetic equipment. The premises could not have been better placed strategically and No. 34 soon became the meeting place for anaesthetists with half an hour to spare. Tea and topical conversation were available and everyone left feeling the better for the proprietor's friendly but dignified welcome.

Charles King and Ivan Magill developed a friendship based on admiration of each other's skills. Magill was working at Queen Mary's Hospital in Sidcup, Kent, using intratracheal insufflation anaesthesia for reconstructive surgery of facial trauma from the First World War. King and Magill joined forces to develop Magill's laryngoscope, originally sold as an intubating spatula for placement of the insufflation catheters. As Magill moved on to wide bore endotracheal tubes, King became involved in the development of the famous Magill red rubber tubes and their connectors. One woman, nicknamed 'Catheter Kate', was particularly adept at making the tubes from coils of rubber tubing bought from a rubber company in Euston Road, cutting the bevel with a pair of scissors and then smoothing the rough edges with an electric iron.

As he became busier, King added highly trained engineers to complement his own skills. He produced reducing valves, endotracheal tubes, forceps, connectors, laryngoscopes and anaesthetic machines in rapid succession. Much of the manufacturing occurred in the Devonshire Street premises, although an increasing amount was subcontracted out to local small instrument manufacturers.

Unfortunately, Charles King was not a businessman and this frequently resulted in cash-flow problems. He approached Coxeter and Son (who manufactured anaesthetic apparatus, including Boyle machines) for help. The financial aid became more and more extensive and in 1926 led to the formation of A.C. King Ltd. Number 34 Devonshire Street continued as before, but with the majority of shares being held by Coxeter.

In October 1932, the Liverpool Maternity Hospital invited Robert Minnitt to investigate the possibility of a nitrous oxide apparatus for use by trained but unsupervised midwives to provide obstetric analgesia. He approached King in July 1933 and they modified a demand-flow McKesson apparatus. The first Minnitt gas–air analgesia apparatus (Figure 3) was used in October of that year, soon followed by a series of modified versions for use in hospital or the home.

In 1939, the British Oxygen Company bought out Coxeter and A.C. King Ltd came under the new management. At the height of the blitz in 1941, 34 Devonshire Street was destroyed by a land mine. King then carried on the business from two parked cars in the street! The Genito-Urinary Company that had premises on the street corner provided a telephone service. Within a week, a grocer's shop opposite became vacant and King moved across the road to open new premises at 27 Devonshire Street.

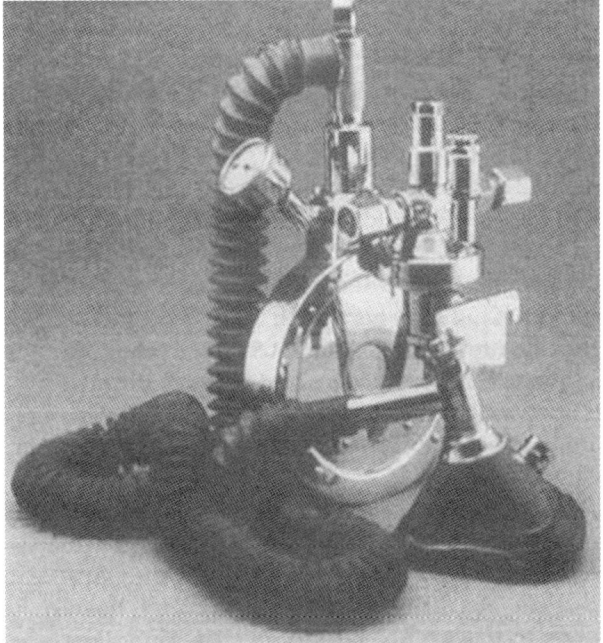

Figure 3. Original Minnit apparatus.

Ralph Waters described King's showroom as a 'Mecca for anaesthetists worldwide'. It was King who located the copy of John Snow's *On Chloroform and Other Anaesthetics* for Waters in 1937 that is now in the Wood Library–Museum of Anesthesiology in Park Ridge, Illinois. King browsed through second-hand bookshops and he purchased his own copy in Paris for two francs. Any visiting doctor was welcome to consult his large collection of anaesthetic textbooks, both historical and current. Later, he gave these books to the libraries of the Royal Society of Medicine and the Royal College of Surgeons. He also built up his extensive collection of equipment, some of it from the earliest days of anaesthesia, by exchanging new apparatus for old, and manufacturing facsimile items he was unable to collect. His demonstrations of anaesthetic apparatus were essential for all anaesthetists training for higher examinations in post Second World War Britain. He also had a series of films and lantern slides, available for hire, which illustrated the various aspects of anaesthetic practice.

Several provincial anaesthetists' societies elected King to honorary membership. In January 1949 he had the rare honour of being elected to honorary fellowship of the Section of Anaesthetics of the Royal Society of

Medicine. This was followed by election to honorary membership of several national societies during a world tour in 1950.

The historical anaesthetic apparatus that he collected over the years became the Charles King Collection and was given to the Association of Anaesthetists of Great Britain and Ireland in 1953. It was originally maintained at his showrooms in 27 Devonshire Street, and later at the Royal College of Surgeons. It formed the nucleus of the museum that was officially opened at the Association of Anaesthetists building at 9 Bedford Square, London on 9 July 1987.

Acknowledgement

Portrait photograph reproduced with kind permission from the Wood Library–Museum of Anesthesiology, Park Ridge, IL, USA.

Further reading

King AC. The history and development of anaesthetic apparatus. *British Medical Journal* 1946; 2: 136–53.

Obituary. A. Charles King. *Anaesthesia* 1966; 21: 439–40.

Wilkinson DJ. A. Charles King: a unique contribution to anaesthesia. *Journal of the Royal Society of Medicine* 1987; 80: 510–14.

CARL KOLLER MEDAL
CARL KOLLER MEMORIAL RESEARCH FUND

Carl Koller (1857–1944)

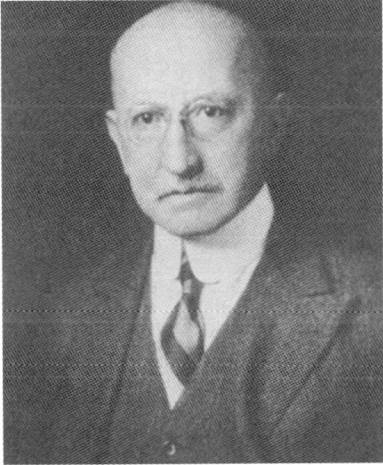

Carl Koller was born in 1857 in Schüttenhofen in Bohemia, which was then in the Austro-Hungarian Empire. His father, a Jewish businessman in Teplitz, moved to Vienna when his wife died and Carl was still a small child. Koller was educated by private tutors, Jesuit fathers and at the local Akademisches Gymnasium. He studied jurisprudence for one year before entering medical school at the University of Vienna in 1876. He graduated in 1882 and served his year of compulsory military training as a medical officer in the Army Reserve.

While he was still a medical student, Koller did original research on the origin of the mesoderm of the chick embryo in the laboratory of Salomon Stricker (1834–98). Koller always regarded this work as his most valuable contribution to science. However, history remembers him for his recognition of the local anaesthetic property of cocaine. Koller's work on cocaine began when Professor von Arldt (1812–87), his teacher in ophthalmology, drew attention to the shortcomings of general anaesthesia in eye surgery and the need for a local anaesthetic. Koller realized that discovery of a local anaesthetic agent might win him one of the coveted university assistantships in ophthalmology. While still a student, he unsuccessfully tested solutions of chloral hydrate, bromide and morphine in the eyes of animals.

It had long been observed that the lips and tongue went numb from chewing coca leaves and with pure cocaine that Albert Niemann (1834–61) first extracted in 1860 at the University of Göttingen, Germany. In 1879, Vasili Konstantinovich von Anrep, at the Pharmacological Institute in Würtzburg, Germany described dilatation of the pupil with topical application of cocaine to the eye, but did not record numbness of the cornea or conjunctiva.

Sigmund Freud (1856–1939), a friend of Koller in Vienna General Hospital, was a budding neurologist and psychiatrist. Freud completed a monograph, *Über Coca*, in the early months of 1884, with high hopes that cocaine might be useful in the treatment of neurasthenia, alcohol and morphine addiction, asthma and other medical conditions. That summer, before setting off on a visit to Hamburg, he asked Koller, who was 18 months his junior, to continue investigations of the effects of cocaine on muscle grip strength when the drug was taken by mouth. Koller and a colleague did this, and the colleague commented on the numbness of his tongue. Koller replied that everyone had noticed that sensation. Then, in a moment of inspiration, he realized that this was the agent for which he had been looking.

He went straight to Stricker's laboratory, where he and Stricker's assistant, Gustav Gärtner (1855–1937), dissolved the cocaine powder in distilled water and trickled it into the eye of a lively frog. After one minute, the frog allowed the cornea of that eye to be touched and injured without any reflex action, whereas its other eye responded to the slightest touch. They repeated the experiment on a rabbit and a dog with the same results. They then took the final step by trickling it into each other's eyes and discovering that they could indent the cornea with a pin head without feeling the slightest touch. In that one afternoon, Koller progressed from observation to proof of local anaesthesia.

Koller was still a poorly paid 26-year-old intern, and could not afford the railway fare to present his findings at the Ophthalmological Society meeting scheduled for 15 September 1884 in Heidelberg, Germany. His friend, Josef Brettauer (1835–1905) from Trieste, Italy read his paper for him and demonstrated the effects of Koller's 2% cocaine solution in the hospital eye clinic. Henry Noyes, a New York ophthalmologist who attended the meeting, wrote an account of the discovery that was published in the New York *Medical Record* on 11 October. Koller himself read a fuller paper before the Vienna Medical Society on 17 October in which he acknowledged the previous descriptions of the analgesic properties of cocaine made by Niemann, von Anrep and others, and credited Freud for introducing him to the drug.

Within three months, Koller's days in Vienna were numbered. Anti-Semitism permeated the whole social structure of Vienna in the 1880s. Koller and Freud had close individual friendships with non-Jews, but Koller was a difficult young man who would not speak diplomatically, even for his own good. He got into an argument with another intern about the removal of a tourniquet from a man's seriously injured finger. The intern hurled an insult at Koller that sounded like 'Impudent Jew'. Koller retaliated with a resounding punch to his ear. Both men had served in the army and, to defend honour they fought a sabre duel the next day in which Koller inflicted face and arm wounds on his opponent. Letters from fellow Jews poured in to congratulate Koller for his stand against the insult. Although he was later pardoned, he knew he had no hope of promotion within the university.

He left Vienna and worked for two years under the famous Dutch ophthalmologist, Cornelius Donders (1818–89), in Utrecht. Then, after consulting with his friends in Vienna, he decided to emigrate to the USA and set off in May 1888 for New York City, where he soon became established. He was elected to the staff of several hospitals including the Mount Sinai Hospital, and spent the remainder of his long life as an eye specialist with increasing reputation and success. He took no further part in the development of local anaesthesia.

Koller received many honours in his later years. He was awarded the Scroll

Table 1. Carl Koller Award winners

Year	Annual Congress	Recipient	Year	Annual Congress	Recipient
1984	Vienna, Austria	Alfred Lee	1994	Barcelona, Spain	Fidel Pages
1985	Rome, Italy	John Bonica	1995	Prague, Czech Rep.	Daniel Moore
1986	Malmo, Sweden	Torsten Gordh	1996	Nice, France	J. Bertil Löfström
1987	Paris, France	Luc Lecron	1997	London, England	Alon Winnie
1988	Mainz, Germany	Sir Robert Macintosh	1998	Geneva, Switzerland	Hans Nolte
1989	Lisbon, Portugal	Philip Bromage	1999	Istanbul, Turkey	Albert Van Steenberge
1990	Bern, Switzerland	Bruce Scott	2000	Rome, Italy	Phulchand Prithvi Raj
1991	Athens, Greece	Ben Covino	2001	Warsaw, Poland	Poul Buckhoj
1992	Brussels, Belgium	Nicholas Greene			
1993	Dublin, Ireland	James Moore			

from the International Anesthesia Research Society in 1927; the Kussmaul Medal of the University of Heidelberg in 1928; the Gold Medal of Honor from the New York Academy of Medicine in 1930; and the Gold Medal of the American Academy of Ophthalmology in 1934.

The American Society of Regional Anesthesia established the Carl Koller Memorial Research Grants to support research related to local anaesthetics, regional anaesthesia in surgery and obstetrics, and pain control. The Carl Koller Award of the European Society of Regional Anaesthesia honours a lifetime of dedication to regional anaesthesia and pain therapy (Table 1). The first award was made in 1984 at the Centenary Meeting of Regional Anaesthesia in Vienna, in the presence of Koller's daughter (Figure 1).

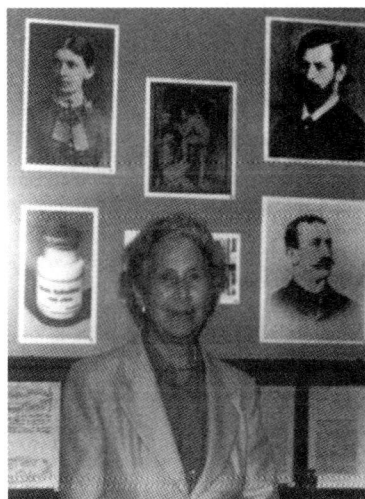

Figure1 . Koller's daughter Hortense Koller Becker (1902–2001) in the Sigmund Freud Museum in Vienna, 1984. The exhibit shows (top) Martha Bernays (Freud's fiancée) and Sigmund Freud, (lower) jar of cocaine crystals and Carl Koller.

Acknowledgement

Portrait photograph reproduced with kind permission from the Wood Library–Museum of Anesthesiology, Park Ridge, IL, USA.

Further reading

Becker HK. Carl Koller and Cocaine. *The Psychoanalytic Quarterly* 1963; **32**: 309–73.

Koller C. Personal reminiscences of the first use of cocain as a local anesthetic in eye surgery. *Anesthesia and Analgesia* 1928; **7**: 9–11.

Wyklicky H, Skopee M. Carl Koller (1857–1944) and his time in Vienna. In: Scott DB, McClure J, Wildsmith JAW (Eds) *Regional Anaesthesia 1884–1984*. Södertälje: ICM AB, 1984: 12–16.

GASTON LABAT AWARD

Louis Gaston Labat (1876–1934)

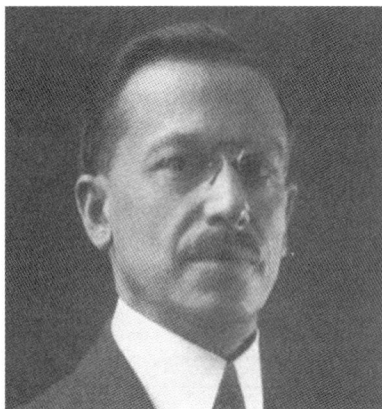

Gaston Labat was born in 1876 in Victoria on Mahe, the largest island of the Seychelles group in the Indian Ocean. Labat's parents, both of French origin, were born in Mauritius and moved to the Seychelles to develop a trading business. After his father drowned in 1883, his mother returned to Mauritius with Labat and two younger sisters. They later joined her brother in Durban, South Africa where Labat was educated in his formative years.

The family returned to Mauritius and Labat completed his schooling at the Royal College of Mauritius in 1894. He took a job as a clerk in a government legal department to earn enough money to marry. The marriage proved unhappy, and in 1907 he left his wife and Mauritius for Portuguese East Africa, now Mozambique, to construct machinery for extracting sugar juice from cane. Labat returned to Mauritius in 1912 and left again in 1914 to complete his baccalaureate degree and register as a medical student at the University of Montpellier in France aged 38. After his transfer to the University of Paris in 1916 he externed at a number of hospitals. From 1918 to 1920, Labat was assistant to Victor Pauchet at several hospitals and at his clinic in Paris. He presented his thesis on paravertebral conduction anaesthesia in surgery of the stomach and intestines and received his doctoral degree in 1920.

Pauchet was a renowned surgeon in France and had a major influence on Labat's medical career. In 1914, Pauchet and Sourdat published the first edition of *L'Anesthésie Regionale* that dealt primarily with the early use of regional anaesthesia. The second edition in 1917 added Pauchet's brother-in-law, Jewels Laboure, as a co-author. After Laboure's death in the First World War, Labat became co-author for the third edition in 1921. In the preface Pauchet described Labat as; 'one of my most devoted assistants, who played the greatest role in the turnaround of this book. His sure hand and anatomical research simplified several technical points.'

The surgeon Charles Mayo of Rochester, Minnesota visited Pauchet in Paris in 1920. After assisting him in an operation, he asked Pauchet's permission to invite Labat, who was looking after the patient at the head of the table, to come to the Mayo Clinic to teach the surgeons his methods of regional anaesthesia. Labat went to the Mayo Clinic (Figure 1) for 12 months as a special lecturer on regional anaesthesia.

One of the most important results of this visit was the publication of Labat's *Regional Anesthesia: Its Technique and Clinical Application* in 1922. This book is outstanding because of the excellence of its illustrations (Figure 2) and its practical instructions on how to perform a wide variety of regional analgesia techniques. It also contains a wealth of useful clinical information

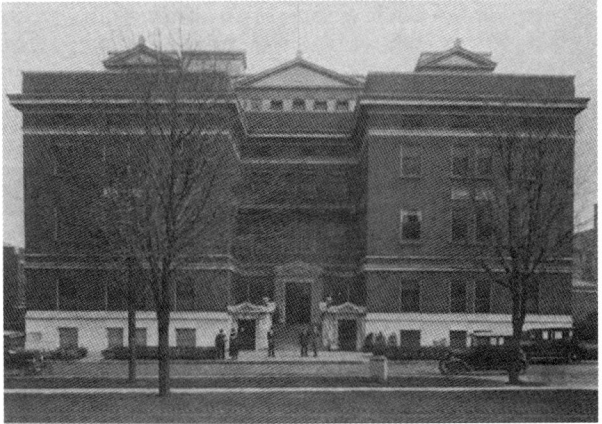

Figure 1. The Mayo Building in Rochester, Minnesota c. 1914. (Reproduced from *Regional Anesthesia* 1992; 17: 249–62.)

about the fine details of the conduct of regional analgesia in the conscious patient. The first edition sold 2500 copies soon followed by a reprint run of 3000 copies and then a further 2000 in 1924. The second edition in 1928 sold 2000 copies and a further 1500 copies in 1930. He published more than 40 articles, mostly on regional anaesthesia.

Labat left the Mayo Clinic to be a clinical professor of surgery at University College of Medicine and Bellevue Hospital in New York City in 1922. He continued to practise anaesthesia during the early 1930s and was certified by the American Board of Anesthesiology in 1934, only to die of a myocardial insufficiency on 1 October that year. Labat's death certificate must be one of the few that lists a physician's occupation as a 'regional anesthetist'.

Labat's name was given to a method of spinal anaesthesia in which he inserted a spinal needle and allowed a predetermined volume of cerebrospinal fluid to flow into an ampoule that contained 50, 80, 100, 120, 150, 200 or 300 mg procaine crystals (Figure 3). For upper abdominal procedures he used 120 or 150 mg procaine with barbotage. Immediately after the drug was injected, he placed the patient in the Trendelenburg position for the duration of the operation and for three hours postoperatively.

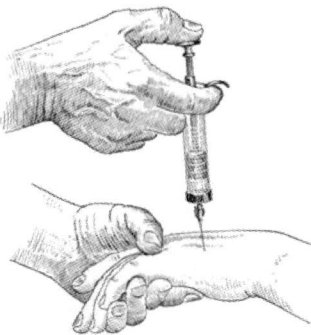

Figure 2. Field block of the hand. (Reproduced from *Regional anesthesia its technic and clinical application*, W.B. Saunders Company, 1923: 326.)

Labat established the original American Society of Regional Anesthesia in 1923. He was its first president, and the majority of its members were neurosurgeons. There were four anaesthetists in the society at that time. Its main objective was to promote the education of residents in regional anaesthesia and pain management. In 1939, the Society merged with the American Society of Anesthesiologists.

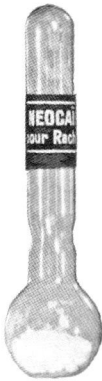

Figure 3. Ampoule containing one accurate dose of sterile crystals for intraspinal block. (Reproduced from *Regional anesthesia its technic and clinical application*, W.B. Saunders Company, 1923: 39.)

However, in 1976 a group of dedicated regional anaesthesia specialists reactivated the separate society. The first annual meeting of the new American Society of Regional Anesthesia was held in Phoenix, Arizona and its membership has grown from 442 in 1977 to more than 7000 in 2002.

The American Society of Regional Anesthesia presents the Gaston Labat Award annually to an individual who has made outstanding contributions to the development, teaching and practice of regional anaesthesia. Recipients of the Gaston Labat Award deliver the Labat Lecture at the annual meeting (Table 1), and comprise a virtual who's who of regional anaesthesia.

Table 1. Gaston Labat lecturers and lecture titles

Year	Lecturer	Title
1977	John J. Bonica	The historical development and current status of regional anesthesia.
1977	Daniel C. Moore	Local anesthetic toxicity.
1978	Sir Robert Macintosh	Gaston Labat: the early years.
1979	Torsten Gordh	On spinal anesthesia: experiences over 40 years.
1980	John Adriani	From Koller to Labat: a historical résumé.
1981	Robert A. Hingson	...development of safe control of obstetric pain in childbirth.
1982	Alon P. Winnie	Nothing new under the sun.
1983	Peere C. Lund	Reflection upon the historical aspects of spinal anesthesia.
1984	Philip R. Bromage	The metamorphosis of regional anesthesia.
1985	J. Alfred Lee	Some foundations on which we have built.
1986	Benjamin G. Covino	One hundred years plus two of regional anesthesia.
1987	Nicholas M. Greene	Challenges and opportunities: the future of regional anesthesia.
1988	D. Bruce Scott	Divided by a common language.
1989	Ronald Melzack	Phantom limbs.
1989	Patrick D. Wall	To what would Gaston Labat be attending today?
1990	Pritvi P. Raj	Pain relief: fact or fancy.
1991	Bertil Lofstrom	The effect of local anesthetics on the peripheral vasculature.
1992	B. Raymond Fink	Towards the mathematization of spinal anesthesia.
1993	Sol Snider	Regional anesthesia for obstetrics.
1994	P.O. Bridenbaugh	Anesthesiology and pain management: medical practice or perception.
1995	Rudolph H. de Jong	Ropivacaine. White knight or dark horse?
1996	Michael J. Cousins	Pain – a persistent problem.
1997	G.E. Thompson	From Pauchet to today – the French connection.
1998	Stephano Ischia	The role of the neurolytic celiac plexus block in pancreatic cancer pain...
1999	L. Brian Ready	Lesson learned from 25,000 patients.
2000	Strichartz G.	Pathways and obstacles to local anesthesia, a personal account.
2001	Cosmo A. DiFazio	New directions in local anesthetic drug design.
2002	J. Anthony W. Wildsmith	No sceptic me, but ...

Acknowledgement

Portrait photograph reporoduced with kind permission from 'Art to Science' by K. Rehder, P. Southorn and A.D. Sessler.

Further reading

Brown DL, Winnie AP. Biography of Louis Gaston Labat, M.D. *Regional Anesthesia* 1992; **17**: 249–62.

Lee JA. Some foundations upon which we have built. *Regional Anesthesia* 1986; **10**: 99–109.

Macintosh RR. Gaston Labat Award acceptance address. *Regional Anesthesia* 1978; **3**: 2–3.

Parallel Lack Anaesthetic Breathing System

John Alastair Lack (1942-)

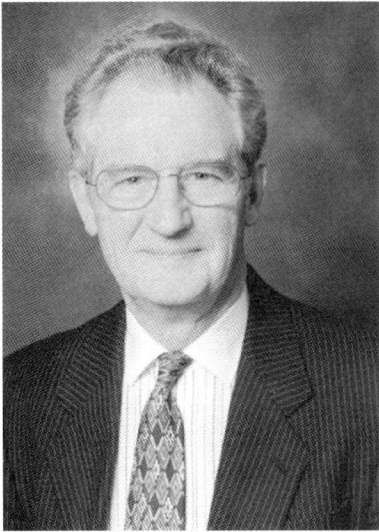

Alastair Lack was born in Cornwall, England in 1942, the son of Charles Lack (later Professor of Pathology at the Royal National Orthopaedic Hospital in London). He was educated at Westminster School, University College and University College Hospital, London where he graduated in medicine and surgery in 1965. He was mildly obsessed with science and technology from medical school days. However, after graduation he was strongly urged by Percy Cliffe at the Westminster Hospital (the pioneer of Clinical Measurement as a science) to obtain a higher specialist medical qualification before taking up a career in medical technology. He therefore trained in anaesthesia at the Westminster Hospital and quickly passed his FFARCS (now FRCA) at the age of 25.

To further his training in the nascent science of computing and engineering in medicine, he was seconded to Imperial College, London in 1969. In 1971 he was awarded its Diploma (DIC) for his thesis on telecommunication of physiological signals. After two years at Stanford University, California as an anaesthetist and assistant professor of anesthesiology, he decided that a rural, service environment would suit him and his family better than an academic career. They returned to England and he was appointed as consultant anaesthetist in Salisbury, Wiltshire in 1974.

Until the mid-1970s, waste anaesthetic gases were allowed to escape freely into the operating room atmosphere, polluting all around and giving rise to the question: 'If the patient can stay awake, Mr. Anaesthetist, why can't you?' Lack demonstrated that the most simple method for getting rid of these gases was simply to duct them to the outside air, and that the positive pressure prevailing in operating rooms was perfectly adequate as the driving force. In 1975 he described a simple copper piping system that terminated at roof level in a Venturi to eliminate back pressures. This became the basis of the British Department of Health's standard design for passive anaesthetic exhaust systems.

However, no scavenging system was available to prevent the escape of waste gases from the patient circuit. Many anaesthetists in Britain were using the Magill breathing system. Lack wanted to achieve two goals; first, to scavenge the waste gases and second, to bring the expiratory adjustable pressure limiting (APL) valve back to the anaesthetic machine where it could easily be reached (Figure 1). At first he took a smooth bore plastic tube back through the flexible corrugated black rubber tube to an exhaust valve mounted above the reservoir bag. However, this decreased the volume of the corrugated outer tube so that some rebreathing could occur with deep tidal volumes and the corrugated rubber was too heavy for a coaxial circuit. The arrival of lighter weight, corrugated plastic tubing in the following year, 1976, facilitated the introduction of the definitive Lack

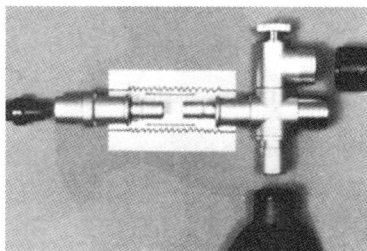

Figure 1. Lack scavenging valve. (Reproduced from *Anaesthesia* 1976; 31: 259–62.)

parallel 'circuit' (Figure 2) in which the rebreathing problem was eliminated.

A by-product of the correspondence that followed the introduction of the original 'circuit' was an investigation into the contribution of different components of the system to the resistance to breathing. There was no standardization of the resistance of expiratory valves and some had extraordinarily high values. Lack and the manufacturers designed a new exhaust valve whose expiratory resistance when fully opened was defined as that just necessary to hold a reservoir bag from collapsing at peak expiratory flow, ie 0.25–0.5 cm water. This design is still in use.

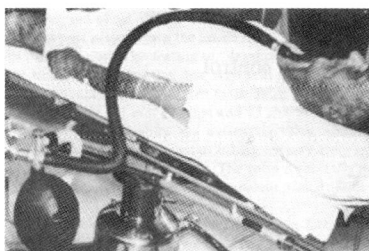

Figure 2. The parallel Lack anaesthetic breathing system. (Reproduced from *Anaesthesia* 1976; 31: 259–62.)

In 1987 Lack co-founded the Society for Computing and Technology in Anaesthesia, of which he was chairman and then president. He was subsequently elected chairman of the World Federation of Technology Societies. In 1990 he developed the concept of iso-resource grouping as a means of coding patients awaiting elective surgery into groups with similar medical conditions requiring similar treatments. He personally wrote a number of widely used computer programs for medical applications, including trainee logbooks, theatre management systems and pharmacokinetic drug models.

Lack was involved in anaesthetic related critical incident analysis for many years. In 1990, he published what became known as the Salisbury severity score for critical incidents. In 1997 he was elected to the council of the Royal College of Anaesthetists. In 2000 he highlighted the importance of the measurement of quality of anaesthetic practice with the publication by the Royal College of Anaesthetists of his book of audit recipes. The book demonstrated how this difficult topic might be approached in a logical fashion.

Further reading

Department of Health and Social Security. *Design guide for Anaesthetic Gas Disposal Systems*, 1986.

Lack JA. Theatre pollution control. *Anaesthesia* 1976; 31: 259–62.

Ooi R, Lack JA, Soni N, Whittle J, Pattison J. The parallel Lack anaesthetic breathing system. *Anaesthesia* 1993; 48: 409–14.

LEE'S 'SYNOPSIS OF ANAESTHESIA'

LEE EPIDURAL NEEDLE

John Alfred Lee (1906–1989)

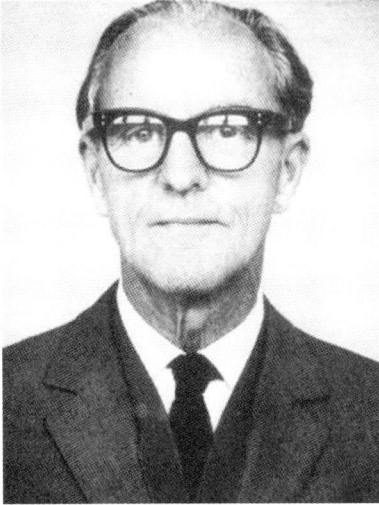

Alfred Lee was born in Liverpool, Merseyside in 1906, the eldest son of a well-known non-conformist minister. He was educated at Taunton School in Somerset. Lee studied medicine at the University of Durham College of Medicine in Newcastle upon Tyne where he graduated (MRCS and LRCP) in 1927 at the age of 21. He spent the next two years as resident medical officer in Newcastle, first at the Princess Mary Maternity Hospital and then at the Royal Victoria Infirmary, appointments that involved giving some anaesthetics. At a time when doctors could go straight into practice after qualifying, he was unusually well qualified when he bought a share of a practice in Southend-on-Sea, Essex. He was appointed as a general practitioner anaesthetist at the Southend Victoria Hospital in 1931, one of the first two hospital anaesthetists to be appointed in the town. He took a similar appointment at the new Southend General Hospital in 1932.

He continued in general practice until the outbreak of the Second World War in 1939 when he joined the Emergency Medical Service (EMS) as a full-time anaesthetist. The EMS looked after both civilian air raid casualties from the London area and wounded servicemen who were evacuated from the various war zones. He somehow found time in 1940 to pass the Diploma in Anaesthetics. He stayed with the EMS until it was disbanded after the end of the war. Lee became a consultant anaesthetist to Southend General Hospital in 1947, often working a 12-hour day, including Saturdays. On Sundays he worked on his writing.

The first edition of his famous book, *A Synopsis of Anaesthesia,* rapidly became a best seller. It was an essential source of clear and concise information for every anaesthetist. Although the early editions had no references or only a few footnotes, later editions were among the most fully referenced anaesthetic textbooks. Lee was the sole author of the first four editions. His Southend colleagues, Richard Atkinson (1926–2001) and Geoffrey Rushman, joined him for later editions and it has officially been translated into six other languages. After Lee died, its title was changed to the eponymous *Lee's Synopsis of Anaesthesia*. Lee wrote many biographical and historical journal articles. He also co-authored three editions of Sir Robert Macintosh's

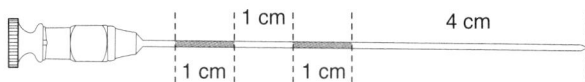

Figure 1. Lee epidural needle with centimetre markings. (Reproduced from *Anaesthesia* 1960; 15: 186.)

Lumbar Puncture and Spinal Analgesia, other regional anaesthesia textbooks and a *History of the Hospitals of Southend-on-Sea*.

Southend was noted for providing excellent tuition in regional analgesia. Lee was one of the few British anaesthetists who practised spinal anaesthesia in the 1950s. Epidural analgesia was gaining in popularity but accidental dural puncture was not uncommon. One of the problems was to know exactly how far the needle had been inserted, because the distance from skin to epidural space varies from less than 3 cm to more than 6 cm. In 1957, Lee designed an epidural needle that reduced the incidence of dural puncture. It had alternating black and metallic markings every 1 cm beginning 4 cm from the needle tip (Figure 1). It could safely be advanced 3 cm through the skin, ie 1 cm from the first black marking, without risk of puncturing the dura or having missed the epidural space. Similarly, in all but exceptionally large patients, if the epidural space was not identified by 6 cm the anaesthetist should stop and try a different angle or different space. He welcomed interested anaesthetists as visitors, but reminded regional enthusiasts that general anaesthesia was equally important and they should maintain a balanced view.

Lee had an amazing depth and range of knowledge and he was also a man of vision. His reputation as a clinician and teacher attracted many overseas students, as well as British trainees. They were allowed time off to study in an era before most departments even considered such 'concessions'. Lee enjoyed using as well as teaching practical skills, such as blind nasal intubation. He even passed his own endotracheal tube under local anaesthesia in preparation for his thyroidectomy under general anaesthesia. He started the first anaesthetic outpatient clinic in Britain in 1948 and the first postoperative recovery ward in a British general hospital in 1955.

Lee was one of the last of the self-taught generation of anaesthetists. He retired from his National Health Service post in Southend in 1971, but he continued to work and teach actively as a locum in Southend and elsewhere until his 80th birthday. He was active culturally as well as professionally. He and his wife loved opera and visited Bayreuth and Munich as well as Glyndebourne. He was also a lifelong supporter of Newcastle United football club.

Lee was made a foundation Fellow of the Faculty of Anaesthetists of the Royal College of Surgeons in 1953. He served on its board and was an examiner for the final FFARCS examination. He was president of the Section of Anaesthetics of the Royal Society of Medicine in 1959; president of the Association of Anaesthetists of Great Britain and Ireland in 1971–3 and elected to Honorary Membership in 1976; and he was the first president of the History of Anaesthesia Society from 1986 to 1988.

He gave the Joseph Clover Lecture of the Faculty of Anaesthetists in 1960 and was awarded the Faculty Medal in 1976. He was the Hickman Medallist of the Royal Society of Medicine in 1976. He received the first Carl Koller Award of the European Society of Regional Anaesthesia in 1984 and the Gaston Labat Award of the American Society of Regional Anesthesia in 1985. He gave the T.H. Seldon Memorial Lecture of the International Anesthesia Research Society in 1986 and continued to attend meetings until his death in 1989.

Acknowledgement

Portrait photograph reproduced with kind permission from the Association of Anaesthetists of Great Britain and Ireland.

Further reading

Lee JA. Specially marked needle to facilitate extradural block. *Anaesthesia* 1960; 15: 186.

Lee JA, Lunn JN. [Editorial]. John Alfred Lee (1906–1989) MRCS, LRCP, MMSA, FFARCS, FFARCSI (Hon). *Anaesthesia* 1989; 44: 631.

Lee JA, Atkinson RS, Davies NJ, Rushman GB. *Lee's Synopsis of Anaesthesia 11th edn* Oxford, UK: Butterworth-Heinemann, 1993.

MJW [obituary]. J.A. Lee MRCS, LRCP, FCANAES, MMSA, DA. *British Medical Journal* 1989; 298: 1639.

THE CRAWFORD W. LONG
MEDICAL MUSEUM

Crawford Williamson Long (1815-1878)

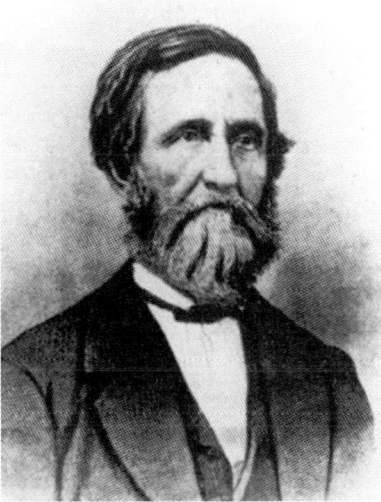

Crawford Long was born in Danielsville, Madison County, Georgia in 1815. His grandfather, who left Ireland for Carlisle, Pennsylvania in approximately 1761, fought in the War of Independence and moved to Madison County, Georgia in 1791. Long's father was a planter, clerk of the Superior Court of Georgia and sat for two terms in the state senate.

Long entered Franklin College, now the University of Georgia, in Augusta aged just 14 and gained an AM in 1835. He taught for one year in the academy that his father had founded at Danielsville and then became apprenticed to George Grant, a doctor in the isolated village of Jefferson, Georgia. The majority of American doctors in the 1830s trained in the apprentice system, and only one in five obtained a medical degree. Long, however, continued his medical training at Transylvania University in Lexington, Kentucky and at the University of Pennsylvania in Philadelphia, where he graduated in 1839. He then took two years of surgical training in New York City and was unusually well qualified when he bought Grant's practice and settled in Jefferson in 1841.

His practice soon extended into the neighbouring counties and towns of Georgia and his home was the favourite social gathering place for the young men of the neighbourhood. The effect of inhaling nitrous oxide was well known in the early 1840s, when wandering charlatans or travelling lecturers gave demonstrations to volunteers in community halls. In January 1842, several of Long's friends saw a demonstration and asked Long to let them have a 'nitrous oxide frolic' in his room. He did not have the apparatus for preparing nitrous oxide, but he offered ether as a substitute. He told them that it would produce equally exhilarating effects, that he had inhaled it himself, and that it was as safe as nitrous oxide.

All the young men inhaled it. They were so pleased with its effect that ether inhalation became fashionable in several counties in that part of Georgia. Long observed that his etherized friends fell and received blows that should have produced pain, but they all assured him that they did not feel the least pain or discomfort from these accidents. He inferred that ether must produce insensibility and that it might be used to prevent pain in surgical operations.

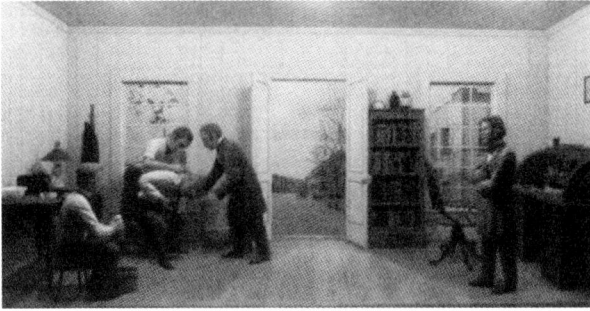

Figure 1. Diorama of the first ether anaesthetic. (Reproduced with kind permission from the Crawford W. Long Medical Museum.)

Two months later, on 30 March 1842, one of the young men, James Venable, agreed to inhale ether from a towel while Long removed a cyst from the back of his neck (Figure 1). He later testified that he experienced no pain and a fellow student who witnessed the operation confirmed this in a sworn statement. Long removed another similar tumour from Venable's neck under ether inhalation on 6 June 1842. He performed six more operations under ether before September 1846, then William Morton gave his public demonstration of ether in Boston on 16 October 1846.

Long's failure to publish his discovery clouded the issue of who had the rightful claim for the discovery of anaesthesia. He explained that he had wished to try etherization in enough cases to be sure that it was the ether, and not the patient's imagination, that produced the anaesthetic state. He also explained that surgical operations were not frequent in a young doctor's country practice. Long eventually published his paper in the *Southern Medical and Surgical Journal* in 1849. He presented a clear statement, with full supporting documentation and affidavits from witnesses, to validate his claim to be the discoverer of ether anaesthesia. His paper remained largely unrecognized until the famous gynaecologist, Marion Sims (1813–83) asserted Long's priority in the *Virginia Medical Monthly* in 1877. Long is rightfully credited with discovering surgical anaesthesia, but that is all. He had no influence on its development, nor did he play any part in its introduction to the world at large.

Crawford Long married Mary Caroline Swain, the 16-year-old daughter of a planter and niece of Governor Swain of North Carolina, on 11 August 1842. They had 12 children, six of whom grew to adulthood. There is a third-party claim that Long used ether to lessen his wife's pains at the birth of one of their daughters on 27 December 1845. That was 13 months before James Simpson used it in Edinburgh on 19 January 1847. This claim came not from Crawford Long himself but from the daughter in question, Frances (Fanny) Long Taylor, who wrote a biography of her father. However, Fanny told only one friend because revealing the information

Figure 2. Crawford W. Long US postage stamp.

would reveal her age. The friend released the information after Fanny's death.

In 1850, Long moved to Athens, Georgia where he and his younger brother bought a practice and drugstore from two retiring physicians. Long continued to administer ether anaesthetics for the rest of his life. During the Civil War he was in charge of Confederate military hospitals in Athens. For this service he received the Southern Cross from the Daughters of the Confederacy. He died of a cerebral haemorrhage, aged 62, while delivering a baby. His last articulate words were; 'Care for the mother and child first.'

On 30 March 1926, the state of Georgia presented a marble effigy of Crawford W. Long in the Statuary Hall at the US National Capitol in Washington DC. The engraving reads; 'My profession is to me a ministry of God'. There are other monuments or memorials in the University of Pennsylvania and in Danielsville, Jefferson and Athens.

Figure 3. Crawford W. Long Medical Museum in Jefferson, Georgia. (Reproduced with kind permission from the Crawford W. Long Medical Museum.)

The United States postal service honoured Long with a red two-cent stamp in the 'Great Americans' series that was released in Jefferson on 8 April 1940 (Figure 2). The Crawford W. Long Medical Museum in Jefferson (Figure 3), 60 miles (100 km) north of Atlanta, was opened in 1957. It houses exhibits on Long, anaesthesia, a typical doctor's office and an apothecary's shop in the 1840s and a 19th century general store. There is also a medical museum at the Crawford Long Hospital in Atlanta.

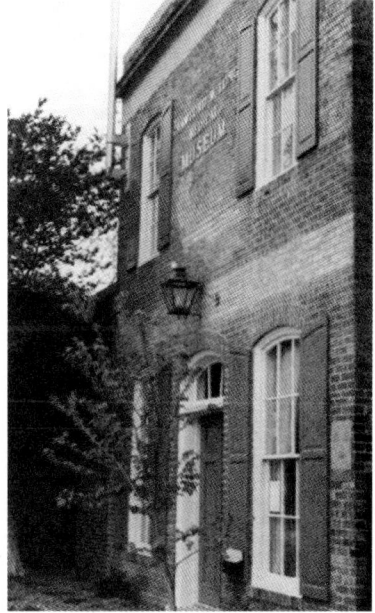

Acknowledgement

Portrait photograph reproduced with kind permission from the Wood Library–Museum of Anesthesiology, Park Ridge, IL, USA.

Further reading

Long CW. An account of the first use of sulphuric ether by inhalation as an anaesthetic in surgical operations. *Southern Medical and Surgical Journal* 1849; 5: 705–13. [Reprinted in: Faulconer A, Keys TE. *Foundations of anesthesiology, Vol. I.* Springfield: Charles C. Thomas, 1965: 310–16.]

Raper HR. A review of the Crawford W. Long centennial anniversary celebrations. *Bulletin of the History of Medicine* 1943; 13: 340–56.

Taylor FL. *Crawford W. Long & the discovery of ether anesthesia.* New York: Hoeber, 1928.

MACINTOSH LARYNGOSCOPE BLADE

Sir Robert Reynolds Macintosh (1897–1989)

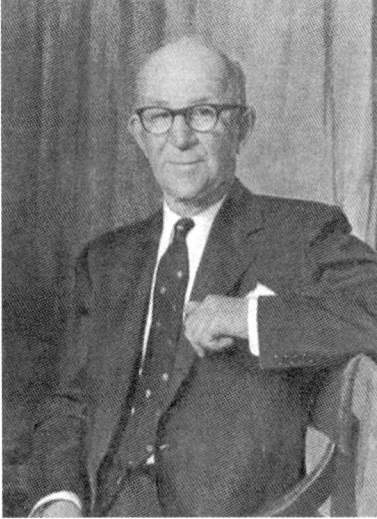

Robert Reynolds Macintosh was named Rew Rawhiti Macintosh when he was born in Timaru, New Zealand in 1897. His father was one of the members of the original All Blacks rugby team. He spent part of his childhood in Argentina where he learned to speak fluent Spanish. He returned to New Zealand in his teens and attended Waitaki Boy's High School in Oamaru. At the outbreak of the First World War he went to England and volunteered as a fighter pilot with the Royal Flying Corps. He was shot down over Germany and taken prisoner. He became fluent in German and escaped several times, but was always recaptured.

He gained the MRCS and LRCP from Guy's Hospital Medical School, London in 1924, and passed the FRCS (Edinburgh) examination in 1927. He started giving dental anaesthetics at Guy's charging one guinea per session, and he became interested in anaesthesia. He founded a private anaesthesia group practice, irreverently known as the Mayfair Gas Company, for the fashionable dental and surgical clinics in the West End of London.

In 1936, Macintosh went to Spain at the request of an American plastic surgeon to provide anaesthesia for maxillofacial surgery in casualties from the Spanish Civil War. He took his own laryngoscope and endotracheal tubes but when he arrived he found that there were no compressed gases. Fortunately, he was familiar with the Flagg can, so he improvised a drawover ether and air vaporizer from a golden syrup tin. This experience led to his appointment of a team to design the more sophisticated Oxford ether vaporizer, the ESO chloroform drawover apparatus, and the Oxford inflating bellows for British armed forces during the Second World War (Figure 1).

Macintosh was the first anaesthetist outside the USA to have a university chair when he was appointed professor at the Nuffield Department of Anaesthetics at the University of Oxford in 1937. Soon after his appointment he took a leave of absence to visit the principal academic departments in Britain and the USA. He was particularly impressed by Ralph Waters's department in Madison, Wisconsin. On his return he appointed both medical and non-medical individuals to his academic staff as the need arose.

They included Edgar Pask and William Mushin (1910–93) who became professors of anaesthesia in Newcastle upon Tyne and Cardiff respectively; Richard Salt who had been Macintosh's technician in London; Hans Epstein, a physicist; and Barbara Duncum, a historian. In the face of university prejudice, Macintosh created an academic department in what was formerly a provincial general hospital.

Macintosh held the rank of Air Commodore during the Second World War, and was adviser in anaesthetics to both the Royal Air Force and the Royal Navy. Early in the war, he and Pask carried out research on self-righting life vests. The Nuffield department trained physician anaesthetists for the British and allied services and many of them became consultant anaesthetists when the National Health Service was inaugurated in 1948.

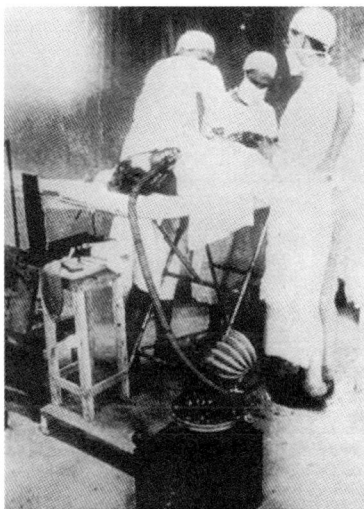

Figure 1. The Oxford vaporizer in use in Burma, 1943. (Reproduced from the Nuffield Department of Anaesthetics.)

Salt was a technician who quickly converted a concept into a mechanical form. One example of his ability was the curved Macintosh laryngoscope blade (Figure 2). Until 1943, the standard laryngoscope blades were straight and were designed to pass beyond the epiglottis. One day, during a tonsillectomy, a surgeon inserted a larger size of Boyle–Davis gag than he had intended. When the mouth was fully opened, the vocal cords came into view. With conventional laryngoscopy it would have been impossible to lift up the epiglottis at that depth of anaesthesia. Macintosh reasoned that it was the relationship between the tip of the blade and the epiglottis that was important. The new curved blade brought the tip into contact with the base of the tongue, which is innervated by the glossopharyngeal nerve, and not with the posterior surface of the epiglottis which is innervated by the superior laryngeal nerve. On the same day, Salt modified the blade of a Boyle–Davis gag and attached a laryngoscope handle to it. After streamlining, the curved blade was manufactured by Medical and Industrial Equipment Ltd.

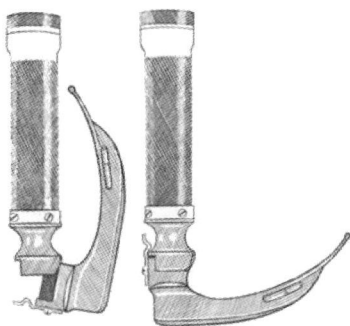

Figure 2. Macintosh laryngoscope. (Reproduced with permission from A Synopsis of Anaesthesia, John Wright, 1947: 95.)

The Nuffield department was noted for regional anaesthesia during the 1940s and 1950s when its use was not generally popular in Britain. Macintosh and Alfred Lee were among the few British anaesthetists who continued to use and teach spinal anaesthesia after two men, Woolley and Roe, became permanently paraplegic after spinal anaesthesia in 1947. Macintosh was an early advocate of autoclaving reusable syringes, needles and

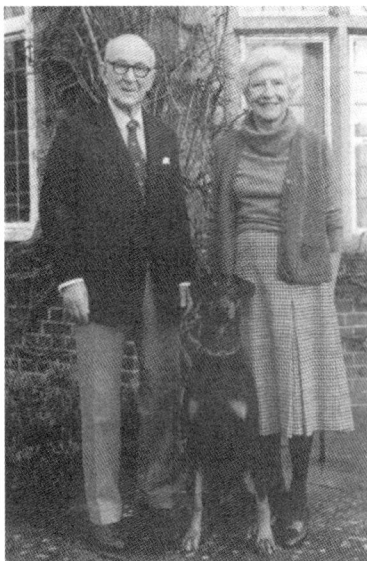

Figure 3. Sir Robert Macintosh aged 90 with Lady Macintosh and their dog Oscar.

ampoules for spinal anaesthesia. He designed a balloon that attached to the hub of the epidural needle and deflated when the tip of the needle reached negative pressure in the extradural space. He and Salt designed the Oxford Tuohy needle with wings to assist with controlling the advancing epidural needle. He was the primary author of four clearly illustrated books on regional anaesthesia

Macintosh was particularly interested in anaesthesia in developing countries in the postwar period. He travelled widely and demonstrated the principles of modern anaesthesia using simple, effective technology. The wartime Oxford vaporizers for ether and chloroform were the forerunners of the Epstein Macintosh Oxford (EMO) for ether and the Oxford miniature vaporizer (OMV) for halothane and trichlorethylene that became important in developing countries and military anaesthesia.

Macintosh received many honours in many countries. He was Hickman Medallist of the Royal Society of Medicine in 1947, and received his knighthood from the Queen in 1955. He celebrated his 90th birthday at a meeting hosted jointly by the Royal Society of Medicine, the Association of Anaesthetists of Great Britain and Ireland and the Faculty of Anaesthetists of the Royal College of Surgeons of England (Figure 3). The following year he fell while exercising his dog, and sustained a head injury from which he died.

Acknowledgement

Portrait photograph reproduced from the Nuffield Department of Anaesthetics, Oxford, UK.

Further reading

ACS. [Obituary]. Sir Robert Macintosh DM, FRCSED, FCANAES, DA. *British Medical Journal* 1989; **299**: 851.

Boulton TB. Professor Sir Robert Macintosh, 1897–1989: personal reflections on a remarkable man and his career. *Regional Anesthesia* 1993; **18**: 145–54.

Macintosh RR. A new laryngoscope. *Lancet* 1943; **1**: 205.

MAGILL FORCEPS

Sir Ivan Whiteside Magill (1888–1986)

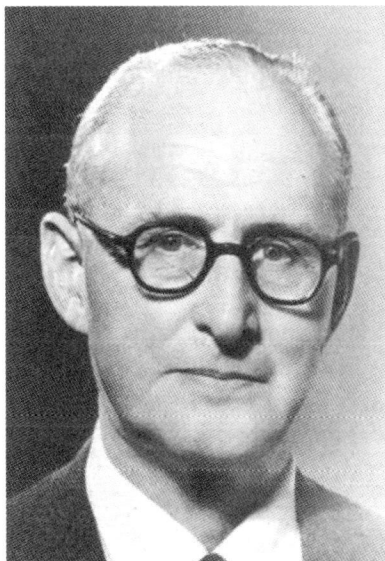

Ivan Magill was born in Larne, County Antrim in Northern Ireland in 1888, the son of Samuel Magill, a draper. He was educated at Larne Grammar School, and graduated in medicine and surgery from Queen's University, Belfast in 1913. He was a rugby forward and boxed for his university as a heavyweight.

He had been resident medical officer at the Walton Hospital in Liverpool for six months at the outbreak of the First World War. He served throughout the war as Captain in the Royal Army Medical Corps (RAMC), and was medical officer to the Irish Guards at the Battle of Loos in northern France. At the end of the hostilities he was posted to the Barnet War Hospital where he gave occasional anaesthetics. His colleagues told him to answer 'anaesthetist' as his current status on an RAMC questionnaire. Early in 1919, this led to his being posted to the Queen's Hospital for Facial and Jaw Injuries at Sidcup in Kent as an anaesthetist. There he met Stanley Rowbotham (1890–1979) and together these two inexperienced young doctors faced some of the most challenging problems in anaesthesia.

Many of the patients had suffered gross facial trauma from the war. The usual anaesthetic was rectal oil ether, a technique that was recommended for operations around the mouth or nose, removal of the tongue and excision of the mandible. Magill found that the patients were often too lightly sedated at the start, too deep during surgery and then slept for up to 24 hours afterwards. The surgeon doing his work often increased the problem of keeping a clear airway. Anaesthesia for these cases intrigued rather than frightened Magill. In London, Sir Francis Shipway (1875–1968) had introduced warm ether endotracheal insufflation – the anaesthetist passed a catheter through the nose for oral operations and used a laryngoscope and forceps to guide it through the larynx. However, the surgeon inhaled ether-laden air as it had bubbled up through the operative field. Magill improved the insufflation technique by passing a Silk's tube alongside the insufflation catheter as a route for exhaled gases. Eighteen months after he arrived in Sidcup, he described the forceps (Figure 1) that became known throughout the world as Magill forceps and how they are used with catheters (Figure 2):

... The forceps are constructed with a bend to clear the field of vision, as in Heath's nasal forceps, the ends of which grasp the catheter representing a cylinder split longitudinally and serrated on the inner surface. Introduction of the catheter into the trachea is carried out with an electrically illuminated speculum... I need hardly add that in operations involving bleeding into the pharynx the fixation of a suitable suction pump to the expiratory nasal tube provides an even clearer field for the surgeon by removing blood without continual swabbing.

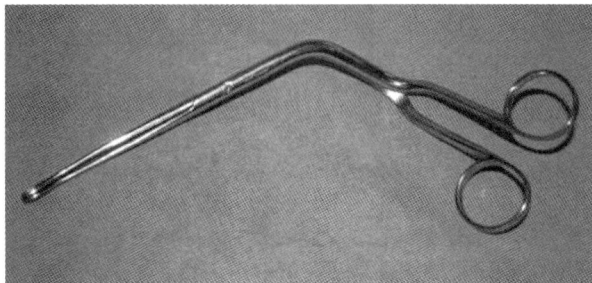

Figure 1. Magill forceps. (Reproduced with kind permission from the Association of Anaesthetists of Great Britain and Ireland.)

He found that Silk's tube sometimes passed blindly into the trachea and this led to his technique of blind nasal intubation. Endotracheal insufflation had many drawbacks and intubation with a single, wide-bore tube had many advantages. In one step, Magill had secured a safe and adequate airway and removed himself from the operative field. He passed the tube via the mouth or nose according to the type of operation, but concentrated on the nasal route because this did not require use of a laryngoscope. He described the ideal position of the patient's head as that of a man 'scenting the air' or, later and more characteristically, 'draining a pint of beer'!

In 1923, he was appointed to the Brompton Hospital in London. Bronchiectasis was gross and tuberculosis was rife. He was a pioneer thoracic anaesthetist and devised several useful items of equipment. These included his combined suction catheter and bronchial blocker with an inflatable cuff, endobronchial tubes to provide one-lung anaesthesia and an intubating bronchoscope. In 1924, he joined the Westminster Hospital where he worked until his retirement from the National Health Service.

Magill was in great demand in private practice. He designed portable apparatus so that he could give a safe anaesthetic in a private house, ill-equipped nursing homes or even 'for four hours in a bathroom in the Ritz [Hotel]'. In 1926, he added nitrous oxide and a dry gas-flow meter to his portable apparatus, suspending the cylinders from a yoke over his shoulders and carrying them under his overcoat. In 1932, he suggested replacement of the dry gas flowmeter by the rotameter to the manufacturer Charles King, and this was done in 1935.

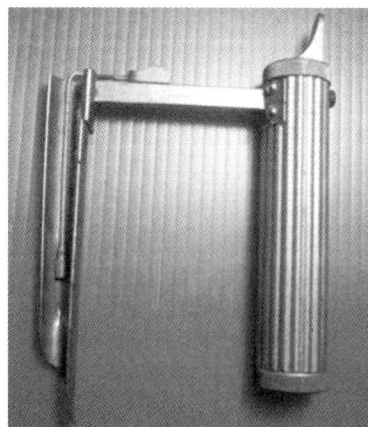

Figure 2. Magill 'intubating spatula'. (Reproduced with kind permission from the Association of Anaesthetists of Great Britain and Ireland.)

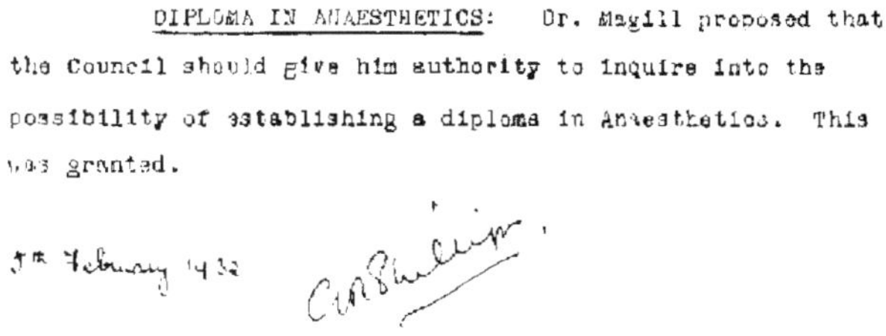
DIPLOMA IN ANAESTHETICS: Dr. Magill proposed that the Council should give him authority to inquire into the possibility of establishing a diploma in Anaesthetics. This was granted.

Figure 3. Royal Society of Medicine minute of Magill's proposal.

In 1931, as senior secretary of the Section of Anaesthetics of the Royal Society of Medicine, Magill proposed to the council that an examination for a Diploma in Anaesthetics should be instituted (Figure 3). However, the Royal Society of Medicine could not initiate this under its charter. The Association of Anaesthetists was therefore constituted in 1932 and the first diploma examination of the conjoint board of the Royal College of Surgeons of England was held on 8 November 1935. It was the world's first qualification in anaesthesia. Magill received his diploma in the same year without examination.

Magill was the President of the Section of Anaesthetics of the Royal Society of Medicine in 1937, and was Hickman Medallist in 1938. The Queen's University of Belfast awarded him an honorary DSc degree in 1945. He was made a Commander of the Royal Victorian Order for services to the Royal Family in 1946, and received a knighthood in 1960. His memorial at Westminster Hospital Medical School is the Magill Department of Anaesthetics.

He stayed in London throughout the Second World War, despite his house being destroyed by a bomb in 1941. He gave his last anaesthetic in 1972 at the age of 84. Magill loved food, drink, Burma cheroots, lively company and practical jokes. He loved fishing, which he also excelled at, and in 1932 he was made a member of the one of the most exclusive fishing clubs, The Houghton, at Stockbridge on the Test. He stalked trout whenever he had time, while his wife sketched. He caught a five-pounder on his 97th birthday and died in his 99th year.

Further reading

Edridge AW [Editorial]. Sir Ivan Whiteside Magill KCVO, DSc (Hon), MB, BCh, BAO, FRCS (Hon), FFARCS (Hon), FFARCSI (Hon), DA. 23 July 1888–25 November 1986. *Anaesthesia* 1987; 42: 231–3.

Magill IW. Endotracheal anaesthesia. *Proceedings of the Royal Society of Medicine* 1929; 22: 83–7.

Magill IW. Forceps for intratracheal anaesthesia. *British Medical Journal* 1920; 2: 670.

MALLAMPATI SCORE

Seshagiri Rao Mallampati (1941–)

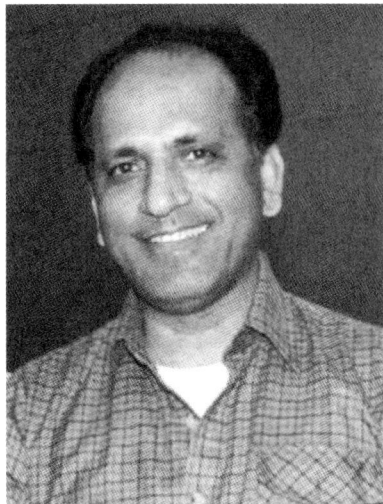

Rao Mallampati was born in Patchalatadi Parru, Andhra Pradesh, India in 1941 and was educated at Andhra Loyola College in Vijayawada and Hindu College in Guntur, Andhra Pradesh. He entered Guntur Medical College in 1963, transferred to Andhra Medical College in 1965 and graduated MB, BS in 1968. After interning at King George Hospital in Visakhapatnam, he spent two years in private general practice before immigrating to the USA in 1971. He completed his residency in anaesthesiology at the Lahey Clinic Foundation and Boston Hospital for Women in 1975, and followed that with a clinical fellowship at Harvard Medical School in Boston, Massachusetts. He became a Diplomate of the American Board of Anesthesiology in 1976 and a Fellow of the American College of Anesthesiology in 1977. He was attending anesthesiologist at the Boston Hospital for Women from 1975 to 1980, at Brigham and Women's Hospital, Boston from 1980 to 1985 and assistant professor of anesthesia at Harvard Medical School since 1985.

Anaesthesia-related morbidity and mortality were two of Mallampati's concerns from the outset of his career in anaesthesia. Although more than one factor may have played a part in these tragic events, the unanticipated difficult airway was a major factor in the majority of cases. Mallampati focused his attention on preoperative airway evaluation to identify patients who would need difficult airway management.

In 1983, he published a letter to the editor in the *Canadian Anaesthetists' Society Journal*. While he was working at the Boston Hospital for Women in the late 1970s, he had encountered difficulty in intubating the trachea of an adult female patient. In spite of adequate muscle relaxation, optimal positioning and appropriate equipment, he just about accomplished orotracheal intubation after four attempts. His subsequent examination revealed that the anatomical features of her head and neck, including the teeth, were normal and mobility of the temporomandibular joints and neck was unrestricted. However, during examination of her upper airway, he noticed that her soft palate was only barely visible when she opened her mouth wide and protruded her tongue. The faucial pillars (palatoglossal and palatopharyngeal arches) and uvula were completely concealed by the tongue, even with maximal protrusion. This concealment of the faucial pillars and uvula by the base (posterior part) of the tongue was the only noteworthy anatomical feature in this case.

Mallampati subsequently made it his practice to see whether the faucial pillars and uvula were visible in every patient. He asked the seated patient to open his or her mouth widely and to protrude the tongue fully. He found that it was generally easy to expose the glottis by direct laryngoscopy in patients whose faucial pillars and uvula

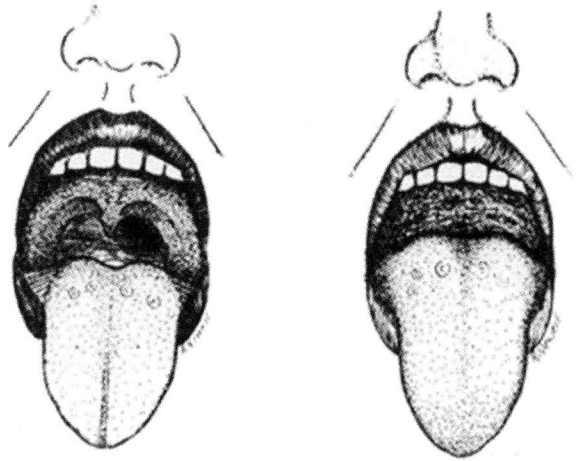

Figure 1. (Left) Class 1: faucial pillars, soft palate and uvula visible, (right) Class 3: only soft palate visible. (Reproduced from *Canadian Anaesthetists' Society Journal* 1985; 32: 429–34.)

were normally visible, but difficult if they were concealed by the tongue (Figure 1). He found that this clinical sign of concealment of faucial pillars and uvula was helpful in predicting the great majority of difficult orotracheal intubations.

Mallampati wondered why it should be difficult to expose the glottis by direct laryngoscopy in patients in whom the faucial pillars and uvula were masked by the base of the tongue. If the tongue, particularly the base, were disproportionately large relative to the capacity of the oropharyngeal cavity, it would obscure the view of the faucial pillars, the posterior part of the soft palate and eventually the uvula. It would also obscure the larynx and render the angle to the larynx more acute. Such an anatomical relation was a simple and useful predictor of difficult orotracheal intubation. He had already started a prospective study, and invited anaesthetists in other centres to do the same, to compare this clinical sign with existing predictors of difficult intubation.

In 1985, Mallampati and colleagues in Boston published their study of 210 patients. They divided their patients into three classes according to which pharyngeal structures were visible:

Class 1: Faucial pillars, soft palate and uvula visible.
Class 2: Faucial pillars and soft palate visible, uvula obscured by base of tongue.
Class 3: Soft palate visible only.

They correlated their view of pharyngeal structures with four grades of laryngoscopy, similar to those of Cormack and Lehane. Their results confirmed that the degree of difficulty in seeing the three pharyngeal structures was an accurate predictor of difficulty when using direct laryngoscopy. Mallampati's simple scoring system soon gained international acceptance.

Class I   Class II

Class III   Class IV

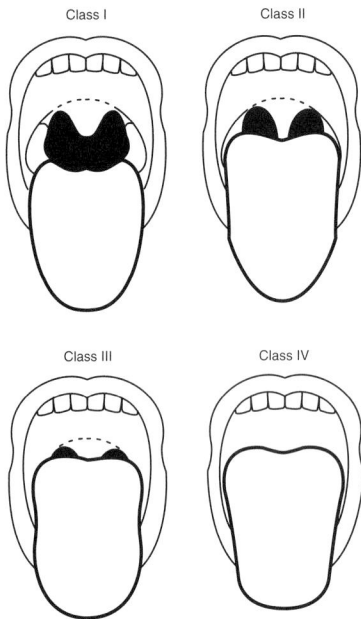

Figure 2. Samsoon and Young's modified classification of visibility of pharyngeal structures. (Reproduced from *Anaesthesia* 1987; 42: 487–90.)

Two years later, Samsoon and Young in Portsmouth, UK added a new Class 4 (Figure 2) to Mallampati's scoring system, in which not even the soft palate was visible. Tracheal intubation had been impossible in seven out of 1980 obstetric patients during 1982–85. They recalled these seven patients and found that six of them had a Class 4 view of pharyngeal structures and Cormack and Lehane's Grade III or IV laryngoscopy. The seventh patient had Grade I laryngoscopy but unsuspected tracheal stenosis. For the same period, tracheal intubation was impossible in six surgical patients from a total of 13,380. Samsoon and Young also found that all these patients had Class 4 airways.

Difficult laryngoscopy and intubation may be predicted in some patients by the external examination of anatomical factors such as a short thick neck, prominent incisor teeth, receding mandible or rigid neck. Despite this, a perfectly normal looking patient may still unexpectedly present the greatest difficulty.

More complex scoring systems and investigations have been suggested, but asking patients to sit and open their mouths for examination of the upper airway is equally important. The clear and simple Mallampati score, modified by Samsoon and Young, has gained worldwide acceptance in clinical practice.

Further reading

Mallampati SR. Clinical sign to predict difficult tracheal intubation (hypothesis). *Canadian Anaesthetists' Society Journal* 1983; 30: 316–17.

Mallampati SR, Gatt SP, Gugino LD *et al*. A clinical sign to predict difficult tracheal intubation: a prospective study. *Canadian Anaesthetists' Society Journal* 1985; 32: 429–34.

Samsoon GLT, Young JRB. Difficult tracheal intubation: a retrospective study. *Anaesthesia* 1987; 42: 487–90.

MANLEY VENTILATOR
PENLON MANLEY MULTIVENT

Roger Edward Wentworth Manley (1930–91)

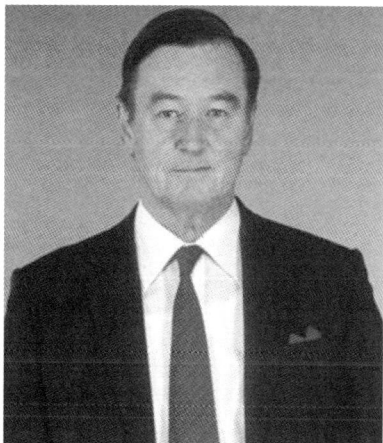

Roger Manley was an anaesthetist, engineer, and inventor. There can hardly be an anaesthetist in Britain from the 1960s onwards who has not used a Manley ventilator. He graduated in medicine and surgery from the Westminster Hospital Medical College, London in 1954 and completed junior appointments in anaesthesia at the Westminster Hospital. He was still only a registrar when he designed his first ventilator in 1961.

When halothane became available in 1956, the early vaporizers were inaccurate at fresh gas below 4 litres per minute. Most anaesthetists therefore used halothane in a high-flow system without carbon dioxide absorption. Anaesthetic techniques that used curare were gaining in popularity but squeezing the reservoir bag occupied the anaesthetist's hands (and occasionally a foot). Anaesthetists welcomed the 'minute volume divider' Manley ventilator. They only needed to set the fresh gas flow on the rotameters as the patient's minute volume and the desired tidal volume on the ventilator. The ventilator automatically divided the minute volume by the tidal volume to set the respiratory rate.

Ventilators were not an integral part of an anaesthetic machine in the 1960s. Manley designed his ventilator to fit on the commonly used Boyle machine (Figure 1). The difference in pressure of the fresh gas between leaving the reducing valves of the machine and leaving the needle valve of the flow meter was more than sufficient to operate the valves of the ventilator. The ventilator did not require an ancillary source of energy.

The ventilator produced inflation by means

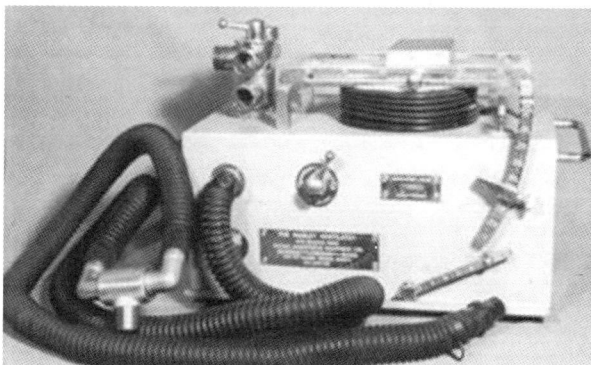

Figure 1. Manley ventilator. (Reproduced with kind permission from the Association of Anaesthetists of Great Britain and Ireland.)

of a variable weight-loaded bellows that delivered a preset volume to the non-rebreathing circuit. Minute volume was set on the rotameters and tidal volume was set by moving the adjustable stop on the curved arm to the appropriate point. The weight on the bar above the bellows could be moved along a graduated scale to give pressures of 8–30 cm water. A tap allowed diversion of the gas flow directly to the patient's lungs for manual ventilation with the reservoir bag. During the expiratory phase, the patient's lungs were open to the atmosphere and fresh gas passed into the large concertina bellows.

A mounting was provided for a Wright respirometer to measure expired volume. There was no electronic low-pressure or high-pressure alarm, but anaesthetists became attuned to audible change if there was a disconnection or obstruction in the circuit. With a disconnection there was no airway resistance and the bellows fell with a 'thump' onto the rubber stopper on the ventilator casing. With obstruction or increased resistance due to coughing, the bellows could not deliver the full tidal volume and there was a rapid 'clunking' noise as the ventilator alternated between inspiratory and expiratory phases.

Thirty years later, Manley approached Michael Dobson in Oxford and John Zorab in Bristol; he knew that they both organized courses for anaesthetists working in developing countries and he needed advice on the most important features to build into a ventilator for that environment. Dobson had worked in Nepal, and Zorab was a past president of the World Federation of Societies of Anaesthesiologists. Their advice was to create a simple, low-maintenance, low-cost, multi-purpose ventilator that would work independently of compressed gas and/or mains electricity. Simplicity was important because nurse anaesthetists or anaesthetic officers give much of the anaesthesia in developing countries. Low maintenance was an important factor because technical support and parts are usually not available

In 1990, less than one year later, Manley returned with a prototype and the course participants showed great interest. Manley published a description of his new ventilator in 1991, but he died before it went into production. Roger Eltringham in Gloucester played a major role in its subsequent development and Penlon undertook its manufacture.

The Manley Multivent (Figures 2 and 3) is simple, robust, and requires no maintenance. It is essentially an automatically powered version of the Oxford inflating bellows. The position of a movable weight is adjusted so that it just delivers the selected tidal volume and the inflation pressure is known from the calibrated scale on the beam. The ventilator may be used

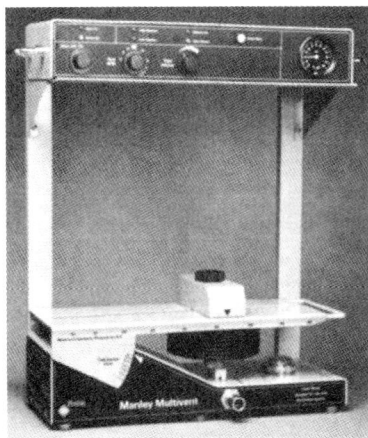

Figure 2. Ether-compatible Penlon Manley Multivent ventilator with electronics arm well above the bellows. (Reproduced with kind permission from Penlon Ltd, England.)

on adults or children for automatic or manual controlled ventilation and also permits spontaneous breathing. It has only two calibrated controls, one for tidal volume and one for frequency. The inspiratory:expiratory ratio is preset to 1:2 over the whole range. It is powered by compressed oxygen or, if this is not available, by compressed air from a small compressor driven by mains electricity or a 12-volt DC car battery.

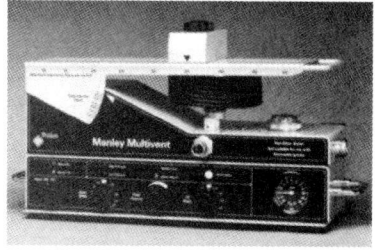

Figure 3. Penlon Manley Multivent ventilator for nonflammable anaesthetics. (Reproduced with kind permission from Penlon Ltd, England.)

If one litre of oxygen per minute is used as the drive gas, it entrains nine litres of air to give a minute volume of 10 litres. The oxygen then enters the patient circuit to give approximately 35% oxygen. The ventilator can be used with the full range of anaesthetic machines with either plenum or drawover vaporizers, and non-rebreathing, partial rebreathing (eg the Bain circuit) or closed circuits with carbon dioxide absorbers. For intensive care units, several ventilators can be powered by mains electricity when it is available, or from a back-up 12-volt DC compressor with a car battery and a battery charger.

The Manley Multivent has made a major contribution to the problem of mechanical ventilation in the developing world. It is now combined with a modified oxygen concentrator, which incorporates an air compressor in the Oxyvent (now renamed the Glostavent) anaesthetic machine. This was just what Manley had hoped for. He would have been pleased with the result.

Roger Manley was a quiet, modest yet practical man. In his later years he was managing director of his own engineering company, advisor in medical engineering to Westminster Hospital and an honorary clinical assistant at the Medical Research Council unit at Northwick Park Hospital, Harrow. His cheerful stoicism was an example to many. Despite having dyslexia, he qualified in medicine and engineering and, although he later suffered a painful and disabling illness, he never lost his enthusiasm and drive. Medicine and anaesthesia will always remain grateful to his foresight and ingenuity.

Acknowledgement

Portrait photograph courtesy of J.S.M. Zorab.

Further reading

Eltringham RJ, Varvinski A. The Oxyvent: an anaesthetic machine designed to be used in developing countries and difficult situations. *Anaesthesia* 1997; **52**: 668–72.

Forward RFM. [Obituary] REW Manley MB, BS, DA, CENG, MIMECHE. *British Medical Journal* 1992; **304**: 1050.

Manley RW. A new mechanical ventilator. *Anaesthesia* 1961; **16**: 317–23.

MAPLESON BREATHING SYSTEMS

William Wellesley Mapleson (1926–)

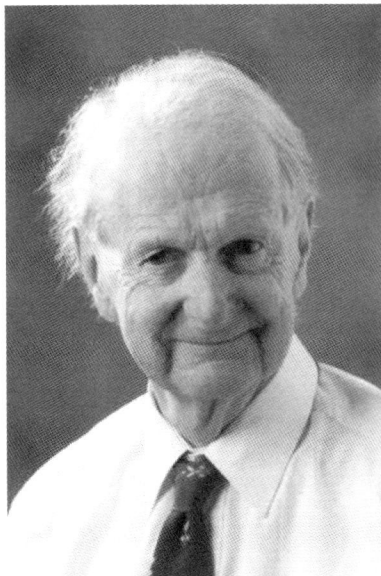

Bill Mapleson was born in London, England in 1926. His father was an insurance clerk and therefore an arithmetician. In 1937 the family moved to Amersham, Buckinghamshire where he took his secondary education at Dr Challoner's Grammar School. There he was blessed with an excellent mathematics and physics teacher, who was also the careers master. When Mapleson was in the sixth form (Grade 11), this teacher told him, 'You will go to the University of Durham and read physics'. Mapleson obligingly did as he was told and never regretted it. He graduated in 1947 and after two years National Service in the Royal Air Force, returned to Durham to do a PhD on point discharge in atmospheric electricity. When that neared completion, he was faced with the awful prospect of earning a living, instead of living off his family or the taxpayer.

Mapleson responded to an advertisement from the Department of Anaesthetics of the Welsh National School of Medicine, now the University of Wales College of Medicine, in Cardiff: 'Wanted: a research assistant/lecturer with a wide knowledge of physics, physiology or pharmacology'. He thought it would be an opportunity to gain some interviewing experience. To his acute embarrassment, he was offered the job and so was faced with making the first real decision in his life. He decided to try it for five years – so far the association has lasted for nearly 50 years. In 1954 he made the second real decision in his life by marrying Doreen Wood, a librarian and fellow enthusiast for amateur theatre.

The head of the department, (later Professor) William Mushin, set Mapleson his first task. This was to measure the neuromuscular blocking action of gallamine triethiodide in volunteers. While Mapleson was waiting for volunteers, Mushin drew the five anaesthetic breathing systems (Figure 1) and said; 'Have a look at these Bill and see if you can work out the conditions needed for the elimination of rebreathing.' Mapleson regarded this as a minor theoretical study, but its publication brought him to the attention of anaesthetists.

He knew nothing of the origins of the systems so, to distinguish them, he just applied the labels A, B, C, D and E. The resulting theoretical analysis was published in the *British Journal of Anaesthesia* in 1954, only his third publication in the field. Within a couple of years, at a meeting of the Section of Anaesthetics of the Royal Society of Medicine, Mapleson was astonished to hear these systems being referred to as the 'Mapleson A', 'Mapleson B' and so on. However, he would like to record his apologies posthumously to Sir Ivan Magill and Jackson Rees for not acknowledging them as the creators of systems 'A' and 'D' (strictly, the later 'F') respectively. A common misunderstanding is that Mapleson classified the breathing systems. He didn't, and actually just labelled them and analysed how they behaved.

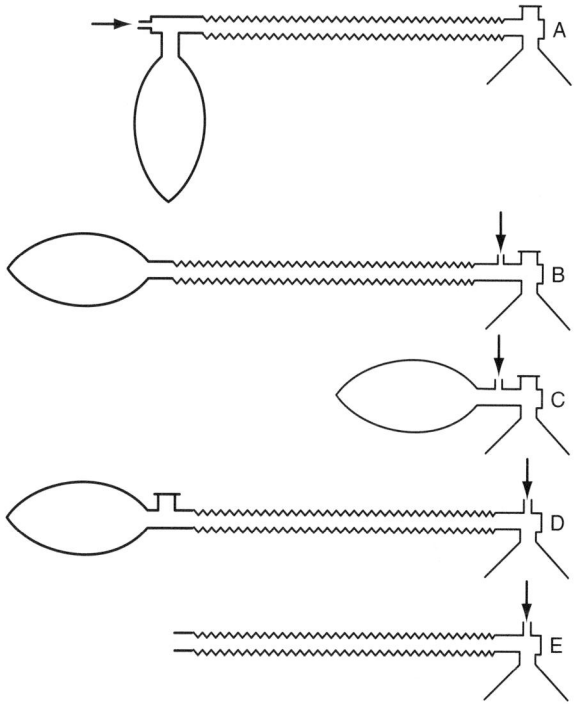

Figure 1. The five semi-closed anaesthetic breathing systems. (Reproduced from *British Journal of Anaesthesia* 1954; **26**: 323–32.)

It was Donald Miller in Stellenbosch, South Africa, who is now senior lecturer and honorary consultant anaesthetist at Guy's Hospital in London, who classified semi-closed breathing systems (Figure 1) into afferent-reservoir systems (A), enclosed afferent-reservoir systems, junctional reservoir systems (B and C) and efferent-reservoir systems (D and E).

Mapleson's main research interests have been in the physiological modelling of the pharmacokinetics of inhaled anaesthetics – a necessary preliminary to his analysis of low-flow anaesthetic breathing systems and the functioning of automatic lung ventilators. More recently he has devised appropriate and sometimes novel statistical analyses for various research projects in the department. However, many anaesthetists in Britain will remember hearing him lecture on pharmacokinetics, using diagrams of his water analogue, and on anaesthetic breathing systems, using animated overhead-projector techniques. He owes a debt of gratitude to Mushin for insisting that he explain everything as clearly as possible and to the statistician Peter Armitage, from whom he picked up the idea of animated overheads. The core material of these lectures has been made into videos with support from Abbott Laboratories Ltd.

All this activity has resulted in over 100 peer-reviewed research papers plus a similar number of other publications, including co-authorship of three editions of *Automatic Ventilation of the Lungs* – which Mapleson's

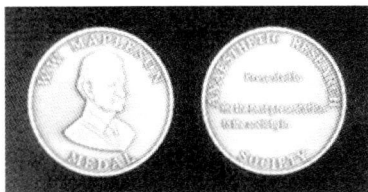

Figure 2. The W.W. Mapleson Medal of the Anaesthetic Research Society.

colleague John Lunn irreverently dubbed 'The Puffing Bible'! He was promoted successively up the academic ladder, reaching a personal chair in the physics of anaesthesia in Cardiff in 1973, after receiving a DSc (Durham) earlier in that year.

Mapleson was a founder member of the British Anaesthetic Research Society in 1958, and in 1999 the Society created the W.W. Mapleson Medal (Figure 2) to be awarded to the presenter of the best paper of each year. He believes this is a reward for his good attendance as he has missed only five of the 127 meetings in 42 years. He was awarded the Pask Certificate of the Association of Anaesthetists of Great Britain and Ireland in 1977 and was elected to Honorary Membership in 1991. He was awarded the Clover Medal of the Faculty of Anaesthetists of the Royal College of Surgeons in 1978 and the Faculty Medal in 1981. He received the Dudley Buxton Medal of the College of Anaesthetists in 1992 and was elected to Honorary Fellowship of the Royal College of Anaesthetists in 1996. He was the Hickman Medallist of the Royal Society of Medicine in 1999.

Although Mapleson officially retired in 1991, he still spends two mornings a week in the department teaching and advising on research. His continued academic work at home makes a total of about thirty hours work per week.

Further reading

Appadurai IR, Horton JN (Eds). *Essays on the first fifty years.* Cardiff, UK: Department of Anaesthetics and Intensive Care Medicine, University of Wales College of Medicine, Cardiff 1997.

Mapleson WW. Circulation-time models of the uptake of inhaled anaesthetics and data for quantifying them. *British Journal of Anaesthesia* 1973; **45**: 319–34.

Mapleson WW. The elimination of rebreathing in various semi-closed anaesthetic systems. *British Journal of Anaesthesia* 1954; **26**: 323–32.

MELZACK AND WALL'S GATE CONTROL THEORY OF PAIN

The gate control theory of pain (Figure 1) stated that pain signals are not carried passively in a direct pathway, but are modulated by other sensory inputs and by psychological factors during their transmission to the brain. Pain signals in both large and small fibres act on target cells and also on some cells in the substantia gelatinosa. Some of the substantia gelatinosa cells have an inhibiting effect on target cells and act as a gate or modulator to onward impulse transmission. The large fibres stimulate the substantia gelatinosa cells and close the gate. Small fibre activity and descending activity from the brain also modulate the gate. The theory provided a plausible physiological mechanism to explain the phenomena of pain. It showed how physiological processes, mental states and social beliefs interacted in the determination of pain experience. The gate control theory is now widely accepted and has given rise to important research on every dimension of pain.

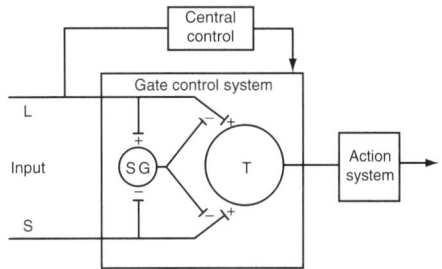

Figure. Gate control theory diagram. L, large-diameter fibres; S, small diameter fibres; SG, substantia gelatinosa; T, first central transmission cells. (Reproduced from *Pain mechanisms: a new theory 1965*; 150: 971–9. Copyright 1965, American Association for the Advancement of Science.)

Ronald Melzack (1929–)

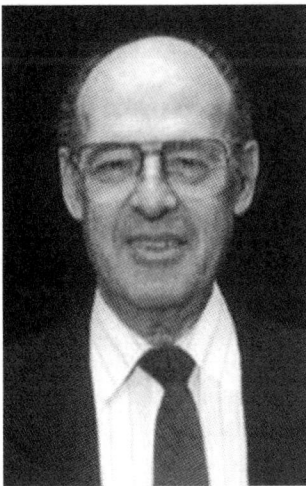

Ronald Melzack was born in Montreal, Quebec in 1929. He graduated in psychology from McGill University, Montreal in 1950, and received his PhD in physiological psychology under D.O. Hebb in 1954. He spent five years carrying out physiological research at the University of Oregon Medical School in Eugene; University College in London, England; and the University of Pisa, Italy. In 1959, he was appointed to the academic staff at the Massachusetts Institute of Technology in Boston where he and Patrick Wall developed the gate control theory of pain.

Melzack returned to McGill University in 1963 where he continued his research on pain. He developed the McGill Pain Questionnaire to measure the multiple dimensions of subjective pain experience with Warren Ferguson. It helps patients and physicians to communicate clearly about pain and provides numerical information for all types of pain research for assessing the relative effectiveness of different forms of therapy. The questionnaire has been translated into numerous languages.

Phantom limb pain fascinated Melzack because it provides a strong argument that central neural mechanisms, rather than peripheral fibres, generate the nerve impulse patterns that produce pain. He developed a new model of brain function in which the concept of a widespread 'neuromatrix' plays a major role in explaining phantom limb pain. The model extends the scope of pain research and theory by incorporating stress-regulation mechanisms as an integral part of the pain process. Prolonged stressors, psychological as well as physical, may produce a variety of disorders and thereby produce the basis for prolonged, chronic pain.

He wrote *The Puzzle of Pain*, which has been translated into seven languages, and he and Wall wrote *The Challenge of Pain* and edited four editions of the *Textbook of Pain*. In 1983, he edited *Pain Measurement and Assessment*, which established his major role in the field of pain measurement. In 1993, he and Dennis Turk edited the *Handbook of Pain Assessment*, which is now the premier book in the field.

Melzack was elected a Fellow of the Royal Society of Canada in 1982 and received the Molson Prize from the Canadian council in 1985. He was elected president of the International Association for the Study of Pain during 1984–87 and honorary president of the Canadian Psychological Association during 1988–89. He was appointed to the E.P. Taylor Chair of Psychology at McGill University in 1986; received an honorary DLitt from the University of Waterloo, Ontario in 1992; and the Prix du Québec (Prix Marie-Victorin) for pure and applied sciences in 1994. The Canadian Anesthesiologists' Society established the Dr Ronald Melzack Pain Research Award in 1997 for two-year postdoctoral fellowships in basic clinical pain research. Melzack was appointed an Officer of the Order of Canada in 1995 and l'Ordre National du Québec in 2000.

Patrick David Wall (1925–2001)

Patrick Wall was born in Nottingham, UK in 1925 and graduated in medicine from Oxford University in 1948. He then went to the USA to start research into mechanisms of pain. He worked briefly at Yale University in New Haven, Connecticut; the University of Chicago, Illinois; and Harvard University in Boston, Massachusetts before settling at the Massachusetts Institute of Technology in Boston, where he met Melzack. Wall claimed that few people read their paper on the gate control theory in *Brain* in 1962, so Melzack and Wall refined their theory and rewrote it for *Science* in 1965. He collaborated with Bill Sweet, an American neurosurgeon, to produce the transcutaneous electrical nerve stimulation (TENS) devices that provided effective treatment for pain and showed that the gate control theory had practical significance.

Wall returned to England in 1967 as professor of anatomy and director of the cerebral functions group at University College, London. He tested his theories on himself, demonstrating pain responses on television by plunging his forearm into iced water that made him grimace, shudder and hyperventilate. He spent some time at the Hebrew University of Jerusalem, Israel after the 1973 Yom Kippur War, where his work with amputees led to further research into phantom limb pain. He founded the journal *Pain* in 1975 and was active in the formation of the International Association for the Study of Pain and the Brain Research Association, forerunner of the British Neuroscience Association. He wrote *Pain: the Science of Suffering* for general readers, and a successful thriller called *Trio: the Revolting Intellectuals Organizations.*

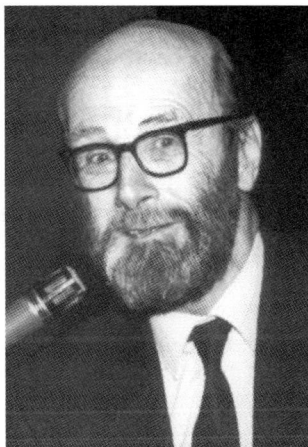

His outspoken anti-authoritarianism sometimes evoked hostile responses and strained relations. Nevertheless, he attracted crowds in the bar at meetings where he could discuss music, culture and politics and he was a great raconteur. He officially retired in 1992, but continued to work and enjoy life until he died in 2001.

He was elected a Fellow of the Royal Society in 1989, having previously been nominated several times for a Nobel Prize. He gave the John Snow lecture at the Association of Anaesthetists Annual Meeting in 1992, and was elected to Honorary Membership in 1998. He was twice awarded Honorary Membership of the Pain Society and was awarded the Queen's Medal of the Royal Society in 2000.

Acknowledgement

The portrait photographs have been reproduced with kind permission from the Wood Library–Museum of Anesthesiology, Park Ridge, IL, USA.

Further reading

MELZACK:

Melzack R. Labat lecture. Phantom limbs. *Regional Anesthesia.* 1989; **14**: 208–11.

Melzack R. The McGill Pain Questionnaire: major properties and scoring methods. *Pain* 1975; **1**: 277–99.

Melzack R, Wall PD. Pain mechanisms: a new theory. *Science* 1965; **150**: 971–9.

Melzack, R, Wall PD. *The challenge of pain 2nd edn.* New York, NY: Penguin, 1996.

WALL:

Charlton E. [Obituary]. Patrick David Wall FRS, DM, FRCP. Honorary member AAGBI, 1925–2001. *Anaesthesia* 2001; **56**: 1202.

Richmond C. [Obituary]. Patrick David Wall. *British Medical Journal* 2001; **329**: 636.

Wall PD, Melzack R. *Textbook of pain, 4th edn.* Edinburgh, UK: Churchill Livingstone, 1999.

Wall PD, Sweet WH. Temporary abolition of pain in man. *Science* 1967; **155**: 108–9.

MENDELSON'S SYNDROME

Curtis Lester Mendelson (1913-)

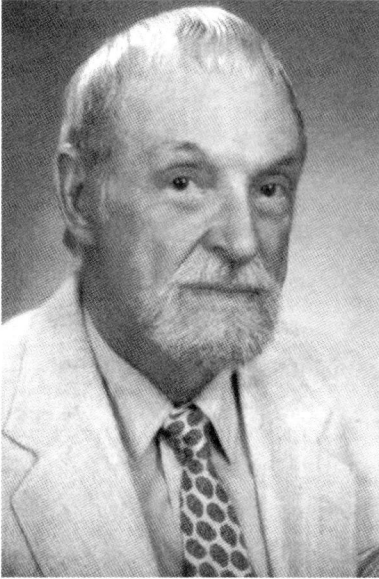

Curtis Mendelson was born in 1913 in New York City, where he attended George Washington High School. He graduated BA from the University of Michigan in 1934 and MD from Cornell University in Ithaca, New York in 1938. After his internship, he completed his residency in obstetrics and gynaecology at the New York Lying-In Hospital. He was on its attending staff during 1945–59, and was a professor at Cornell University from 1950 to 1959.

Although Mendelson was an obstetrician, his name is well known to anaesthetists. The acid aspiration syndrome that he described in 1946 was quite different from the asphyxia, atelectasis, pneumonia or lung abscess that followed aspiration of solid material. Mendelson's interest in acid aspiration began with a case that presented as an acute asthmatic attack and culminated in pulmonary oedema. The clue to its aetiology came some time later when he himself inhaled a small amount of gastric juice.

Mendelson retrospectively analysed 66 cases of aspiration of gastric contents during obstetric anaesthesia in New York Lying-In Hospital from 1932 to 1945. In all cases the anaesthetic was a mixture of nitrous oxide, oxygen and ether; tracheal intubation was not mentioned. There was no suspicion of aspiration in the delivery room in 21 cases; these patients received various lung diagnoses and none died. Of the 45 patients who were seen to aspirate, the aspirated material was solid in five patients, three of whom developed massive atelectasis (Figure 1) and two of them died.

The 40 patients who aspirated liquid had a reaction that Mendelson likened to an acute asthmatic attack and none died. The actual moment of aspiration often escaped notice. Cyanosis, dyspnoea and tachycardia developed but not massive atelectasis or mediastinal

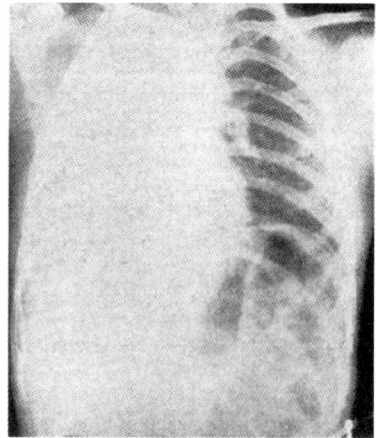

Figure 1. Massive collapse of right lung and mediastinal shift from obstruction by undigested food. (Reproduced from *American Journal of Obstetrics and Gynecology* 1946; 52: 191–205.)

shift. Auscultation revealed numerous wheezes, râles and rhonchi. Patients were critically ill during the acute episode but stabilised in 24–36 hours. Recovery was usually complete with an afebrile and uncomplicated course. Early chest x-rays (Figure 2) showed no mediastinal shift but irregular, soft, mottled densities that cleared in 7–10 days.

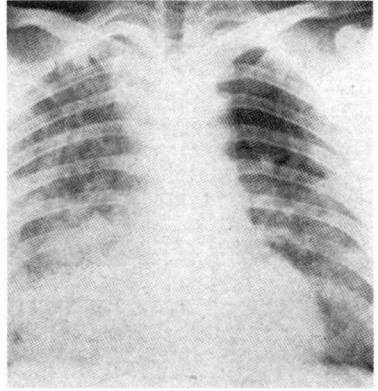

Figure 2. Scattered soft, mottled confluent densities after aspiration of liquid gastric contents. (Reproduced from *American Journal of Obstetrics and Gynecology* 1946; 52: 191–205.)

Mendelson suspected that gastric acid was the cause of this syndrome and experimented by instilling various materials into the lungs of anaesthetized rabbits. He tested 20 mL of distilled water, normal saline, one-tenth normal hydrochloric acid, plain or neutralized liquid vomitus, and plain or neutralised vomitus containing undigested food obtained from parturient patients. Solid undigested food invariably produced the same picture of obstruction as is seen in humans. Complete obstruction caused suffocation and incomplete obstruction produced massive atelectasis. Hydrochloric acid or unneutralized liquid vomitus caused immediate cyanosis and laboured respiration, and chest x-rays showed irregular soft mottled shadows. Death occurred in anything from minutes to hours, and the trachea was filled with pink frothy sputum. Distilled water, normal saline or neutralized liquid vomitus caused a brief period of cyanosis and laboured respiration; full recovery occurred within a few hours with no significant chest x-ray changes.

Mendelson presented this paper at the New York Obstetrical Society in December 1945. Paluel Flagg was an invited discussant. He expressed surprise at the absence of an anaesthetist on the programme, because aspiration of gastric contents is largely an anaesthetic problem. Mendelson explained that obstetrical general anaesthesia, except for Caesarean section, was treated as 'a step-child lacking authoritative guidance'. There were no dedicated obstetrical anaesthesia services or anaesthetists. Busy general surgical schedules took preference and it was not unusual for the least qualified anaesthetist to be dispatched to the delivery room.

Mendelson was director of the Antepartum Cardiac Clinic at New York Lying-In Hospital for 15 years when rheumatic fever was still quite common in children. He saw girls with valvular heart disease as they reached adulthood and became pregnant. He got deeper into cardiology and helped to pioneer open-heart surgery during pregnancy. He presented a successful case of antepartum mitral valvotomy to the International Heart Association in 1954 and wrote several papers on cardiac conditions during pregnancy. His book *Cardiac Disease in Pregnancy* was published in 1960.

Mendelson foresaw the dominance of health maintenance organizations and insurance companies over the medical profession. Despite a very busy private practice, a full teaching schedule, writing and research projects, he

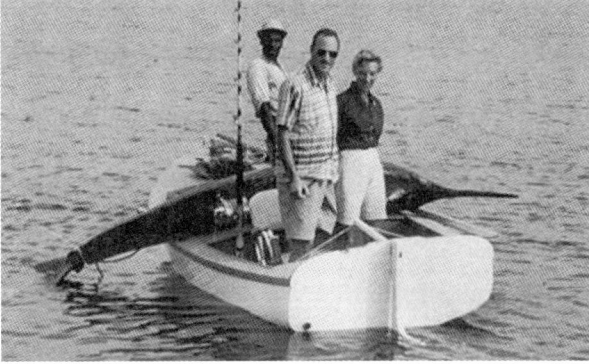

Figure 3. Mendelson with his 12-feet-long, 498-pound blue marlin at Green Turtle Bay, Bahamas, 1958.

decided – to the disbelief of his colleagues in New York City – to give it all up. Mendelson had a pilot's licence with single and multi-engine land and sea ratings. In 1959, when he was 46 years old, he and his wife rented a small one-engine plane and flew towards the West Indies. They landed on the Abaco Islands in the Bahamas to get new supplies and felt that they had found paradise. He officially obtained a one-year leave of absence from his hospital to work as a gynaecologist at Green Turtle Bay Clinic in Abaco. He actually became an 'Out-Island' doctor as director of the local clinic, where he carried on a general practice. He also performed veterinary medicine and minor dentistry. In 1961 New York Lying-In Hospital accepted his resignation with regret.

He and his wife continued to write at Green Turtle Bay. His wife, a dietician, wrote *Nutrition and Health*, which has run to nine editions. In addition to the work and plane trips between the islands, he pursued his hobbies of fishing and swimming. In 1958, Mendelson made worldwide fishing history by catching a 12-foot, 498-pound, blue marlin in a 10-foot skiff (Figure 3). He was later Bahamian representative on the International Game Fishing Association and captain of the Bahamian Team in the International Tuna Tournaments, and was featured in a centrefold-type action photograph in the *National Geographic* in February 1967. He was a member of the English Channel Swimming Association and made his first attempt aged 55, but had to give up after five hours owing to rough seas. The following year he started from France and could see the white cliffs of Dover when hypothermia forced him to give up after 12 hours. Curtis Mendelson served the inhabitants on his paradise island until 1990 when, at the age of 77, he moved to West Palm Beach in Florida where he still lives today.

Further reading

Carlsson M, Lindskog G, Hammarskjöld F. The man behind the syndrome: Curtis Mendelson, he left his career for a life as a village physician on the Bahamas. *Läkartidningen.* 1998; **95**: 400–1.

Mendelson CL. *Cardiac disease in pregnancy: medical care, cardiovascular surgery and obstetric management as related to maternal and fetal welfare.* Philadelphia, PA: F.A. Davis, 1960.

Mendelson CL. The aspiration of stomach contents into the lungs during obstetric anesthesia. *American Journal of Obstetrics and Gynecology* 1946; **52**: 191–205.

MILLER LARYNGOSCOPE BLADE

Robert Arden Miller (1906–1976)

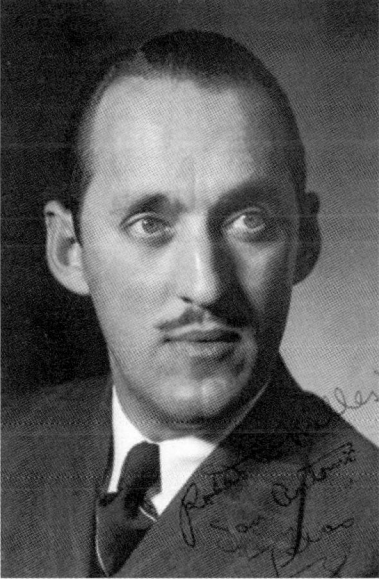

Robert Miller was born in Williamsport, Pennsylvania in 1906. He graduated from the University of Pittsburgh, Pennsylvania in 1925 and obtained his MD degree from the Eclectic Medical College in Cincinnati, Ohio in 1929. After interning in the Grace Hospital in Detroit, Michigan he went into general practice until 1936, when he settled in San Antonio, Texas and devoted all his time to anaesthesia. He joined the American Society of Anesthetists and International College of Anesthetists in 1936 and was a member of the American Board of Anesthesia in 1941. He served as a Captain in the US Army from 1940 to 1942.

Doctors in the 19th century tried to see the larynx using natural light. In 1829, Babington of Guy's Hospital, London used a spatula with a mirror attached that his colleagues, Bright and Hodgkins, named the 'speculum laryngis' or laryngoscope. Alfred Kirsten in Germany designed the first direct laryngoscope in 1895. Chevalier Jackson (1865–1958) performed his first bronchoscopy in 1899 and published a book on tracheobronchoscopy, oesophagoscopy and gastroscopy in 1907, which also popularized direct laryngoscopy. He designed a laryngoscope in 1913 that anaesthetists used for many years, although the electric cords that ran from a large dry battery were inconvenient and even dangerous. One fatality resulted from the explosion of anaesthetic vapour. Ivan Magill in London designed a rigid U-shaped laryngoscope with self-contained batteries in the handle in the mid-1920s that became popular in Britain. The handle was L-shaped with a vertical stem onto which the blade fitted to lie parallel to the handle. Paluel Flagg designed a rigid L-shaped laryngoscope in 1928 and this was modified by Goldman in Britain and Guedel, Waters and Lundy in America. The more convenient folding laryngoscopes were introduced in the 1940s.

By 1941, when Miller described his adult laryngoscope blade, most specialist anaesthetists were familiar with the advantages of endotracheal intubation. It was being used more frequently, especially with the widespread use of closed-circuit cyclopropane anaesthesia. Miller's contribution was to make several changes in the design of the laryngoscope to make laryngoscopy and intubation easier and more certain. This was the year before the

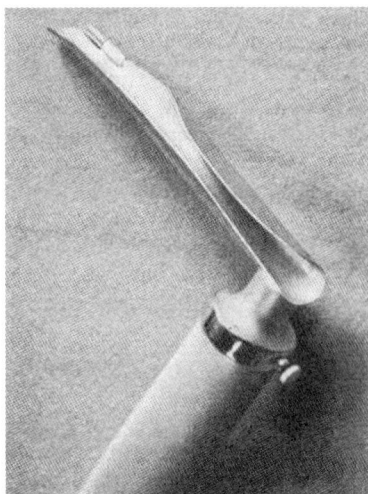

Figure 1. Miller's long, narrow laryngoscope blade, 1941. (Reproduced from *Anesthesiology* 1941; 2: 317–20, with permission from Lippincott Williams & Wilkins.)

introduction of curare and more than a decade before suxamethonium (succinylcholine).

Miller emphasized that 'proper depth of anaesthesia with adequate relaxation' was necessary to facilitate intubation. He described patients who were typically difficult – those with a deep throat, thick tongue or prominent upper incisors - in whom damage to the teeth might occur from undue pressure. He considered an 'unnamed anaesthetist's laryngoscope' was too thick at the base and this increased the danger of trauma to the teeth. The tip was frequently incorrectly shaped to lift the epiglottis, and the blade was often too short. The curve of the blade was too near the tip, while its flat bottom tended to push the tongue into the floor of the mouth. These factors did not facilitate adequate exposure of the larynx in difficult patients.

Miller designed his new model by making it longer than the old-style medium-sized blade (Figure 1). It was rounded on the bottom, smaller at the tip and had an extra curve beginning about two inches from the end (Figure 2). The internal diameter of the base was shallow, but permitted the passage of a size 38 French catheter. Therefore, the mouth did not need to be opened as widely as with the older type of blade, which allowed more anterior movement of the mandible. The small round end of the blade when pressed against the tongue made a channel through which the larynx was exposed. He found the length of the blade to be satisfactory for all patients except infants, so only one blade was required for ordinary use. He recommended using a moulded quarter-inch lead plate to protect the teeth from any accidental pressure and extending the stress to the maxillae.

Miller recommended the usual technique of intubation with his new laryngoscope. The anaesthetist might notice that the mouth did not open as widely as with other blades and that consequently there was not as large an area for manipulation. He suggested the use of

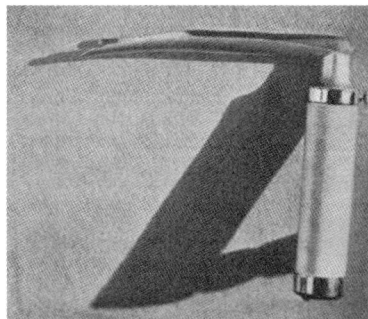

Figure 2. Round bottom of blade, curve two inches from small, narrow tip. (Reproduced from. *Anesthesiology* 1941; 2: 317–20, with permission from Lippincott Williams & Wilkins.)

a stylet rather than forceps when inserting a large, cuffed tube through the mouth. When a smaller tube could be used, he considered the nasal route to be easier. When the nasal tube was well lubricated and passed through the nose into the pharynx, the cords could easily be seen through the laryngoscope and the tube could usually be inserted by rotating it, with or without the aid of forceps. He compared the features of other laryngoscope blades with those of his design.

Other blades	Miller blade
High base	Shallow base
Flat bottom	Round bottom
Wide end	Narrow end
Curve at tip	Curve two inches back
Large and medium sizes	One size (used in all patients except infants)

In 1946, Miller developed a lighter, thinner, folding paediatric laryngoscope with a similarly curved infant blade (Figure 3), particularly for use in neonatal resuscitation. He knew that some anaesthetists and obstetricians could intubate infants blindly by palpating the epiglottis with the finger and passing the tube into the trachea through the mouth. This method was often time-consuming and if it failed the vocal cords had to be exposed. He advocated intubating under direct vision from the start, using a size 12 French tube with a wire stylet. He designed the infant laryngoscope blade to allow the tube to pass outside the blade rather than inside the channel of the straight-bladed varieties.

Miller was in private anaesthesia practice in San Antonio, Texas from 1936. He was a golfer and pilot and was the chairman of public relations for the Texas State Medical Society from 1940 to 1945. According to his American Society of Anesthesiologists biographical file, he made 52 speeches for the Texas Society on socialized medicine – whether for or against is not stated.

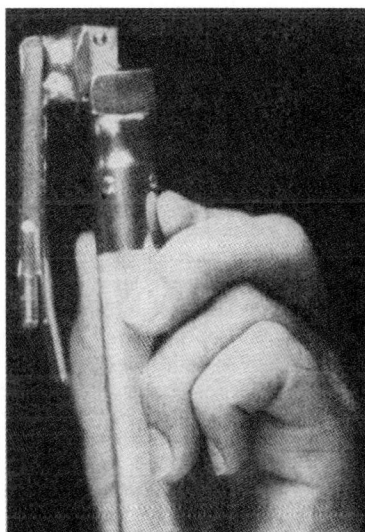

Figure 3. Miller infant laryngoscope. (Reproduced from *Anesthesiology* 1946; 7: 205–6, with permission from Lippincott Williams & Wilkins.)

Acknowledgement

Portrait photograph reproduced with kind permission from the Wood Library–Museum of Anesthesiology, Park Ridge, IL, USA.

Further reading

Gillespie NA. *Endotracheal anesthesia, 2nd edn.* Madison, WI: University of Wisconsin Press, 1948.

Miller RA. A new laryngoscope. *Anesthesiology* 1941; 2: 317–20.

Miller RA. A new laryngoscope for intubation of infants. *Anesthesiology* 1946; 7: 205–6.

MINNITT GAS AND AIR APPARATUS

Robert James Minnitt (1889–1974)

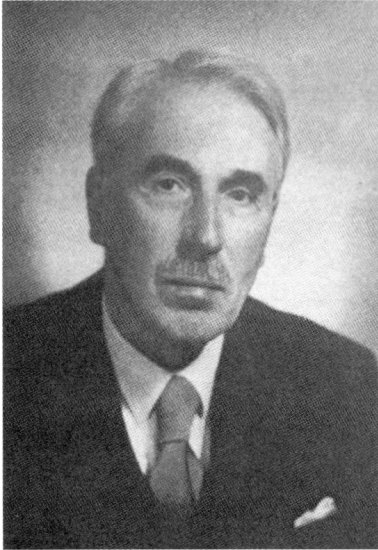

Robert Minnitt was born in 1889 in Preston, Lancashire. His grandfather and father were vicars and he initially felt called to serve in the Church, but after one year at Trinity College, Cambridge he decided that he could serve more usefully in medicine. He graduated from Liverpool Medical School in 1915 and his research into the use of insulin and glucose in shock led to his MD degree in 1925. Like most anaesthetists of that era, he was a general practitioner as well as being an honorary anaesthetist to the David Lewis Northern Hospital, Liverpool Royal Infirmary and the Liverpool Maternity Hospital.

Minnitt dedicated himself to the relief of pain during labour, so that giving birth was 'but a sleep and a forgetting'. James Simpson had introduced ether and chloroform anaesthesia in 1847 for pain relief in childbirth and 'twilight sleep', which was a combination of morphine and scopolamine, had been available since 1902. However, only doctors could administer these drugs and the majority of women depended on midwives who were not authorized to use them.

The National Birthday Trust Fund (Trust) was inaugurated in 1928 and the British College of Obstetricians and Gynaecologists (BCOG) in 1929. The Prime Minster's wife, Lucy Baldwin, joined the Trust with a particular interest in pain relief in labour. The Trust raised money so that some London hospitals could support a resident anaesthetist, but analgesia in hospitals did not help women delivering at home with a midwife. The Ministry of Health showed little interest and most doctors were not interested because there was no financial advantage in providing pain relief.

Minnitt wanted a method of pain relief that could safely be used by midwives either in hospital or in the home. He attended a discussion at the Royal Society of Medicine in 1933 on the use of nitrous oxide and oxygen for obstetric pain relief, but nitrous oxide and air seemed more practical. Within two months, he and Charles King produced an adaptation of an 'on demand' McKesson oxygen therapy apparatus that delivered 45% nitrous oxide in air (Figures 1 and 2). It had an automatic valve that shut off the flow of nitrous oxide when the patient did not inhale. The gas was self administered; the patient held the mask and, if she started to lose consciousness, the mask fell from her face and the gas ceased to flow.

The first 'gas and air' analgesia was administered at Liverpool Maternity Hospital on 16 October 1933. A four-month study at that hospital and at Wellhouse Hospital in Barnet, Hertfordshire confirmed its effectiveness. The only abnormality that Minnitt found in a later study was a reduction in maternal blood oxygen content; umbilical vein blood did not show any 'marked variation' and the second stage of labour was within normal limits. Minnitt wrote that this 'was not a terminus, but a thoroughfare to greater possibilities for painless labour'. He was hailed in the press as the man who killed the agony of childbirth.

A serious difficulty arose within nine months. Many midwives had been using gas and air under 'medical direction', but without a doctor present. Objections were raised and the Central Midwives Board insisted upon 'personal medical supervision', so progress stopped. In July 1934, the matter was taken up by (now Lady) Baldwin and Lord Knutsford of the Trust.

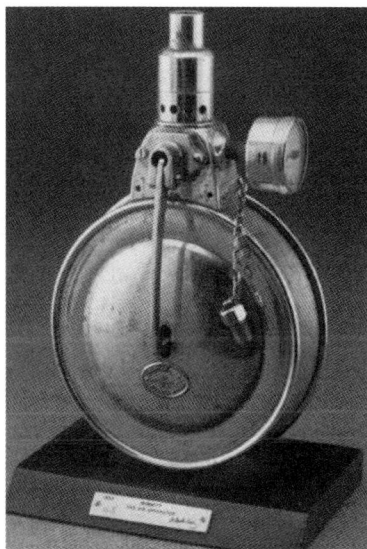

Figure 1. Minnit gas and air apparatus, 1933, which was mounted on a nitrous oxide cylinder. The patient breathed a mixture of nitrous oxide from a small rubber bag in the metal drum, and air was entrained from several small holes on the apex of the machine. The outlet was divided into two channels, one for air and one for nitrous oxide. (Reproduced with kind permission from the Association of Anaesthetists of Great Britain and Ireland.)

The BCOG was about to investigate the use of analgesics in labour in 36 hospitals throughout Britain and Ireland at the request of the Trust. Its report in January 1936 led to Central Midwives Board regulations that governed the training required for an unsupervised midwife to administer analgesic drugs and gas and air with a recognized apparatus (Figure 3). Minnitt's course of four lectures covered the history of drugs, description and demonstration of apparatus, the theory and practice of administration of gas and air analgesia, and the rules and regulations for its use by midwives. He and a member of the Medical Board examined each candidate in the presence of the nursing instructor and the hospital granted a certificate. He lectured all over

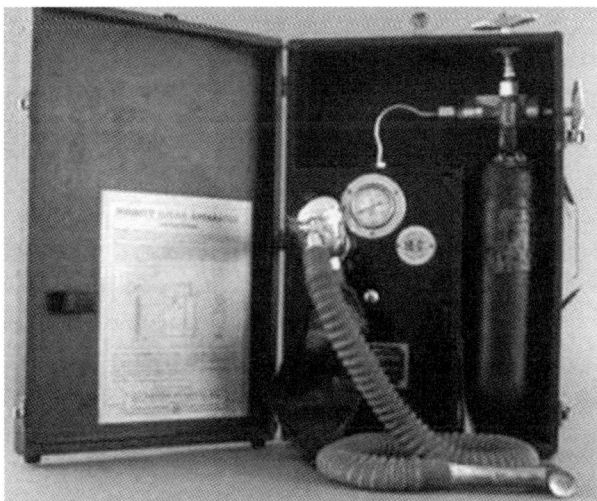

Figure 2. Standard Minnitt gas and air apparatus, 1939. (Reproduced with kind permission from the Association of Anaesthetists of Great Britain and Ireland.)

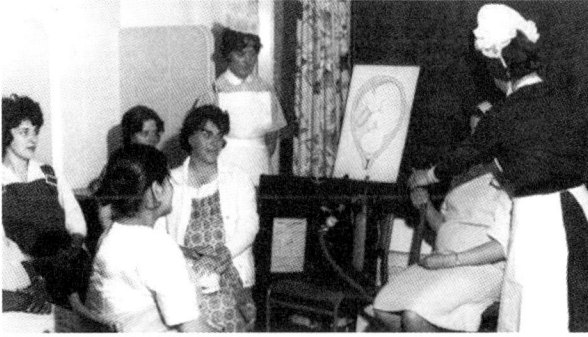

Figure 3. Midwives class at St Thomas's Hospital, London. (Reproduced from St Thomas's Hospital, London.)

the country, prepared filmstrips on the administration of gas and air and published a monograph on *Gas and Air Analgesia* in 1938. He strongly advocated antenatal tuition for patients so that they were familiar with the apparatus when they went into labour.

Trichloroethylene and air inhalers in the 1950s and Entonox (premixed 50:50 nitrous oxide and oxygen) in 1963 gradually superseded Minnitt's gas and air machines. Authorization for the use of gas and air was withdrawn in 1970. The modern era of obstetric management was dawning, with almost all births taking place in hospital and specialist obstetrical anaesthetists providing 24-hour epidural services for pain relief.

Minnitt was an influential teacher of safe and scientifically based anaesthesia. He became the first lecturer in anaesthesia at the University of Liverpool in 1933, the first anaesthetist to be a member of the faculty of medicine, and his efforts contributed to the establishment of the University Department of Anaesthesia. Minnitt, with John Gillies (1895–1976) of Edinburgh, published a widely used *Textbook of Anaesthetics* in 1944.

Minnitt was president of the Section of Anaesthetics of the Royal Society of Medicine in 1943 and was its Hickman Medallist in 1950. He was the first anaesthetist to be elected to Honorary Fellowship of the Royal College of Obstetricians and Gynaecologists. He was elected to Honorary Fellowship of the Royal Society of Medicine and the Faculty of Anaesthetists of the Royal College of Surgeons. He was elected to Honorary Membership of the Association of Anaesthetists Great Britain and Ireland in 1961 and received MSc (Hon) from Liverpool University in 1967.

Minnitt's concept of traditional principles of practice caused him to resign his hospital appointments at the inauguration of the National Health Service in 1948, but he maintained a small private general practice.

Acknowledgement

Portrait photograph reproduced with kind permission from the Association of Anaesthetists of Great Britain and Ireland.

Further reading

Minnitt RJ. Self-administered analgesia for the midwifery of general practice. *Proceedings of the Royal Society of Medicine* 1934; **27**: 1313–18.

O'Sullivan EP. Dr Robert James Minnitt 1889–1974: a pioneer of inhalational analgesia. *Proceedings of the Royal Society of Medicine* 1989; **82**: 221–2.

Williams AS. *Women & Childbirth in the Twentieth Century*. Stroud, UK: Sutton Publishing, 1997: 124–46.

THE ETHER DOME

William Thomas Green Morton (1819–1868)

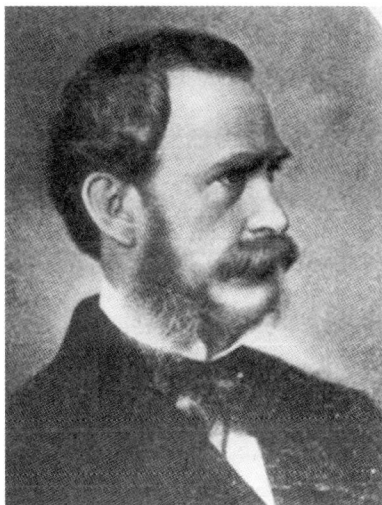

William Morton was born in 1819 in Charlton, Worcester County, Massachusetts. His family moved to North Charlton in 1827 for Morton to receive better schooling. Aged 13, he was boarding with a local doctor when he announced his intention of studying medicine. He lacked funds, but a small legacy on his twenty-first birthday in 1840 enabled him to study dentistry in Baltimore, Maryland.

His funds ran out and in May 1841 he returned north and continued his studies under Horace Wells (1815–48) in Hartford, Connecticut. He practised briefly at nearby Farmington while continuing to receive instruction from Wells. In 1843, Morton opened a practice in Boston, Massachusetts. Wells joined him, but the enterprise was not profitable and Wells returned to Hartford.

In Hartford on 10 December 1844, Gardner Colton (1814–98), a travelling popular science lecturer gave a public demonstration of the effects of nitrous oxide inhalation. Wells observed a man bang his shin while under its influence without any recollection of pain. Wells realized that nitrous oxide might allow painless tooth extraction. The next day, Colton administered nitrous oxide to Wells while another dentist, John Riggs (1810–85) painlessly extracted one of Wells's wisdom teeth. Wells and Riggs subsequently administered the gas for 16 dental extractions.

Meanwhile, in March 1844, Morton became a medical student in Boston under Charles Jackson (1805–80) – a well-recognized doctor, chemist and geologist. Morton lived in Jackson's home with access to his extensive library. In July, after talks with Jackson, he started experimenting with ether, but in late summer a 'breakdown' caused him to live with his in-laws in Farmington.

In November, Morton returned to Boston and enrolled at Harvard Medical School. In January 1845, Wells visited Morton who obtained permission from John Collins Warren (1778–1886), senior surgeon at Massachusetts General Hospital, for Wells to demonstrate a tooth extraction in front of his class. Although the patient claimed that he felt no pain, he cried out during the extraction and the demonstration was a fiasco. Within months, Wells abandoned his dental practice and later became a chloroform addict. In 1848, he was jailed in New York for spattering a prostitute with sulphuric acid and he committed suicide a few days later.

NEW AND VALUABLE DISOVERY. We noticed yesterday the discovery of a new preparation by Dr Morton which is intended to alleviate the sufferings of those who are forced to undergo painful operations in surgery and dentistry, as well as to facilitate the work of operators. The effect of this new discovery is to throw the patient into a state of insensibility and while unconscious any operation can be performed without occasioning pain. We are told by a gentleman of the highest respectability that he witnessed an experiment of the use of this most extraordinary discovery at the rooms of Dr Morton one evening this week. An ulcerated tooth was extracted from the mouth of an individual without giving him the slightest pain. He was put into a kind of sleep, by inhaling a portion of this preparation, the effects of which lasted for about three quarters of a minute, just long enough to extract the tooth. This discovery is destined to make a great revolution in the arts of surgery and surgical dentistry.

Figure 1. First news item of ether anaesthesia in the Boston *Daily Evening Transcript*, 2 October 1846.

Morton's practice was flourishing by the summer of 1845 and he had established a factory to manufacture false teeth. In order for the dentures to fit properly, he first had to extract all the old roots. He tried intoxicants, opium and mesmerism to make it less painful, but none was effective.

His search continued into 1846 and his medical studies were eventually crowded out. He revived the ether experiments that included anaesthetising a goldfish, his pet spaniel, two dental assistants and himself. All recovered without ill effect, but the results were inconclusive. Even though Morton thought he had been etherized deeply enough to have a painless tooth extraction, he was discouraged. In September, he conferred with Jackson and obtained information about highly rectified sulphuric ether.

On the afternoon of 30 September 1846, Eben Frost came to Morton with a painful wisdom tooth. Frost agreed to breathe ether from an ether-saturated handkerchief and within five minutes the tooth was painlessly extracted. News of the event appeared in Boston newspapers over the next two days (Figure 1). Other successful extractions followed in the next two weeks. Morton's use of ether in his dental practice attracted the attention of the young Boston surgeon Henry Jacob Bigelow (1818–90). He called on Morton, and passed on details to Warren, who arranged for Morton to demonstrate his new discovery.

Morton gave the first public demonstration in the 'ether dome' of the 1821 Bulfinch Building (Figure 2) of Massachusetts General Hospital on 16 October 1846. He was late arriving, owing to last-minute modifications to his glass inhaler (Figure 3). Warren removed a vascular tumour from the left side of the neck of a young printer and journalist named Gilbert Abbott (1825–55), with surgeons, other prominent doctors and medical students in the audience. The operation took five minutes and the patient showed no evidence of pain, although he moved slightly toward the end of the operation. Warren remarked to his audience; 'Gentlemen, this is no humbug'.

George Hayward carried out another painless operation under Morton's anaesthesia the following day. Ethical arguments then arose as to whether Morton should be allowed to continue providing anaesthesia in the hospital because he was not medically qualified. Also, he refused to divulge the composition of the anaesthetic agent. The difficulties were

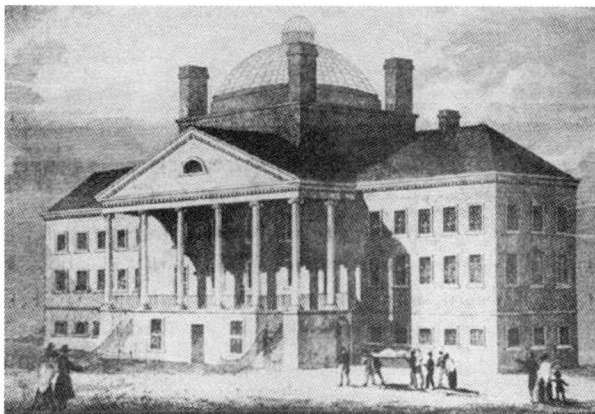

Figure 2. Bulfinch Building, opened in 1821, surmounted by the ether dome.

finally overcome when Morton was not allowed to give a third anaesthetic until he admitted that the characteristic odour was that of ether. Bigelow announced the discovery in the 18 November 1846 issue of the *Boston Medical and Surgical Journal.*

News of Morton's discovery spread rapidly throughout the world. It was used on 19 December in London, England and Dumfries, Scotland, and on 21 December for an amputation by Robert Liston at University College Hospital, London. Mesmerism had never been reliable and when Liston finished he remarked; 'This Yankee dodge beats mesmerism hollow'. Ether was used throughout Europe and as far away as South Africa and Australia by the summer of 1847.

Morton's reputation was marred by his attempt to patent his mysterious 'letheon'. He spent much of the remainder of his life fighting legal battles to obtain recognition and financial reward. In 1847, the French Academy of Medicine awarded the Monthyon prize of 5000 Francs jointly to Jackson and Morton, but Morton refused to take his share, saying that the discovery was entirely his. Jackson claimed that his telling Morton about highly rectified ether before Morton used it proved his claim to priority. Several plans to give Morton financial support brought honour to Morton but no riches and he died in poverty.

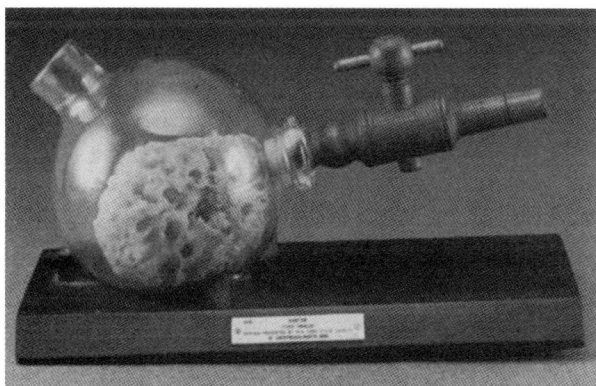

Figure 3. Replica of Morton's vaporizer. (Reproduced with kind permission from the Association of Anaesthetists of Great Britain and Ireland.)

Long, Wells and Jackson all contributed to the discovery of surgical

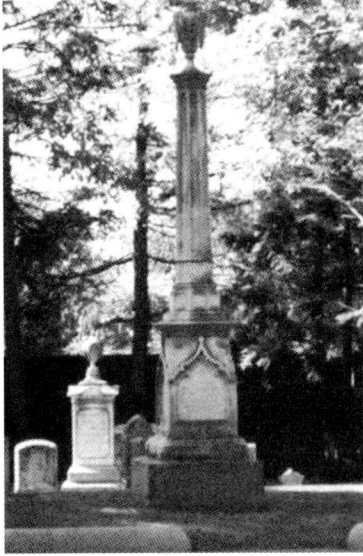

Figure 4. Morton's tombstone in Mount Auburn Cemetery, Boston.

anaesthesia. It was Morton who searched for an anaesthetic and conducted experiments with ether. He gave the first public demonstrations on patients and he convinced the surgical world of its value. Bigelow composed the inscription on Morton's tombstone (Figure 4) in Mount Auburn Cemetery, Boston:

> Before Whom, in All Time, Surgery
> was Agony;
> By Whom, Pain in Surgery was averted;
> Since Whom, Science has Control of Pain.

Acknowledgement

Portrait photograph reproduced with kind permission from the Wood Library–Museum of Anesthesiology, Park Ridge, IL, USA.

Further reading

Bigelow HJ. Insensibility during surgical operations produced by inhalation. *Boston Medical and Surgical Journal* 1846; **35**: 309–17. (Reprinted in Faulconer A, Keys TE. *Foundations of anesthesiology, vol. I.* Springfield, IL: Charles C. Thomas, 1965: 286–95.)

Ford WW. William Thomas Green Morton. *The Bulletin of the Boston Public Library* 1946; October: 287–302.

Rice NP. *Trials of a public benefactor.* New York, NY: Pudney & Russell, 1859. (Facsimile reproduction under the auspices of the Australian Society of Anaesthetists, 1995.)

MURPHY EYE

Francis John Murphy (1900–1972)

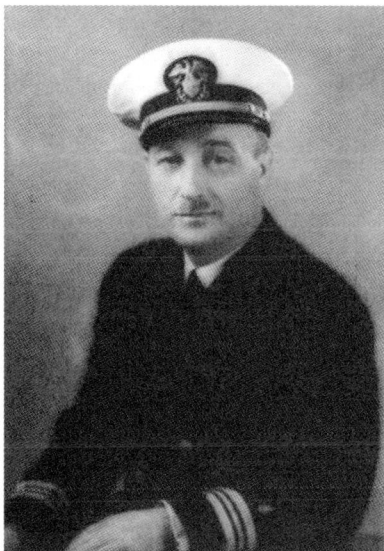

Frank Murphy was born in Oldham, South Dakota in 1900. He attended high school in High River, Alberta, Canada and graduated from the University of Alberta in Edmonton in 1923. He then went to McGill University College of Medicine in Montreal, Quebec. He graduated in medicine with a Masters in surgery in 1925 and completed two years of internship and residency at Montreal General Hospital. He was chief of anesthesia at Harper Hospital in Detroit, Michigan from 1930 to 1946 and was certified as a specialist by the American Board of Anesthesiology in 1939. During the Second World War he served in naval hospitals from 1942 to 1946 and held the rank of Lieutenant Commander in the US Navy. He moved to San Francisco in 1946 as chief anesthetist and associate clinical professor at the University of California hospitals.

Anaesthetists who administered endotracheal anaesthesia in the 1920s usually insufflated the anaesthetic agent by a plenum system through a narrow-bore catheter. Exhalation took place either freely around the catheter or through an auxiliary tube. Catheters of this size did not accommodate to-and-fro breathing and were not suitable for closed-circuit anaesthesia when cyclopropane became available in 1934. Larger diameter tubes became unsatisfactory after repeated sterilization.

In 1940, Murphy had been practising anaesthesia for about 10 years when he became dissatisfied with existing endotracheal tubes and began to design his own. He provided a vivid picture of the challenge of endotracheal anaesthesia in his day, which contrasts markedly with its routine use nowadays. He listed nine characteristics for the ideal endotracheal tube:

(i) Sufficient flexibility to accommodate itself to the pharynx and larynx.
(ii) Sufficient elasticity to prevent irritation to the parts through which it passes.
(iii) Sufficient body to resist the compression to which it would ordinarily be subjected in use.
(iv) Resistance to kinking when bent at a moderately acute angle.
(v) Ease of sterilization (preferably by heat).
(vi) Durability in spite of repeated sterilizations.
(vii) Ease of insertion.

(viii) Adequate diameter of lumen in relation to outside diameter.
(ix) Availability in a sufficient range of sizes.

Murphy knew that the tube for to-and-fro breathing had to be large enough for inhalation and exhalation without marked resistance. He believed the best size was the largest that the patient's larynx could comfortably accommodate. There would be little or no leakage and the use of inflatable cuffs would be unnecessary. Leakage around a slightly undersized catheter could be prevented by packing the throat with a gauze roll.

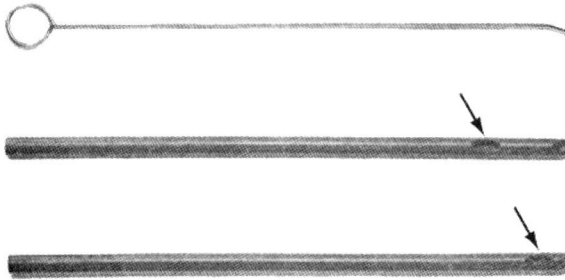

Figure 1. Two views of Murphy straight oral tube with two eyes and stylet. (Reproduced from *Anesthesia and Analgesia* 1941; 20: 102–5, with permission from Lippincott Williams & Wilkins.)

In 1940 he designed straight tubes (Figure 1) for oral intubation, using ordinary stock urethral catheters and rectal tubes. The length was 41 cm for all size catheters (from size 34 to 40 French) with smooth surfaces inside and outside. The tip was the 'whistle' type to make introduction between the vocal cords easy and minimize the danger of trauma. There were two lateral 'eyes' in addition to the opening at the distal end of the tube. The total area of the openings was much greater than the cross section of the lumen so that breathing would not be affected if one or more of the eyes became obstructed with mucus. A suitable connector joined the proximal end of the tube to the tubing from the anaesthetic machine.

The high quality stock from which he made these tubes offered considerable resistance to compression. The wall was thin so maximum internal diameter was possible. The tubes could be bent at a fairly acute angle without kinking, and they were extremely durable. He used a smooth bronze or steel stylet to hold the tube rigid during intubation under direct vision. The smooth inner surface of the tube enabled the anaesthetist to pass an ordinary small urethral type catheter for aspiration of fluid or mucus. This permitted aspiration from the distal end of the tube and avoided smearing its inner wall with mucus that would effectively decrease the diameter of its lumen.

The tube was cleaned after use with soap and water and a long wire-handled bottlebrush was used to clean the lumen. The tube and stylet were then boiled or autoclaved and were assembled with a suction catheter in a sterile canvas envelope ready for use. Murphy had used the same tube almost daily for over one year before repeated sterilizations softened the rubber enough to render it unsatisfactory for further use.

Murphy's curved nasal tubes were moulded (Figure 2) – they were not cut from straight rubber tubing that had been stored in a coil (eg the

Magill red rubber tubes). They retained their shape in spite of repeated sterilization. The tubes were 31cm long with whistle-tip ends and one lateral eye. The maximum catheter size was 36 French. The tube was inserted to its full length with the proximal end flush with the external nares, and a metal angle piece connected it to the tubing from the gas machine. Murphy believed that the whistle-tip facilitated intubation, whereas the straight bevelled tip of the Magill tube frequently caught on the vocal cord and either directed the tube to one side or caused it to kink in the pharynx.

Figure 2. Murphy curved nasal tube with one eye. (Reproduced from *Anesthesia and Analgesia* 1941; 20: 102–5, with permission from Lippincott Williams & Wilkins.)

Although the materials that Murphy used for endotracheal tubes 60 years ago have long been obsolete in most countries, the Murphy eye lives on. In 1957, Murphy moved from San Francisco to St Vincent's and the Deaconess Hospitals in Billings, Montana. He had an interest in cattle ranching and retired in 1970 to live on a ranch at Spirit Lake, Idaho.

Acknowledgement

Portrait photograph reproduced with kind permission from the Wood Library–Museum of Anesthesiology, Park Ridge, IL, USA.

Further reading

Magill IW. Technique in endotracheal anaesthesia. *British Medical Journal* 1930; 2: 817–19.

Murphy FJ. Two improved intratracheal catheters. *Anesthesia and Analgesia* 1941; 20: 102–5.

Waters RM, Rovenstine EA, Guedel AE. Endotracheal anesthesia and its historical development. *Anesthesia and Analgesia* 1933; 12: 196–203.

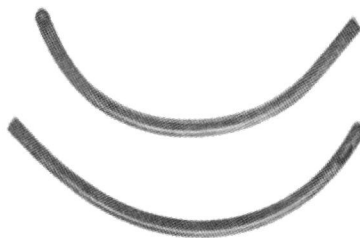

NUFFIELD DEPARTMENT OF ANAESTHETICS

Lord Nuffield (1877-1963)

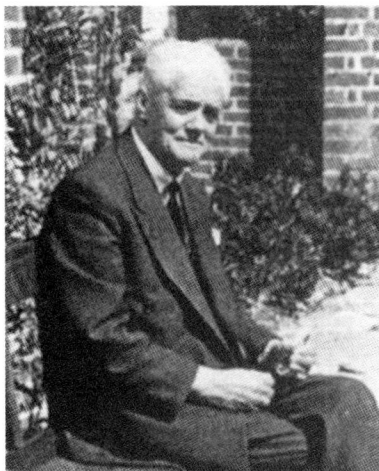

Lord Nuffield, who was born William Richard Morris in 1877, was 20 years senior to Sir Robert Macintosh. His father was a farm labourer. Nuffield's modest formal education was restricted to the village school at Cowley on the outskirts of Oxford. He left school when he was 15 to be an apprentice in a bicycle repair shop. After one year, he asked for a wage increase. When this was refused, he left to make his own bicycles, then motorcycles and finally cars. He produced the first Morris Oxford car in 1913 and became one of the first British industrialists to introduce mass production methods. He was an extremely hardworking, naturally gifted mechanical engineer and Morris Motors Ltd. prospered after the First World War. He introduced the famous MG sports car, bought out other British car manufacturers and became a multimillionaire. He made his first philanthropic benefaction in 1926 for a chair of Spanish studies at Oxford University.

When Huntercombe Golf Club (between Oxford and London) was in financial difficulties, he bought it, and he and his wife made their home in its residential quarters. Doctors from Guy's Hospital in London, including Macintosh, frequently spent weekends there. Nuffield and his wife usually joined the doctors for dinner in the Club's dining room and he became involved in their discussions on a wide variety of medical problems.

It so happened that Nuffield's teeth had been neglected when he was young. He had two terrifying nitrous oxide anaesthetics for multiple extractions and had vivid nightmares of prolonged suffocation throughout his life. Without these two experiences, he might never have thought of endowing a chair of anaesthetics at Oxford. In the early 1930s, Macintosh gave Nuffield intravenous Evipan (hexobarbitone) for a minor operation. Nuffield slept afterwards, then looked at his watch and enquired why the operation had been postponed. The contrast between this and the nightmares of prolonged suffocation were so striking that he often referred to the 'magic' of this experience.

During the British Medical Association's annual meeting in Oxford in 1936, the Regius professor of medicine at Oxford University stressed how fitting it would be for Oxford to become a postgraduate medical centre.

Afterwards, he appealed to Nuffield for one million pounds to establish clinical chairs in medicine, surgery and obstetrics. On the following Saturday evening, during dinner at Huntercombe, Nuffield mentioned this proposition. Macintosh, who was sitting next to him, remarked; 'I see they have forgotten anaesthetics again'. Nuffield apparently ignored the remark.

Within days, Nuffield not only informed the University that he was in favour of a postgraduate medical centre, but said that he would increase the endowment to two million pounds to include a chair of anaesthetics. Nuffield was surprised when the Regius professor called on him at Huntercombe to tell him that the University was deeply grateful, but felt it would be wrong to expose the University and Nuffield to ridicule by creating a chair of anaesthetics. Two weeks later, when the Regius professor telephoned to inquire when he could announce the benefaction, Nuffield said he understood that the university had declined his offer. Acceptance of the chair of anaesthetics with professorial status for the appointee was a condition for endowment of the other three chairs. It was all or none. The University accepted Nuffield's conditions rather than lose everything.

The doctors at Huntercombe only knew that Nuffield had won the battle. It was only later that Nuffield said that he had told the University that Macintosh would take the chair. Nuffield had not consulted Macintosh, who was briefly embarrassed. He and his partners in the Mayfair Gas Company were comfortably busy in London's West End. Macintosh saw no advantage to an academic life for which he might not be suited and neither he nor his wife wanted to leave London. However, if he did not accept the post, he knew Nuffield would think he had let him down. His London colleagues happily agreed to keep his place in their partnership open for one year if he took the chair. Macintosh moved to Oxford in 1936 and the Nuffield chair of anaesthetics in Oxford was inaugurated in 1937. It was the first chair of anaesthetics in Europe and the first fully endowed chair of anaesthetics in the world.

Macintosh had earlier pointed out that no anaesthetist had the academic background to justify professorial status in an ancient university. Nuffield replied that this would apply to the first incumbent and probably the second, but he was confident that the third would hold his own (Figure 1). Macintosh's instinct for the essence of

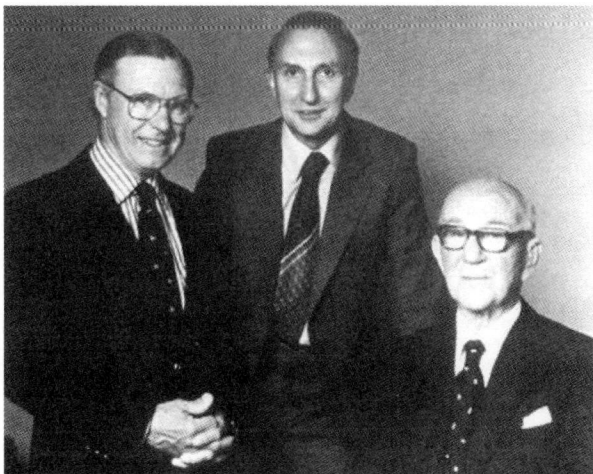

Figure 1. The first three professors: (Left to right) Professor A. Crampton Smith (1965–79), Sir Keith Sykes (1980–91)and Sir Robert Macintosh (1937–65). (Reproduced from the Nuffield Department of Anaesthetics.)

the professorial role overcame any insufficiency of his scholarship. His successor, Alex Crampton Smith, already had an academic record when he was appointed in 1965. The third professor, Keith Sykes, more than fulfilled Nuffield's prediction and was knighted shortly before his retirement in 1991.

Despite his great wealth, Lord Nuffield remained personally frugal and in later life devoted his energies to the philanthropy. He gave away £30 million (more than £300 million pounds or nearly half a billion US dollars at present day values), two-thirds of which was devoted to advancing medical science and patient care. Before the Second World War, he donated a Both respirator, known as an 'iron lung', to every hospital in Britain that requested one. He gave £11,000 to the faculty of anaesthetists of the Royal College of Surgeons in 1951 for research and teaching, and in 1962, his generosity helped to establish the first Australian chair of anaesthesia at Sydney University.

Lord Nuffield was appointed a baronet in 1929, a baron in 1934 and a viscount in 1938. He was elected to Honorary Membership of the Association of Anaesthetists of Great Britain and Ireland in 1936. He was elected to Honorary Fellowship of the Royal College of Surgeons in 1948, the Faculty of Anaesthetists in 1953 and the Royal College of Obstetricians and Gynaecologists in 1956.

Acknowledgement

Portrait photograph reproduced from the Nuffield Department of Anaesthetics.

Further reading

Andrews PWS, Brunner E. *The life of Lord Nuffield; a study in enterprise and benevolence.* Oxford, UK: Blackwell, 1955.

[Anonymous]. Benefactions of Lord Nuffield. *British Medical Journal* 1963; 2: 553.

Beinart J. *A history of the Nuffield Department of Anaesthetics, Oxford 1937–1987.* Oxford, UK: Oxford University Press, 1987.

NUNN'S APPLIED RESPIRATORY PHYSIOLOGY

John Francis Nunn (1925–)

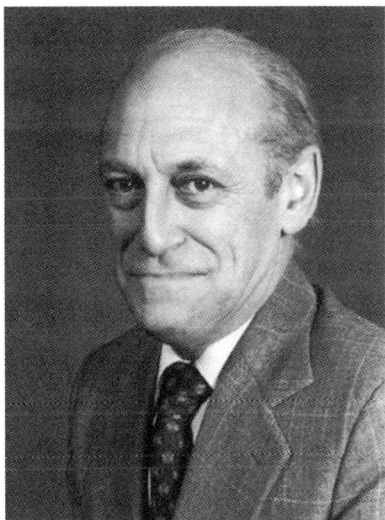

John Nunn was born in 1925 in North Wales. After four years at Wrekin College, he entered Medical School at the University of Birmingham in 1943 and graduated in June 1948. Within 24 hours of graduation, he had departed for Spitsbergen in the Arctic Ocean as medical officer and surveyor to a Birmingham University geological expedition (Figure 1). They worked in total isolation for two months, half way between the Arctic Circle and the North Pole.

House physician posts followed and he then married Sheila. Soon after the wedding, they left to work for three years in the Malayan Medical Service, where Nunn was posted to Penang to give anaesthetics. Equipment was sparse in 1949 and the only anaesthetic options were spinals, or chloroform and ether on the open mask. However, after some time he found a tracheal tube, which he passed blindly by the nasal route as there was no intubating laryngoscope. There was no other anaesthetist and he taught himself from Alfred Lee's *A Synopsis of Anaesthesia* and then Minnitt and Gillies's *A Textbook of Anaesthetics*.

He soon acquired a Macintosh laryngoscope, a Boyle's apparatus and then a Coxeter–Mushin circle absorber system. Neuromuscular blocking agents were introduced and finger-stalls were used to make cuffed tracheal tubes. Nunn was now totally committed to the practice of anaesthesia, but had still never met another anaesthetist since arriving in Malaya. The next stage was to start training Malayan graduates, one of whom later took the Nuffield Prize in the primary FFARCS examination.

This idyllic existence ceased abruptly in 1953, when Nunn returned to England and immediately

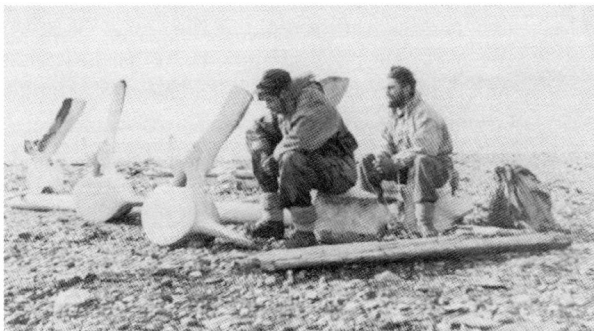

Figure 1. John Nunn (on the right) with the late Brian Baker seated on whale vertebrae on the coast of Spitsbergen in 1948.

took the two-part Diploma in Anaesthetics, without having received any formal training apart from a one month secondment to Singapore General Hospital in 1952. He became a registrar and then senior registrar in Birmingham. This was an anticlimax and he became increasingly dissatisfied with the prevailing ignorance of respiratory physiology in relation to anaesthesia. He bade farewell to the National Health Service and in 1955 became a PhD student under Ken Donald, who was a reader in medicine in Birmingham and gave Nunn every encouragement to study the effects of anaesthesia on the respiratory system. In January 1957, Nunn was appointed Leverhulme research fellow under Ronald Woolmer (1908–62), the first British Oxygen professor of anaesthesia in the newly established research department at the Royal College of Surgeons in London, where facilities were outstanding. Nunn collaborated with Dennis Hill, the physicist, and was granted his PhD in 1958 for his thesis '*Factors influencing the arterial carbon dioxide tension during anaesthesia*'.

Around 1959, the polarograph became a practical possibility for measuring arterial PO_2, and Nunn commenced clinical studies with an international team comprizing Tony Coleman (later professor in Durban, South Africa), Norman Bergman (later professor in Portland, Oregon) and, for three months, Armen Bunatyan (professor in Moscow, Russia). The Leverhulme Research Fellowship continued until 1964, but his clinical attachment was transferred from the Whittington Hospital, Highgate to the Royal Postgraduate Medical School, Hammersmith.

Nunn's experience as a lecturer and demonstrator on the basic science course at the Royal College of Surgeons highlighted the lack of a suitable textbook that dealt with the respiratory problems confronting anaesthetists. About the same time, Professor Cecil Gray of Liverpool invited Nunn to contribute chapters to *Modern Trends in Anaesthesia*. This led to close links with Butterworths, the publishers, whose head office was then within a stone's throw of the Royal College of Surgeons. The time was ripe for a book on applied respiratory physiology in relation to anaesthesia and Nunn started work on it in 1963.

A crucial event occurred in 1964 when John Goligher, professor of surgery in Leeds, invited Nunn to visit the University of Leeds with a view to becoming the foundation professor of anaesthesia. What the University of Leeds offered could not be refused. The Nunn family moved north in time for the start of the academic year and four golden years in Leeds. Amongst the staff Nunn recruited, were two future presidents of the Royal College of Anaesthetists (Alastair Spence and Cedric Prys-Roberts) and four professors of anaesthesia (Spence in Glasgow and then Edinburgh; Prys-Roberts in Bristol; Graham Smith in Leicester; and Richard Ellis in Leeds). He established day-release courses for both primary and final FFARCS examinations, a post-fellowship practical laboratory course and a two-week intensive course for groups of 14 undergraduates at a time. A series of senior registrars joined the university department for instruction in clinical research.

In 1968, Nunn was appointed head of the division of anaesthesia of the Medical Research Council. The division grew to about 25 people, the majority of whom were basic scientists. Fourteen of the anaesthetists employed in the Clinical Research Centre and Northwick Park Hospital in Harrow, Middlesex became professors.

The multitude of activities in Leeds had put Nunn's proposed book on hold until he moved to Northwick Park. The first edition finally appeared in 1969 under the title of *Applied Respiratory Physiology, with Special Reference to Anaesthesia*. The second edition was published in 1977, without reference to anaesthesia in the title to reflect its broader scope of applications. A term as dean of the faculty of anaesthetists of the Royal College of Surgeons (1979–82) delayed the third edition until 1987. The fourth edition, eponymously renamed *Nunn's Applied Respiratory Physiology*, followed on schedule in 1993 (Figure 2) after Nunn's retirement in 1991. Thereafter, Andrew Lumb, Nunn's last research fellow at Northwick Park from 1988 to 1991, took over authorship of the fifth edition in 2000. Meanwhile Nunn was enjoying his retirement, pursuing his other interests of Egyptology, geology, gardening and model engineering.

Nunn's awards include an MD (honours) and a DSc (by thesis) from the University of Birmingham, honorary doctorates from the Universities of Turin and Uppsala, and Honorary Fellowships of the Royal College of Anaesthetists in 1993, the Irish Faculty of Anaesthetists, the Australian and New Zealand College of Anaesthetists in 1984, and the Royal Society of Medicine in 1992. He was awarded the Dudley Buxton Medal of the Royal College of Anaesthetists in 1968, the Sir Ivan Magill Gold Medal of the Association of Anaesthetists in 1988, and the Excellence in Research Award of the American Society of Anesthesiologists in 1991. He received the Richardson Award of the Geologists' Association in 1999 and in 2001 he was elected to the Fellowship of the Geological Society of London.

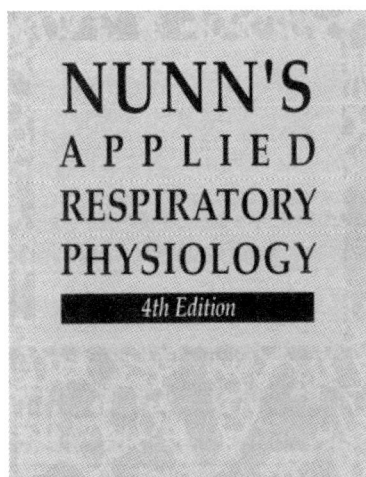

NUNN'S APPLIED RESPIRATORY PHYSIOLOGY
4th Edition

Figure 2. Cover of the fourth edition of *Nunn's Applied Respiratory Physiology*.

Further reading

Nunn JF. *Ancient Egyptian medicine*. London, UK: British Museum Press, 1996.

Nunn JF. *Applied respiratory physiology, 3rd edn*. London, UK: Butterworth, 1987.

Nunn JF. Development of academic anaesthesia in the UK up to the end of 1998. *British Journal of Anaesthesia* 1999; 83: 916–32.

Nunn JF. Evolution of the atmosphere. *Proceedings of the Geologists Association* 1998; 109: 1–13.

PASK CERTIFICATE OF HONOUR

Edgar Alexander Pask (1912–1966)

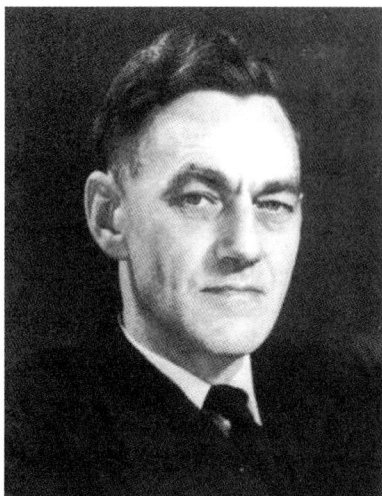

Edgar Pask was born in 1912 in Derby, Derbyshire. He won an open scholarship from Rydal School in Colwyn Bay, North Wales to Downing College, Cambridge, where he obtained a first-class honours degree in the natural sciences tripos. He completed his clinical studies at The (now Royal) London Hospital, graduated in medicine and surgery in 1937, and became interested in anaesthesia during house appointments at The London. He was appointed house anaesthetist at the Radcliffe Infirmary, Oxford and in 1940 he became junior assistant to Professor Macintosh and obtained the Diploma in Anaesthetics.

He volunteered for service with the Royal Air Force (RAF) in 1941. He undertook research, which frequently necessitated dangerous experiments on human subjects, at the physiological laboratory at Farnborough, Hampshire (later the Institution of Aviation Medicine). His investigations started with the design of immersion suits for pilots of Merchant Ship Fighter Units who might have to survive exposure. He used Tropal, a new synthetic material, and barrage balloon fabric and tested them in actual conditions of wind chill and the sea. When he tested one version in Sullum Voe in Shetland, swimming in the suit made him too hot while the observers were so cold they had to give up. He also had himself parachuted into the sea off Shetland in another version.

Pask volunteered to be deeply anaesthetized on several occasions in April 1943 to compare different methods of artificial respiration. Anaesthesia was induced with 500 mg of 10% thiopentone, and was maintained with ether through a cuffed endotracheal tube. Forced hyperventilation with seven or eight breaths of 15% ether produced respiratory arrest so that the efficiency of Shafer's method, Sylvester's method, Eve's rocking method, and the mouth-to-mouth method of artificial respiration could be studied during the next two hours.

Pask also carried out experiments that involved his exposure to very low oxygen levels (under 7%) in an attempt to discover whether RAF crews could survive if they bailed out of an aircraft at high altitude. He then related the effects, especially on his level of consciousness, to actual descents. He concluded that 35,000 feet (10,600 metres) was the greatest height from which escape by parachute could be made without oxygen with any chance of survival. He risked his life on every occasion.

Pask's best known work at Farnborough relates to the design of flotation jackets. It was discovered that, although the 'Mae West' inflatable jacket kept unconscious subjects afloat, they sometimes drowned because it did

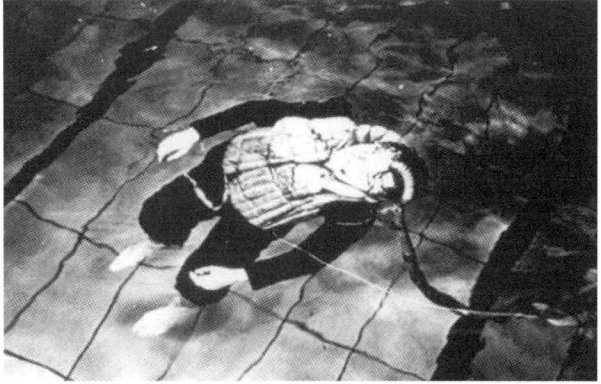

Figure 1. Lifejacket experiment. Pask is floating, fully anaesthetized. (Reproduced from the Nuffield Department of Anaesthetics.)

not keep the head out of the water. Instead, it often turned the individual face-down. Again, the only way to test improved prototypes was on unconscious volunteers. Pask and Macintosh, who was adviser in anaesthetics to the RAF, designed a coaxial breathing system. Pask was anaesthetized, immersed in the pool and allowed to float or sink freely to determine whether different jackets would keep his head above water. The anaesthetic delivery system remained buoyant, while Macintosh controlled the EMO anaesthetic machine on the poolside or on a table in the pool (Figures 1 and 2). The results were recorded on film and formed the basis of Pask's Cambridge MD thesis. Macintosh later remarked that it was probably the first time that such a degree had been given to a man who was deeply unconscious during the all important parts of the research! Recognition of Pask's bravery was shown when he was appointed OBE (Military Division) in 1944.

After the war, Pask was appointed reader in anaesthetics at the Newcastle division of the University of Durham. The appointment was delayed so that he could first spend time with Ralph Waters in Madison, Wisconsin and with Wilder Penfield, neurosurgeon at the Montreal Neurological Institute in Canada. He took up his post in 1947 and was awarded a personal chair in 1949, thus becoming only the second professor of anaesthetics in the UK. His research produced innovations in lung ventilator design and helped him write many papers and deliver several prestigious

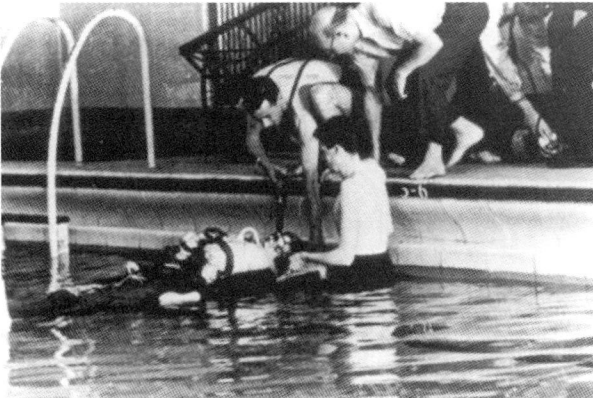

Figure 2. Pask is the subject; Macintosh is in bare feet at the poolside. (Reproduced from the Nuffield Department of Anaesthetics.)

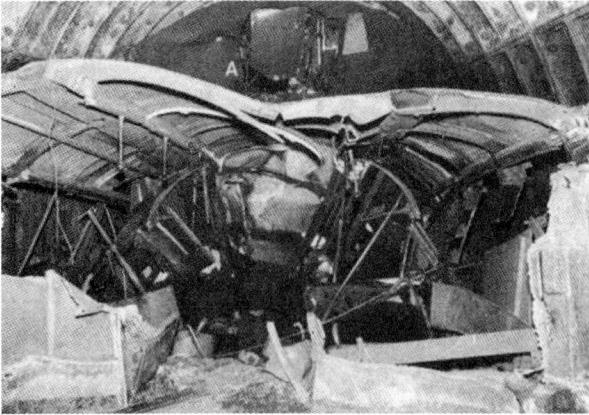

Figure 3. Wreckage of front coach in the Moorgate disaster. (Reproduced from *Anesthesia* 1975; **30**: 666–76.)

lectures. An established chair was created in 1959.

Pask had a charismatic personality. He was able to inspire all who worked with him and to instil into them the same principles of utter dedication and care that were his own hallmarks. This influence ensured that several of his staff later attained great distinction. He was meticulous and gained a reputation for asking challenging questions combined with requests for evidence to support any statement made. His incisive mind allowed him to make great contributions and he was much sought-after as a member of committees.

The Association of Anaesthetists of Great Britain and Ireland created the illuminated 'Pask certificate of honour' in 1975, following the Moorgate underground railway disaster in London in which a six-car underground train crashed into the end of a blind tunnel (Figures 3 and 4). No national honour had been awarded in recognition of the gallantry of Philip Finch, an anaesthetic registrar from St Bartholomew's Hospital, during the immediate rescue operations. The certificate honours 'those who have rendered distinguished service, either with gallantry in the performance of their clinical duties, to the specialty of anaesthesia as a whole, or to the Association itself, either in a single meritorious act, or consistently and faithfully over a long period'. The Pask Certificate has been awarded more than 80 times; five times for gallantry at civilian disasters, including the Moorgate disaster, and once to the Ministry of Defence for the contribution of the 14 Defence Service anaesthetists who were on active service in the 1982 Falklands War.

Pask was a founder member of the Faculty of Anaesthetists of the Royal College of Surgeons and became vice-dean. He was the third recipient of the John Snow Medal of the Association of Anaesthetists of Great Britain and Ireland in 1946; president of the Section of Anaesthetics of the Royal Society of Medicine in 1964–65; and a Member of Council of the Association from 1955 to 1966. His sudden death after a heart attack at his home in 1966 followed a spell of deteriorating health.

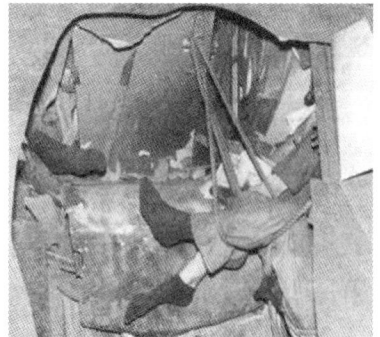

Figure 4. Close-up of Fig 3: ten people were trapped in this space; five were rescued alive. (Reproduced from *Anaesthesia* 1975; **30**: 666–76.)

Acknowledgement

Portrait photograph reproduced with kind permission from the Association of Anaesthetists of Great Britain and Ireland.

Further Reading

Beinart J. *A History of the Nuffield Department of Anaesthetics, Oxford 1937–87.* Oxford, UK: Oxford University Press, 1987: 52–4.

Boulton TB. *The Association of Anaesthetists of Great Britain and Ireland 1932–1992 and the development of the specialty of anaesthesia.* London, UK: The Association of Anaesthetists of Great Britain and Ireland, 1999: 734–45.

Finch P, Nancekievel DG. The role of hospital medical teams at a major accident. *Anaesthesia* 1975; **30**: 666–76.

QUINCKE SPINAL NEEDLE

Heinrich Irenaeus Quincke (1842–1922)

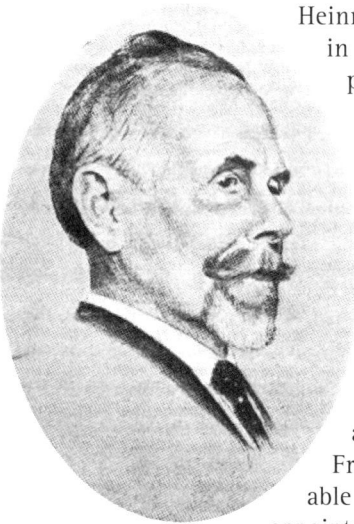

Heinrich Quincke was born in Frankfurt-an-der-Oder in Germany in 1842, the son of a distinguished physician. The family later moved to Berlin, where Quincke completed high school in 1858. He studied medicine at Berlin, Wurzburg and Heidelberg Universities under some of the best medical scientists and teachers of the day. New chemical and microscopic methods of studying disease were appearing and Quincke found himself in an intellectual environment conducive to energetic work and innovation.

He served for three years (from 1867 to 1870) as an assistant to his former teacher, Friedrich Frerichs, in Berlin. He must have made a considerable impression on his colleagues because he was appointed professor and chairman of internal medicine in Bern in 1873 at the early age of 30. He became professor and chairman of internal medicine at Kiel in 1878 and a colleague of the famous surgeon August Bier.

Quincke was an astute observer, an excellent teacher and a master in internal medicine and clinical neurology. His contributions to the medical literature include his classic description of Quincke's oedema (angioneurotic oedema) and his introduction and promotion of lumbar puncture as a diagnostic and therapeutic clinical procedure.

Many doctors, from the Italian Marcello Donato in 1586 onwards, had recorded the sudden onset of painless, non-itchy oedema that tends to migrate to areas with loose skin without affecting the general condition of the patient before Quincke published his description in 1882. The term Quincke's oedema first appeared in 1902 in a paper by Felix Mendel from Berlin. This eponym then entered the medical language all over the world, but there is no explanation as to why Quincke's name was given to the syndrome, except that he was a well-known professor.

Quincke's great contribution was his introduction of lumbar puncture, which he first described in 1891. Twenty years earlier in Berlin he had used it experimentally in animals to study the anatomy and physiology of cerebrospinal fluid in dogs, and he later studied the communication between the subarachnoid space in the brain and spinal cord. Tait and Gaglieri of San Francisco, California wrote that; 'To Quincke is due the credit of having demonstrated the innocuousness of subarachnoid lumbar puncture, its facility of execution and the harmlessness of the withdrawal of a considerable amount of cerebrospinal fluid.'

Quincke presented his first communication on lumbar puncture to the Tenth Congress on Internal Medicine at Weisbaden, Germany on 8 April 1891. He performed the puncture by inserting a fine needle with a stylet through the lumbar intervertebral space. He reported 10 cases – the earliest from 1889 but most from 1891. Some of the reports were of hydrocephalus and one each of meningitis, pneumonia, cerebral haemorrhage and cerebral tumour. He performed repeated punctures, some under chloroform anaesthesia and instituted prolonged drainage. He always recorded the condition of the cerebral spinal fluid. He was the first to examine the constituents of the fluid and to record the manometric pressures at the beginning and end of the puncture. He counted the cells and measured the specific gravity and the total protein concentration. He also identified bacteria and noted the decrease in sugar content in the fluid in cases of purulent meningitis. His clinical results were disappointing, but his long-term vision of the diagnostic potential of lumbar puncture was of greater importance.

By the time Quincke published his paper on lumbar puncture in individuals with hydrocephalus in September 1891, he had performed 22 punctures on 10 additional patients – five children and five adults. In this paper he acknowledged the work of Walter Wynter (1860–1945) in England, who described lumbar puncture using a Southey tube with a rubber drainage tube to release pressure in four cases of tuberculous meningitis in the *Lancet* in June 1891. Wynter's first patient, in 1889, was a three-year-old boy with meningitis secondary to an inner ear infection. The other three patients were an 11-year-old girl, a two-year-old boy and a 13-month-old girl, all of whom had tuberculous meningitis. The procedure resulted in only temporary relief of the symptoms and all four died.

It is not clear how and when the simple, bevel-point spinal needle became known as the Quincke needle. Quincke himself described only a fine needle with a stylet. When Bier performed his series of six spinal anaesthetics in 1898, he merely wrote; 'Quincke's lumbar puncture is done in the usual manner. A very fine hollow needle is selected. After the dural sac has been entered, the stylet, which occludes the lumen of the needle, is withdrawn...'. Labat described a set of five spinal needles in *Regional Anesthesia* in 1922; these ranged in length from 20 to 120 mm and diameter from 0.6 to 1.0 mm but he did not name them. In 1966, Richard Schorr at the Sheppard Air Force Base, Texas reviewed the history of spinal needles. Among the earliest were those designed before 1910 by Corning in the USA, Bier in Germany and Barker in England (Figure 1). Next came the Labat, Greene and Pitkin needles in the 1920s (Figure 2), each with its distinctive bevelled point. Lemmon

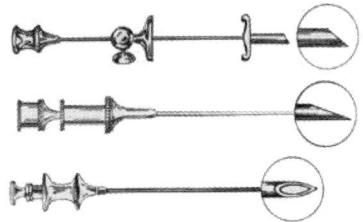

Figure 1. (Top to bottom) Corning, Bier, Barker spinal needles. (Reproduced from *Anesthesia and Analgesia* 1966; 45: 509–13, with permission from Lippincott Williams & Wilkins.)

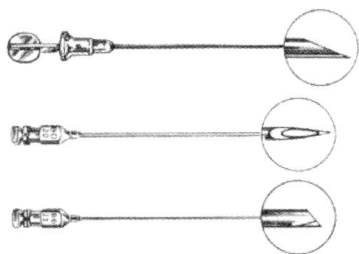

Figure 2. (Top to bottom) Labat, Greene, Pitkin spinal needles. (Reproduced from *Anesthesia and Analgesia* 1966; **45**: 514–19, with permission from Lippincott Williams & Wilkins.)

and Tuohy described their needles (Figure 3) for continuous spinal anesthesia in the early 1940s. Whitacre described his 20-gauge, pencil-point needle with side orifice in 1951, with the object of reducing the incidence of post-spinal headache. Schorr also illustrated Brace and Levy needles, which appeared in the 1950s, but he made no mention of a Quincke needle.

Quincke later developed lumbar puncture in neurological diagnosis and treatment. He recorded occasional sixth cranial nerve paralysis after withdrawal of cerebrospinal fluid. His surgical colleague, August Bier, combined the pharmacological local anaesthetic effect of cocaine with lumbar puncture to produce the first spinal anaesthetic in 1898. Quincke remained in Kiel for 30 years, refusing positions offered to him at Königsberg in Lithuania and Vienna in Austria. He retired in 1908 and died in 1922 at the age of 80 in Frankfurt-am-Main.

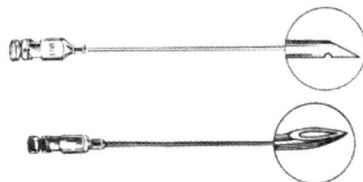

Figure 3. (Top) Lemmon (bottom) Tuohy continuous spinal needles. (Reproduced from *Anesthesia and Analgesia* 1966; **45**: 514–19, with permission from Lippincott Williams & Wilkins.)

Acknowledgement

Portrait photograph reproduced from *The Founders of Neurology, 2nd edn*, Charles C. Thomas, 1970: 500.

Further reading

Hägermark Ö. Mannen bakom syndromet: Heinrich Quincke. *Läkartidningen* 1983; 80: 4429–30.

Hiller F. Heinrich Quincke (1842–1922). In: Haymaker W, Schiller F (Eds) *The Founders of Neurology, 2nd edn.* Springfield, IL: Charles C. Thomas, 1970: 499–503.

Schorr RM. Needles: some points to think about Parts I, II. *Anesthesia and Analgesia* 1966; 45: 509–13, 514–19.

RAE (Ring, Adair and Elwyn) Endotracheal Tubes

Wallace Harold Ring (1932-)

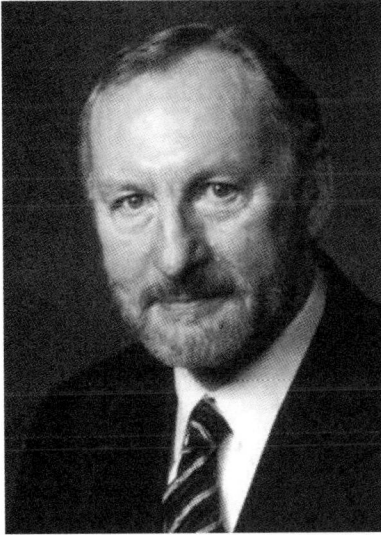

Wallace Ring was born in 1932 in Chicago, Illinois, the son of working class parents. His father worked as a joiner for the Pullman Company. In 1945, at the end of the Second World War, his father quit the railroad and the family moved to Boulder, Colorado. Ring completed high school in Boulder and received a joint-honour scholarship to the University of Colorado in Denver. After a three-year accelerated programme, he was admitted to the University of Colorado School of Medicine, receiving his Bachelor of arts in 1954 and his Doctorate of medicine in 1957. Upon completing a one-year internship at Denver General Hospital, he entered the US Air Force School of Aviation Medicine. He was then sent for a two-year tour of duty as liaison medical officer to the post-war German Luftwaffe, stationed at Fürstenfeldbruck, West Germany.

After discharge from active service in 1960, he trained in anaesthesia at the University of Utah School of Medicine in Salt Lake City. He completed his training in 1962 and accepted a faculty appointment as instructor in ancsthesiology for the next three years. He then entered private practice at Primary Children's Hospital in Salt Lake City where he limited his practice to paediatric anaesthesia.

While still at the University of Utah, Ring met James Sorenson who was just starting a new company, the Sorenson Research Company, and was looking for innovative ideas. The company's first product was a device Ring had patented and which Sorenson called the Ring retractor (Figure 1). This was an adaptation of the McIvor and Crowe–Davis mouth gags for holding the mouth open during oral surgery. The new retractor enabled an endotracheal tube to be placed between the tongue depressor and the tongue. During a short relationship with the Sorenson Research Company (later Abbott), Ring was named on about 12 patents that were issued either in his name or shared with others. One was for a new intravenous catheter system, marketed as the Intrafusor. Another one, which was sold by a different company, was a replacement for both McIvor and Crowe–Davis gags. This novel device, the Ring gag, incorporated a pivoted bow that allowed greater adjustability for placement.

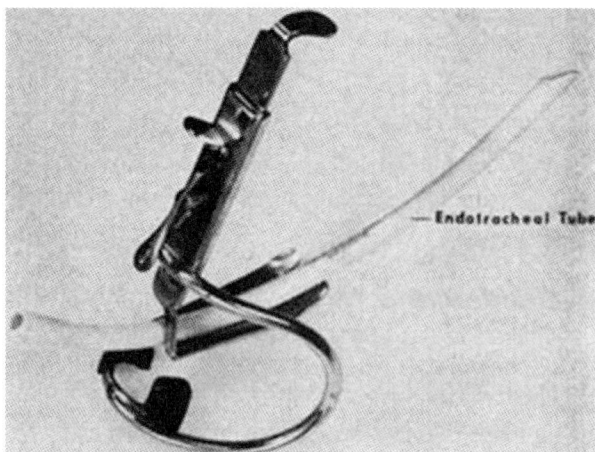

Figure 1. View of Ring's modified blade in a Crowe–Davis gag. (Reproduced from *Anesthesiology* 1963; 24: 740–1, with permission from Lippincott Williams & Wilkins.)

In the early 1960s, Ring joined the committee on mechanical equipment of the American Society of Anesthesiologists. He was also a member of both the American National Standards Institute (ANSI) and the International Standards Organization. Later, he served as consultant to the Federal Drug Administration (FDA), as chairman of a panel of the Bureau of Medical Devices and Diagnostic Products and as a member of the FDA's advisory committee on good manufacturing practices.

Richard Elwyn returned to Denver from a fellowship at Boston Children's Hospital with a clever trick. Elwyn would place a pipe cleaner inside the lumen of a Portex plastic, uncuffed, endotracheal tube and bend it into a desired shape. He then autoclaved it at a high temperature, which hardened the tube into the preset shape (Figure 2). The original softness of the tube could be partially recovered by soaking it in hot water immediately before use. These tubes, with the distal end bent into a 'hockey stick' shape, were of enormous benefit for intubating neonates with Pierre–Robin syndrome.

Ring began receiving comments from users of the Ring retractor who found it clumsy because the endotracheal tube would kink as it exited from the mouth. He also noticed in his own practice that the Y-piece attached to the endotracheal tube connector obstructed the surgeon's view during surgery. A similar solution to Elwyn's presented itself. He created a bend in the endotracheal tube where it exited from the Ring retractor. The tube then lay along the chin and the connector and Y-piece were placed at a convenient distance from the mouth.

Such preformed oral tubes were useful for many other surgical procedures and preformed nasal tubes could be moulded to lie along the forehead (Figure 3). For this idea to be practical, these tubes had to have predetermined lengths, and a direct correlation between the required diameter and appropriate length soon became apparent. Elwyn suggested providing two 'eyes' or portals on every tube. The tubes' distal ends were bevelled on the left, with one eye on the right side opposite the bevel, and one above the bevel on the left side. These eyes provided a tube that could be inserted

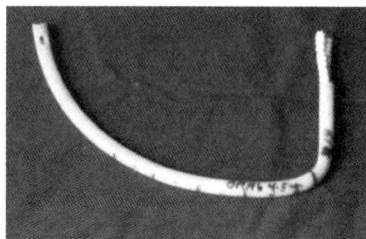

Figure 2. Pipe cleaner in tube to fix desired shape during autoclaving.

into the right main stem bronchus while still ventilating both lungs. Several sets of these tubes of all sizes were built from Portex tubes and pipe cleaners and a clinical trial proved their feasibility.

At one of the ANSI meetings, Ring met David Sheridan who was looking for original ideas for his new National Catheter Company. Sheridan made the tubes and Wallace Ring, John Adair and Richard Elwyn (anaesthetists at Primary Children's Hospital) kept careful records of the next 10,000 intubations performed with preformed tubes. Tracheal tube diameter for uncuffed paediatric tubes had to be precise to achieve a snug but not tight fit

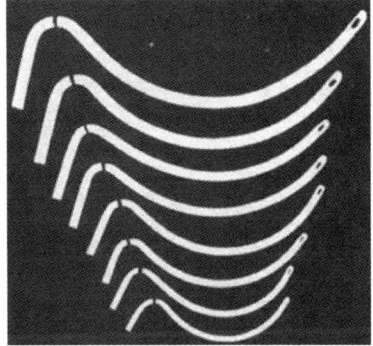

Figure 3. Series of RAE nasal tubes from 3.5 to 7.0 mm internal diameters. (Reproduced from *Anesthesia and Analgesia* 1975; **54**: 273–4, with permission from Lippincott Williams & Wilkins.)

within the trachea. This study demonstrated that the best predictor for tracheal tube diameter was the patient's actual age, regardless of patient size, weight or other characteristics. Sheridan agreed to market the tubes; a paper was published and the new RAE tubes took their name from the initial letters of Ring, Adair and Elwyn.

Shortly thereafter, Ring and Adair left paediatric practice and, with Harry Wong, opened Utah's first freestanding surgical centre. It was also one of the first in the USA. Four years later this facility was enlarged and three years after that it was sold to American Medical International.

After this sale, Ring left private practice to become a corporate medical director for Becton–Dickinson, a multinational manufacturer of medical devices, where his name appeared on another three patents before his retirement in 1996.

Further reading

Ring WH. Modification of Crowe–Davis gag. *Anesthesiology* 1963; **24**: 740–1.

Ring WH. A new device for exposure of the oropharynx. *Archives of Otolaryngology* 1972; **96**: 86–7.

Ring WH, Adair JC, Elwyn RA. A new pediatric endotracheal tube. *Anesthesia and Analgesia* 1975; **54**: 273–4.

JACKSON REES MODIFICATION OF THE T-PIECE SYSTEM

Gordon Jackson Rees (1918–2001)

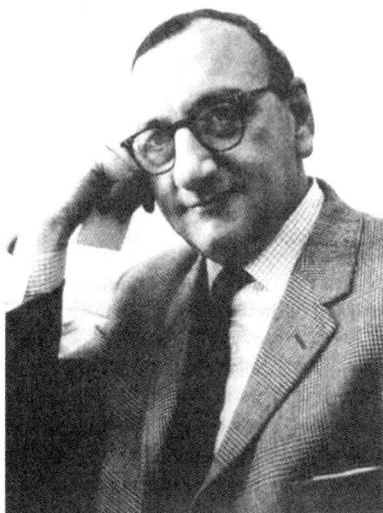

Jackson Rees was born in 1918 in the small market town of Oswestry, Shropshire on the Welsh border. His ancestors had farmed in that region for many generations. He attended Oswestry School, which was founded in 1407 by Henry IV to provide education for both English and Welsh boys and to promote harmony between them.

In 1942, six months after graduating in medicine from Liverpool University, he was drafted into the Royal Air Force (RAF) and served as a medical officer in Africa. Many recruits had very bad teeth; in fact many were edentulous. This introduced the problem of holding a tight seal with an anaesthesia mask. This he solved by designing an intra-oral cheek support – the subject of his first publication.

At the end of the war he remained in the RAF, but he was disenchanted with general duties and sought an appointment to a service hospital. All these appointments were hotly contested, but there was a shortage of juniors wishing to serve in psychiatry or anaesthesia. Neither appealed to him greatly but he chose anaesthesia as being the lesser evil and had the good fortune to be seconded to the Nuffield department in Oxford for an intensive course of training under Robert Macintosh.

In October 1947, Cecil Gray was appointed reader in the Liverpool University department of anaesthesia and invited Jackson Rees to join the department as a demonstrator – thus began a lifelong association. A short time later Gray received a visit from a distinguished and outspoken paediatric surgeon, Isabella Forshall, who demanded that she be assigned a full-time paediatric anaesthetist. Gray agreed and recommended Jackson Rees, who was again faced with what seemed an unattractive choice. Gray persisted and Jackson Rees became, in the words of Forshall's successor, Peter Rickham, 'The first paediatric anaesthetist in Europe'.

Forshall was very supportive of Rees as he strove to improve the anaesthesia management of their young patients. They became close colleagues and friends, each with a great respect for the other's skills. This was a period when great strides were being taken in the development of paediatric surgery. Many new operative approaches to diseases of infancy and childhood were being perfected and their success was dependent on progress in anaesthesia management. Endotracheal intubation for paediatric patients was gaining acceptance. Controlled ventilation during surgery, however, was a new concept that had rarely been applied to infants and children.

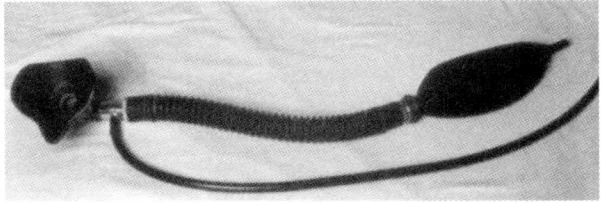

Figure 1. The Jackson Rees modification of Ayre's T-piece, marketed by Medical Industrial Equipment (MIE) Ltd in England, with a Rendell-Baker–Soucek mask. (Image courtesy of D.J. Steward.)

Jackson Rees first mentioned his modification of Ayre's T-piece system in 1950 (Figure 1):

'Artificial ventilation may be carried out by attaching a double-ended bag (BLB type) to the exhaust tube, the open end of which is fitted with a vulcanite tap. This tap can be adjusted so that the intermittent pressure applied to the bag expels the amount of gas required to maintain the equilibrium of the system.'

Philip Ayre travelled from Newcastle upon Tyne to Liverpool in the early 1950s to see Jackson Rees and to discuss his modification of the T-piece system. Ayre was not enthusiastic. He was convinced that the length of the expiratory limb was important in determining the system's performance and did not approve of any alterations. Rees, however, had already decided that the flow rate of fresh gas was of greater importance and persisted in his use of the modified T-piece system for controlled ventilation. This circuit was soon widely used throughout the world. It remains the circuit of choice for many paediatric anaesthetists.

Initially, Rees used ether anaesthesia with his system during controlled ventilation. He turned off the ether at regular 20-minute intervals until the child just started to move and then re-introduced the agent. In this way he maintained a light level of anaesthesia and ensured that the child rapidly awoke at the end of the operation. He noticed that with this technique:

'Babies appear to be in much better condition post-operatively than those in whom spontaneous ventilation was allowed to continue throughout the operation, or in whom deeper levels of anaesthesia were attained.'

Thus, the Jackson Rees technique of light general anaesthesia with controlled ventilation, using the modified T-piece was born. Later, the use of the neuromuscular blocking drug (d-tubocurarine) and nitrous oxide instead of ether allowed further perfection of the technique in neonates and infants.

The use of hand ventilation allowed the adoption of high ventilatory rates with sustained low levels of expiratory pressure. Jackson Rees taught this method to generations of trainees and it became recognized as a part of the Jackson Rees technique. In particular, infants benefited from this pattern of ventilation, which was later shown to maintain lung volume and improve gas exchange.

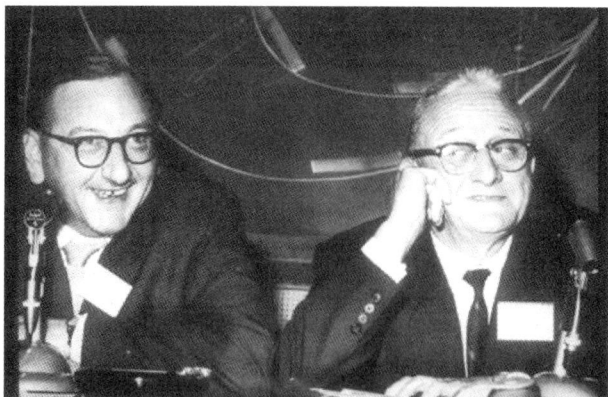

Figure 2. Jackson Rees (left) during an animated debate with Digby Leigh (1904–75) in Toronto, 1964. (Image courtesy of D.J. Steward.)

When confronted by a problem, clinical, technical or medico-legal, Jackson Rees pursued the answer with great vigour and enthusiasm. He was a great clinician, a great thinker and a highly entertaining speaker (Figure 2). Colleagues enjoyed his friendship over many years. One of them wrote this chapter when Jackson Rees was nearing the end of his days, telephoning him from Los Angeles, California most weekends to review the writing. They had many good laughs. He retained his sense of humour and intense interest in his specialty to the very end.

Acknowledgement

Portrait photograph reproduced with kind permission from the Wood Library–Museum of Anesthesiology, Park Ridge, IL, USA.

Further reading

Bush GH. An appreciation of Dr. Gordon Jackson Rees FRCA, FRCP, FRCPCH: pioneer of paediatric anaesthesia. *Paediatric Anaesthesia* 2001; 11: 379–81.
Rees GJ. Anaesthesia in the newborn. *British Medical Journal* 1950; 2: 1419–22.
Rees GJ. Paediatric anaesthesia. *British Journal of Anaesthesia* 1960; 32: 132–40.

RENDELL-BAKER–SOUCEK MASK

Leslie Rendell-Baker (1917–)

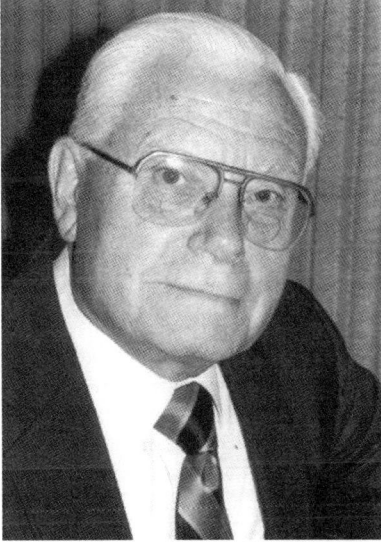

Leslie Rendell-Baker was born in 1917 in St. Helens in Lancashire, UK. His father, grandfather and three uncles were all electrical power engineers. By 1930 they were certain their industry would soon be nationalized and that medicine offered a better career. Leslie took their advice. After completing his education at Ashville College in Harrogate, Yorkshire he entered Guy's Hospital Medical School in London in 1935, graduating in medicine and surgery in 1941.

When Hitler invaded Poland on 1 September 1939, Britain declared war on Germany. Heavy bombing of London was anticipated and all elective surgical patients were sent to hospitals 20–30 miles outside the city. When Rendell-Baker complained about the lack of anaesthetic training, arrangements were made for students to receive ample experience at Orpington Hospital in Kent. He continued to give anaesthetics as a house surgeon in the Guy's sector hospitals and received coaching from the hospitals' anaesthetist William Mushin. In 1942, Rendell-Baker joined a Royal Army Medical Corps Field Dressing Station and his unit became the Forward Surgical Unit in a beach group for the D-Day invasion of Normandy.

In April 1945, facing predictions of one million casualties from the assaults on Japan, he accepted an offer of anaesthesia training at the 29th British General Hospital in Hanover, Germany. He wrote to the director of anaesthetics at Guy's Hospital, who was also advisor in anaesthetics to the Ministry of Health, requesting a trainee post on his demobilization from the army. Guy's obtained grants for Rendell-Baker and seven other ex-servicemen to meet staffing needs for the inauguration of the National Health Service in 1948.

Rendell-Baker found that clinical experience at Guy's was hard to obtain because teaching medical students took precedence. Access to good paediatric equipment and experience was limited, except when the cardiac anaesthetists, who routinely used curare and controlled respiration, provided anaesthesia for Alfred Blalock. He was visiting from The John Hopkins University in Baltimore, Maryland to demonstrate the Blalock–Taussig operation on children with tetralogy of Fallot. However, weekly round-robin quiz sessions on chapters in standard textbooks provided excellent preparation for the Diploma in Anaesthetics which Rendell-Baker obtained in 1947.

The following year, he was appointed senior assistant to Mushin, now at the Cardiff Royal Infirmary in Wales. His job was to organize the clinical services for all the hospitals in Cardiff. Anaesthesia equipment was extremely poor so Mushin followed Macintosh's example in Oxford by appointing a technician and providing a fully equipped workshop.

Mushin passed on a request from the editor of the *Lancet* to Rendell-Baker for an annotation on two papers on anaesthesia for open chest surgery. One advocated spontaneous respiration with constant positive pressure, the other insisted that controlled respiration was essential. While writing the annotation, Rendell-Baker discovered references for positive pressure anaesthesia dating back to the German literature of 1904–05. He and Mushin found more interesting data and insights and wrote their classic book *The Principles of Thoracic Anaesthesia, Past and Present* in 1953, followed in 1959 by *Automatic Ventilation of the Lungs.*

In 1955, Rendell-Baker won a Fulbright award as assistant professor at the University of Pittsburgh, Pennsylvania. He moved to Case Western Reserve University's Lakeside Hospital in Cleveland, Ohio in 1957. At that time it was impossible to interconnect apparatus made by different manufacturers. There were three sizes of tracheal tube connectors, four sizes of facemask fittings, two sizes of breathing tubing and none of the paediatric facemasks could be used with adult equipment. Rendell-Baker became involved in standards for anaesthesia equipment through two Case Western colleagues who were officers of the American National Anaesthesia Standards Committee Z79.

In 1960, a new professor of paediatric surgery at Case Western forbade tracheal intubation for his neonatal hernia repairs, fearing that tracheitis with the need for tracheotomy might follow clumsy attempts at intubation. The facemasks available at that time fitted poorly and had a large dead space. In the absence of a workshop and technician, Rendell-Baker hammered soft aluminium to make low dead-space facemasks that were satisfactory but flattened the babies' noses. Donald H. Soucek DDS, a Case Western dental graduate, who was rotating through anaesthesia as a resident, suggested using a dental technique in which a casting of the palate ensures that dentures fit firmly in the patient's mouth.

The paediatric surgeon approved intubation of a limited number of babies and children and, with Soucek's skilled help, face castings were made (Figures 1 and 2). Next, masks were modelled in wax to provide a mould cavity into which liquid latex was poured. When the latex dried, the mask fitted

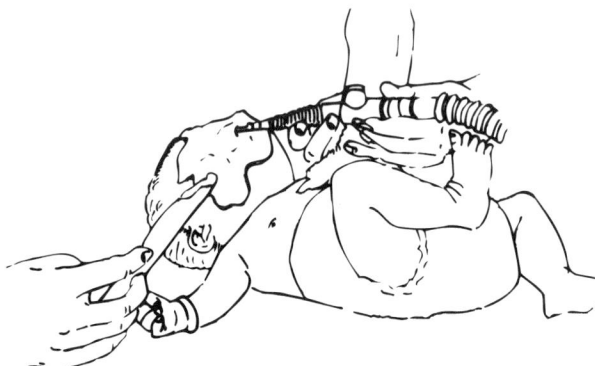

Figure 1. Alginate impression material followed by a supporting layer of plaster of Paris being applied to the face.

the soft tissue of the baby's face, providing a good seal with minimal dead space and without an inflated rim. Prototype latex masks were made in four sizes; Size 0 for premature babies, Size 1 for neonates, Size 2 for 2–3 year olds and Size 3 for 3–6 year olds. The original intention was to produce the masks only in clear plastic. However, the dis-

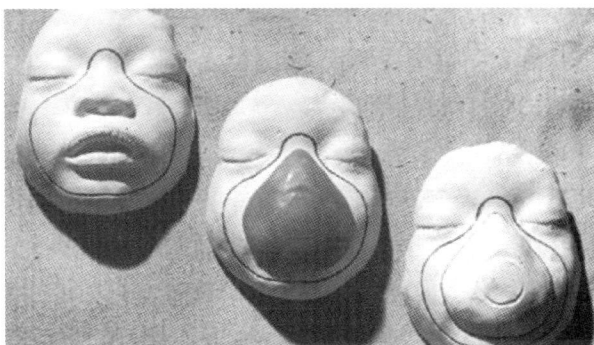

Figure 2. (Left) margin of future mask marked on cast of baby's face, (centre) thin layer of softened red wax moulded over tip of nose and mouth, (right) positive model of face from inner surface, onto which the mask was moulded.

tributors initially insisted on black conductive rubber versions (Figure 3), even though by then anaesthetic agents were non-flammable. All incorporated the newly adopted adult standard 22 mm female connector fitting.

In 1962, Rendell-Baker moved to Mount Sinai Hospital in New York City as director of the department of anesthesiology and was appointed chairman of committee Z79. Mount Sinai Hospital became closely associated with nationwide efforts to improve the safety of anaesthesia equipment by producing standard breathing system fittings, non-toxic tracheal tubes, safe ethylene oxide sterilization and a safe layout of the controls and safety features on anaesthesia apparatus.

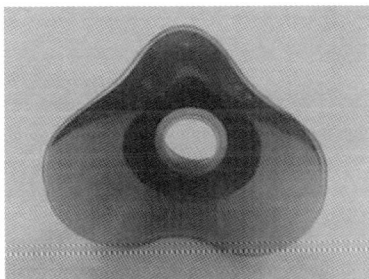

Figure 3. Rendell-Baker–Soucek paediatric face mask.

In 1979 he left Mount Sinai Hospital and joined the staff of Loma Linda University in Southern California. In 1981 he became a founder member and chairman of the American Society for Testing and Materials Subcommittee D10.34, which evolved standard colours for user-applied syringe labels and a standard test of the legibility of text on labels. From 1983 he has been a member of the Association for Advancement of Medical Instrumentation Committee on human factors engineering.

Further reading

Mushin WW, Rendell-Baker L. *The principles of thoracic anaesthesia, past and present.* Oxford, UK: Blackwell Scientific Publications, 1953. (Re-issued in 1991 by the Wood Library–Museum of Anesthesiology, Park Ridge, IL as: *The Origins of Thoracic Anaesthesia.*)

Rendell-Baker L, Soucek DH. New paediatric face masks and anaesthetic equipment. *British Medical Journal* 1962; 1: 1690.

Soucek DH, Rendell-Baker L. The design of experimental latex paediatric face masks in 1961. In: Atkinson RS, Boulton TB (Eds) *The History of Anaesthesia.* London, UK: The Royal Society of Medicine Press, 1989: 328–33.

LACTATED RINGER'S INJECTION USP

HARTMANN'S COMPOUND SODIUM LACTATE SOLUTION BP

Sydney Ringer (1834–1910)

Sydney Ringer was born in Norwich, East Anglia in 1834 and grew up in a nonconformist environment of hard work, sobriety and good behaviour. His father died when he and his brothers were young. After an apprenticeship to a local doctor, friends and relatives provided funds for his training as a medical student at University College and University College Hospital in London. He gained a Bachelor of medicine in 1860, obtained the higher degree of Doctor of medicine in London in 1863, and was elected FRCP London in 1870.

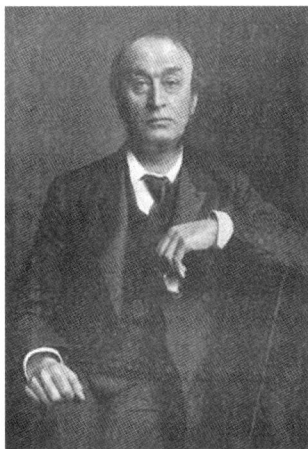

At the beginning of his career, Ringer devoted himself to clinical medicine and became one of the most astute clinicians of his time. He rapidly built up a reputation as a scientific physician and expert diagnostician. Ringer was elected professor of materia medica and therapeutics and later professor of medicine and clinical medicine, in the University of London. He and his wife lived a busy life at 15 Cavendish Place – a fashionable district for London consultants. For 30 years he devoted all the time not occupied by lectures, hospital visits and private patients to experimental investigations in the laboratories of the hospital and college. Clinical medicine was his profession and livelihood; scientific investigation was his hobby. In clinical practice he was a shrewd observer but was cautious in advancing theories that he could not test. In the laboratory, he only tested theories that he could confirm or reject.

On one occasion in 1882, Ringer used a saline solution that his laboratory assistant had prepared with tap water instead of distilled water for experiments on frog hearts. Ringer noticed a difference in effect from his previous published experiments. He knew that tap water contained traces of inorganic substances and analysed the water supplied by the New River Water Company. His results were:

Constituent	Parts per million
Calcium	38.3
Magnesium	4.5
Sodium	23.3
Potassium	7.1
Combined carbonic acid	78.2
Sulphuric acid	55.8
Chlorine	15.0
Silicates	7.1
Free carbonic acid	54.2

Ringer then added various salts to 0.75% sodium chloride to find which would maintain healthy contractions of the isolated frog's heart for the longest period of time. Saline alone or saline with added potassium chloride, sodium bicarbonate or both did not sustain contractility. When a calcium salt was added to any of these solutions, contractility was sustained, but only if calcium and potassium were present in the correct proportions. He formulated Ringer's solution, which permitted laboratory study of the normal function of many tissues and organisms and he reported the influence of various inorganic constituents of solutions on frog hearts in 1882. The great physiological importance of his work was recognized 20 years later with the knowledge and understanding of diffusion and dissociation of ions in biology.

Ringer was also one of the earliest investigators in to the effects of anaesthetics on involuntary muscle, cardiac muscle and the circulation. He carried out these investigations with Dudley Buxton (1855–1931), a young colleague at University College Hospital, who became president of the Society of Anaesthetists in 1907–08. They showed that the vitality of involuntary muscle in the frog persists longer after ether than after chloroform. His later work that was relevant to anaesthetists dealt with the action of pilocarpine and atropine on the frog's heart, and on the antagonism between pilocarpine and muscarine.

Ringer retired from the hospital staff in 1900. He and his family eventually left Cavendish Square for Lastingham on the North Yorkshire moors, where he died in 1910. His greatest honour was his election to the Fellowship of the Royal Society in 1889. In 1912, his only surviving daughter endowed the Sydney Ringer Lecture that is given biennially at University College Hospital and is based on medical research carried out in the laboratories of its medical college or hospital.

Alexis Frank Hartmann (1898–1964)

Alexis Hartmann was born in 1898 in St Louis, Missouri, the grandson, son and father of physicians. He enrolled at the Washington University School

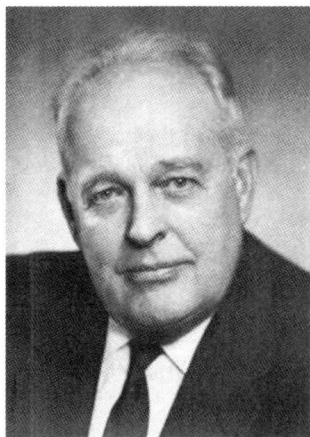

of Medicine in St Louis, Missouri and received his MD degree in 1921 at the age of 23.

As a student, he was influenced by the biochemist Philip Shaffer, and early in his hospital career by William Marriott (1886–1936) who made original contributions to the biochemistry of diseases of children. Hartmann interned at the St Louis Children's Hospital and spent the whole of his professional life in the hospitals of his native city. He devoted himself simultaneously to biochemistry and the clinical practice of paediatrics, bringing the laboratory to the child's bedside. In 1932, he modified Ringer's solution by adding sodium lactate to combat acidosis in his young patients.

Constituent	Hartmann's solution BP (mmol/L)	Lactated Ringer's solution USP (mmol/L)
Sodium	131	130
Potassium	5	4
Calcium	2	1.5
Chloride	111	109
Lactate	29	28

Hartmann and Milton Senn found that one-sixth molar sodium lactate solution was isotonic and could be heat sterilized without decomposition. The lactate was metabolized in the liver, making sodium free to combine with available anions, and reducing the amount of chloride. Curiously, in Britain the modification is called Hartmann's solution after the American, while in America it is called Lactated Ringer's injection after the Englishman.

Hartmann excelled as a researcher, clinician and teacher. When Marriott left for the University of California in 1936, Hartmann succeeded him as physician-in-chief to the St Louis Children's Hospital and Professor of Pediatrics in the university. More than 20 of his students became professors of paediatrics around the world. The Pediatric Section of the American Medical Association awarded Hartmann the first Abraham Jacobi Prize Award in 1963 in recognition of outstanding achievements in paediatrics. The editorial board of the *The Journal of Pediatrics,* on which he served for many years, dedicated the June 1964 issue to him as a *festschrift.* He died of cancer later that year at the age of 66.

Acknowledgement

Portrait photograph of Ringer reproduced with kind permission from The Wellcome Library, London; of Hartmann reproduced with kind permission from *The Journal of Pediatrics* 1964; **64:** 783–92.

Further reading

RINGER:

Anonymous [Obituary]. Sydney Ringer, M.D., F.R.C.P., F.R.S. *British Medical Journal* 1910; **2**: 1384-6.

Ringer S. Concerning the influence exerted by each of the constituents of the blood on the contraction of the ventricle. *The Journal of Physiology (London)* 1880/82; **3**: 389-93.

Ringer S. A further contribution regarding the influence of the different constituents of the blood on the contraction of the heart. *The Journal of Physiology (London)* 1883/84; **4**: 29-42.

HARTMANN:

Hartmann AF, Senn MJE. Studies in the metabolism of sodium *r*-lactate. II. Response of human subjects with acidosis to the intravenous injection of sodium *r*-lactate. *Journal of Clinical Investigation* 1932; **11**: 337-44.

Lee JA. Sydney Ringer (1834-1910) and Alexis Hartmann (1898-1964). *Anaesthesia* 1981; **36**: 1115-21.

White PJ. Alexis F. Hartmann, Sr. *The Journal of Pediatrics* 1964; **64**: 783-92.

EMERY A. ROVENSTINE LECTURE

Emery Andrew Rovenstine (1895-1960)

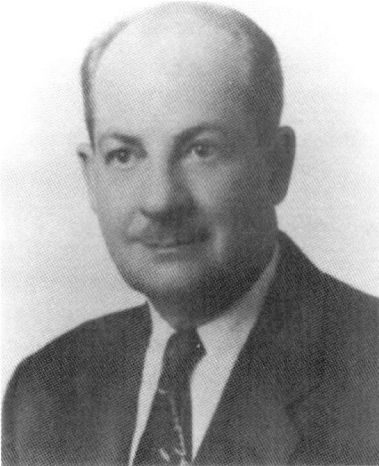

Emery Rovenstine was born in 1895 in Atwood, Indiana where his parents kept the village store. He graduated with a Bachelor of arts from Wabash College in Crawfordsville, Indiana in 1917, served in the US Army for three years and was a high school teacher for a further three years. He then entered Indiana School of Medicine in Indianapolis where he played basketball. His matches were refereed by Arthur Guedel. He graduated in medicine in 1928 and entered general practice with part-time anaesthesia in La Porte, Indiana. Guedel had sparked Rovenstine's interest in anaesthesia and Rovenstine took a course with Elmer McKesson (1881-1935) in Toledo, Ohio. His interest deepened and, on Guedel's advice, he became one of Ralph Waters first two residents at the University of Wisconsin in Madison. He began his formal anaesthesia training in 1930 and, as assistant professor from 1932 to 1934, he assisted Waters in early cyclopropane studies on animals, friends and then patients.

Meanwhile, the chief surgeon of the New York University (NYU) division at Bellevue Hospital, New York City recognized that development in anaesthesia needed doctors who specialized in anaesthesia and he was looking for someone to do this at Bellevue. Nurse anaesthetists, controlled by surgeons and the hospital administration, were providing general anaesthesia and surgery residents gave spinal anaesthetics without supervision. The chief surgeon sought advice from Waters, the only academic anaesthetist in the United States. He recommended Rovenstine who had the necessary missionary zeal to develop the Bellevue programme.

Rovenstine was appointed assistant professor of surgery and arrived at Bellevue in January 1935 to an empty office. The department of surgery had four divisions, each with its own residents, interns, students and one nurse anaesthetist. Anaesthesia was in a primitive state, not only in equipment, but also in status and standard of patient care. Before Rovenstine arrived, patients had a very superficial physical examination and little or no preoperative laboratory work. Many of the patient's charts had only name, address, complaint and diagnosis – surgery often started before the chart was written. Rovenstine took over administration from the superintendent of nurses with a mandate to create and head a Bellevue Department of Anesthesia. He trained interns and residents, organized the service without respect to the four surgical divisions and eventually replaced the nurse anaesthetists with specialist anaesthetists.

Rovenstine attended surgical rounds in each of the divisions to make friends and to assure the surgeons that anaesthetists could contribute to pre- and postoperative patient care. His clinical accomplishments soon persuaded the commissioner of hospitals to promote a change from nurse technician anaesthesia to residency training for physicians. In 1937, Rovenstine became the first Professor of Anesthesia at NYU and the second in the USA. In 1938, the Committee on Graduate Education accepted his proposal for a three-year course with integration of basic sciences and a clinical discipline, leading to a degree of Doctor of Medicine in Medical Science. The first year was exclusively basic sciences with emphasis on physiology and pharmacology. The second and third years were devoted to clinical anaesthesia in Bellevue under university supervision with a core programme of lectures and seminars, journal clubs, examinations, laboratory work and preparation of a thesis. The weekly morbidity–mortality conferences, to which Rovenstine made a significant contribution, were well attended by practising anaesthetists from the metropolitan area. He also fostered and conducted clinical research, improved anaesthetic techniques and devised pieces of anaesthetic equipment.

Rovenstine was anxious to serve in the Second World War but hospital and school authorities declared him essential so he remained in a teaching capacity. He organized an accelerated training programme to produce '90-day wonders' who provided anaesthesia service to the military, and served as a consultant to military hospitals in the area.

The Bellevue programme was one of the outstanding anaesthesia programmes from 1935 to 1950 despite political and organizational problems, surgeons' initial resistance, scarcity of available residents, an overwhelming workload and a World War. The number of residents rose from seven to 27 during 1943–48. Many men and women went from Bellevue to fill teaching positions elsewhere, taking with them lots of Rovenstine's teaching ideas and techniques.

Rovenstine established *Anesthesiology* in 1940 with Henry Ruth, Ralph Tovell, Paul Wood and Ralph Waters and organized the first postgraduate assembly (PGA) in anaesthesiology of the New York State Society of Anesthesiologists (NYSSA) in 1945. His idea for the PGA came from a conversation he had on a flight from Chicago to New York with an ophthalmologist who told him of his specialty's meetings that emphasized basic sciences as well as clinical practice. Rovenstine adopted this format, inviting physiologists, pharmacologists and surgeons to speak in the early years until anaesthesia produced its own leading investigators. He continued this pattern until Lewis Wright (1894–1974) succeeded him as PGA chairman in 1948.

A three-part profile of Rovenstine in the *New Yorker* magazine in 1947 provoked antagonism from within the medical profession. This resulted in Rovenstine being reprimanded and punished by the General Medical Council by having probationary status imposed by the New York Society of

Table 1. Emery A. Rovenstine lecturers and lecture titles

Year	Lecturer	Title
1962	Francis D. Moore	Hemorrhage.
1963	Julius H. Comroe, Jr	The regulation of respiration – 1963.
1964	Eugene Braunwald	The control of cardiac function.
1965	Louis Lasagna	The principles and pitfalls in evaluation of new drugs.
1966	Emanuel M. Papper	Regional anesthesia – a critical assessment of its place in therapeutics.
1967	Arthur C. Guyton	The regulation of cardiac output.
1968	Hermann Rahn	Evolution of gas transport mechanisms from fish to man.
1969	Niels A. Lassen	Cerebral circulation and the anesthetist.
1970	Robert D. Dripps	The physician and society.
1971	Julius Axelrod	Biochemical factors in the inactivation and activation of drugs.
1972	Stuart C. Cullen	Factors influencing education in anesthesiology.
1973	William W. Mushin	The decline and fall of the anesthesiologist?
1974	Otto K. Mayrhofer	Acupuncture-analgesia . . . modern practice of anesthesiology?
1975	H. C. Churchill-Davidson	Clinical observation.
1976	Francis D. Moore	Anesthesia and surgical care.
1977	James E. Eckenhoff	A wideangle view of anesthesiology.
1978	William K. Hamilton	Stress and anesthesia.
1979	Leroy D. Vandam	Anesthesiologists as clinicians.
1980	M.T. "Pepper" Jenkins	Responsibility for the future.
1981	Ephraim S. Siker	A measure of worth.
1982	Solomon G. Hershey	The Rovenstine inheritance: a chain of leadership.
1983	Arthur S. Keats	Cardiovascular anesthesia: perceptions and perspectives.
1984	Eugene A. Stead, Jr	The physician: education and training.
1985	John Lansdale	Anesthesiology: the search for identity.
1986	Edward R. Annis	New challenges – new opportunities.
1987	John F. Nunn	Balancing the risks with the new gases.
1988	John D. Michenfelder	Neuroanesthesia and the achievement of professional respect.
1989	Thomas F. Hornbein	Lessons from on high.
1990	Robert K. Stoelting	Clinical challenges for the anesthesiologist.
1991	Alan R. Nelson	Medicine 2000: expectations, realities and values.
1992	Nicholas M. Greene	The changing horizons of anesthesiology.
1993	Betty J. Bamforth	Learning from our past.
1994	Lawrence J. Saidman	What I have learned after nine years and 9000 papers.
1995	Ellison C. Pierce, Jr	40 years behind the mask: safety revisited.
1996	David E. Longnecker	Is anesthesiology on course for the 21st century?
1997	Michael J. Cousins	Pain: the past, present, and future of anesthesiology.
1998	Francis M. James, III	Who will lead us?
1999	Carl C. Hug, Jr	Patient values, Hippocrates, science and technology.
2000	James F. Arens	Rovenstine legacy: forty years later in Y2K.
2001	Glenn W. Johnson	ASA: education, science, and advocacy – past, present and future.

Medicine and being declined permission to speak at an American Medical Association meeting in Chicago. About 1948 he began to slow down his pace and became involved in medical missions of the Unitarian Service Commission and the World Health Organization. He died in 1960 after a long illness.

Rovenstine received the International Anesthesia Research Award in 1937. He was president of the American Board of Anesthesiology for two terms; president of the American Society of Anesthesiologists in 1943–44; president of the American Society of Regional Anesthesia in 1947; and received the Distinguished Service Award of the American Society of Anesthesiologists in 1957. The Emery A. Rovenstine memorial lecture honours Rovenstine's dedication to education and research that helped anaesthesia to develop in stature and recognition and is the highlight of the American Society of Anesthesiologists annual meeting (Table 1).

Acknowledgement

Portrait photograph reproduced with kind permission from the Wood Library–Museum of Anesthesiology, Park Ridge, IL, USA.

Further reading

Anonymous. We salute . . . Emery A. Rovenstine, B.A., M.D., D.Sc. *Anesthesia and Analgesia* 1960; **39**: 24–6.

Cullen SC. Emery A. Rovenstine. In: Volpitto PP, Vandam LD (Eds) *The genesis of contemporary American anesthesiology*. Springfield, IL: Charles C. Thomas, 1982: 71–87.

Rovenstine EA. Anesthesia: organization for teaching. *Anesthesia and Analgesia* 1937; **16**: 318–22.

RUBEN VALVE

Henning Ruben (1914–)

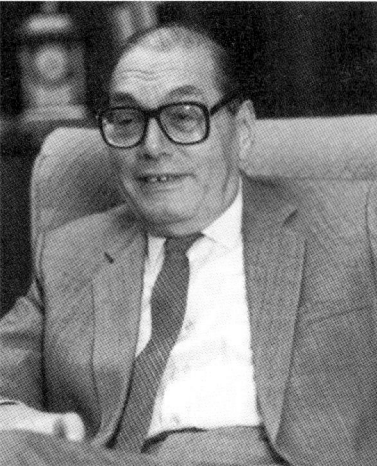

Henning Ruben is a remarkable man who once met is never forgotten. He was born in 1914 in Copenhagen, Denmark, the eldest son of an orthodox Jewish family. He completed high school in 1933 and graduated DDS from the Royal Dental College. He was a professional dancer for some time, touring the Danish provinces with a well-known Danish singer. He was also an outstanding athlete and won a bronze medal for fencing in the 1939 European Championships when he was part of the Danish national team. His talents as a magician, illusionist, mind-reader and member of the Danish Magic Circle were not only entertaining but significant for his future career in anaesthesia.

Ruben graduated in dentistry in 1938 and then undertook medical studies at the University of Copenhagen, supporting himself by his dental practice. Because of his underground activities in the Second World War, in 1943 he was forced to flee occupied Denmark at night in a fishing boat. He went to Sweden, where he worked as a hospital dentist in Stockholm. He returned to Denmark with the 'Danish Brigade' just before VE Day in 1945 and graduated in medicine in January 1946.

Anaesthesia in Denmark was an underdeveloped medical field in those days. Having been introduced to anaesthesia in Stockholm where it was more advanced, he had become fascinated by its combination of physics, physiology and pharmacology and wanted to return there for further study. Strict limitation of foreign exchange prevented this until 1947 when he was invited by the Swedish Society of Illusionists to their meeting in Stockholm. The society even paid for all his travel expenses. He gave a brilliant performance to a packed concert hall. While he was in Stockholm, he introduced himself at Sabbatsberg Hospital and St Ericks Hospital as a student of anaesthesia. Mission accomplished, he went home to Copenhagen.

He returned to Stockholm in 1948 to study neuroanaesthesia, then visited the major anaesthesia centres in Britain before taking up posts in Copenhagen; first at Gentofte Hospital, and later at the Finsen Institute where he became head of department in 1953 and later professor of anaesthesia in the University of Copenhagen. Although his first main interest in anaesthesia was pharmacology, Ruben is better known for his ingenious yet simple inventions.

In 1948, Ruben saw a diagram of the Stephen–Slater non-rebreathing valve. He tried to make a copy but misinterpreted the diagram and produced a different valve that could be used to provide positive end-expiratory pressure. Manual controlled ventilation required two hands, so he designed another valve (with the help of a watchmaker) which only required one hand. This valve contained two springs made from watch balances and rubies, which automatically closed the expiratory port when the bag was compressed (Figure 1). The Ruben valve was later made by the Ambu Company, Denmark, with whom he had a lasting association. The early Ambu valves used the same principles, as did the E-valves that appeared in 1960 in which he substituted silicone membranes for the valve discs and springs. By 1982, more than one million of these valves were in use. The valves became so ubiquitous that a confused anaesthetist once addressed Ruben as Dr Valve!

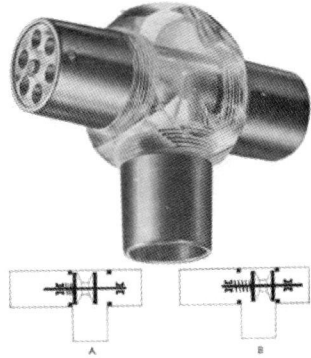

Figure 1. Ruben valve. (A) inspiratory position. (B) expiratory position. (Reproduced with permission from *A synopsis of anesthesia*, 5th edn, John Wright and Sons, 1964: 98.)

Ruben described a simple automatic syringe pump in 1954 for controlled delivery of drugs in a small volume of liquid (Figure 2). Expensive motor driven syringes were used in the laboratory, but Ruben designed a cheap one for clinical use. Two steel springs provided the motive force that was transmitted to the plunger of the syringe by a T-shaped bar. A wind-up alarm clock regulated the speed of injection through the winder shaft with a constant angular velocity and a variable radius pulley.

The most brilliant yet simple invention was that of the first self-inflating bag-valve-mask in 1954. When the Danish truck drivers who brought gasoline to the service stations went on strike, transport of oxygen came to a standstill. By the time the strike was called off, almost no oxygen was left in some hospitals. In case of a lack of compressed oxygen in the future, Ruben designed a self-inflating bag. He went to his bicycle mechanic who welded four bicycle spokes together, then manipulated them into an anaesthetic reservoir bag to produce a globe-shaped frame that kept the bag expanded. When manual compression of the bag was interrupted, their re-expansion refilled the bag. Later models had a different frame and eventually had a simple lining of foam rubber. A Ruben valve was used as an inflating valve and an air inlet valve was added to the tail of the bag to produce the Ambu bag (Figure 3).

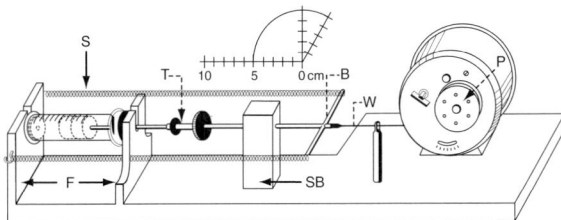

Figure 2. Ruben's mechanical syringe pump. S = spring, F = frame, T = threaded tube, SB = supporting bracket, B = T-shaped bar, W = flexible wire, P = pulley on winder shaft.

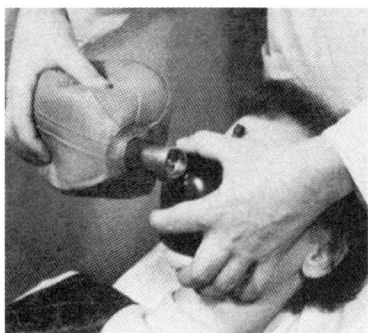

Figure 3. Self-inflating bag with Ruben valve. (Reproduced from *Canadian Medical Association Journal* 1959; **80**: 44–5.)

In 1957, Ruben constructed the first manikin for proper resuscitation training. A member of the local Red Cross who was a painter and modeller helped to make the head, and his bicycle mechanic and watchmaker friend helped with the airway mechanism. It had normal facial anatomy and the airway mechanism allowed lung inflation with forward movement of the jaw and backward tilt of the head. He used it for teaching mouth-to-mouth respiration and demonstrated it at major anaesthesia meetings on both sides of the Atlantic. Modifications were added in 1960 for training in closed-chest cardiac massage.

Ruben managed to create and maintain an anaesthetic department where all categories of staff were happy to work. He was extremely kind towards everybody, maintained his sense of humour and delegated responsibility without losing contact. His was completely free from prejudice towards any problem – human, practical or scientific. He retired from the University Hospital in Copenhagen in 1984.

Ruben was president of the Danish Society of Anaesthetists in 1963–65 and received its Prize of Honour in 1966. He was elected to Honorary Membership of the Association of Anaesthetists of Great Britain and Ireland in 1976 and of the European Resuscitation Council in 1990. He is a Fellow by election of the Royal College of Anaesthetists.

Further reading

Baskett PJF. Citation for Henning Ruben, MD, FFARCS for Honorary Membership of the European Resuscitation Council. *Resuscitation* 1994; **28**: 181–2.

Ruben H. Anesthesia and resuscitation equipment I happened to be involved with. In: Rupreht J, van Lieburg MJ, Lee JA, Erdmann W (Eds) *Anaesthesia essays on its history*. Berlin: Springer-Verlag, 1985: 65–8.

Ruben H. Multipurpose anesthesia valve [in Danish]. *Nordisk Medicin* 1953; **50**: 1242–3.

SANDERS INJECTOR

Richard Douglas Sanders (1906–1977)

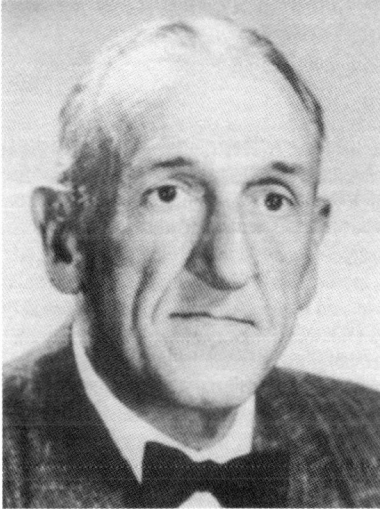

Doug Sanders was born in the tiny village of Erin, Tennessee in 1906. His father was a dentist who also administered anaesthetics. His mother was a professional whistler. He attended Ogden High School and Ogden College in Bowling Green, Kentucky and graduated from the University of Louisville Medical School in 1928. After interning at Louisville General Hospital, he practised family medicine and anaesthesia in Kentucky during the Great Depression from 1929 to 1937. One writer described Sanders as 'an imposing figure of a man, well over six feet tall, with a long, chiselled face and lantern jaw. ... In his leather jacket and bow tie, he resembled a Norman Rockwell sketch of a country doctor.'

He became a skilled clinical anaesthetist with staff appointments at several Louisville hospitals. From 1937, he devoted his time entirely to anaesthesia and his reputation and practice flourished. He was inducted into the US Army in 1942 as a Captain and was appointed chief of the anesthesiology and operating room section at its Valley Forge General Hospital near Philadelphia, Pennsylvania in 1943. This was the army's primary centre for maxillofacial surgical reconstruction of facial injuries in wounded soldiers. Without any formal training, Sanders faced the same challenge of maintaining a clear airway that Ivan Magill had faced during maxillofacial cases in England after the First World War.

Sanders addressed the problem by flattening the tubular blade of the traditional Chevalier Jackson laryngoscope for better exposure of the larynx and designing the first nylon-armoured latex endotracheal tube (Figure 1). He had to master the art of moulding and dipping raw latex in order to make the flexible, non-compressible cuffed tube. After numerous failures, he produced a soft and durable latex rubber cuff on an aluminium mould by repeated manual dipping and drying. He then visited a condom factory to get ideas for a production line. He set up a motorized over-

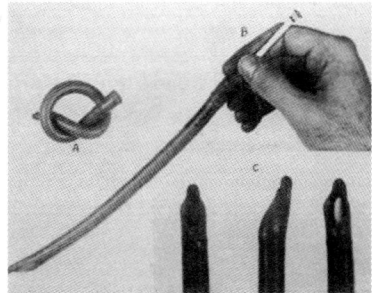

Figure 1. Latex armoured (nylon spiral) endotracheal tube. (A) non-kinking; (B) stylet in place; (C) details of the tip. (Reproduced from *Anesthesiology* 1947; 8: 57–61, with permission from Lippincott Williams & Wilkins.)

head rail in his basement that immersed the moulds into latex at one point and into a drying oven a few feet further along. He gave samples of his cuffed tubes to colleagues and soon received orders from across the USA. Much to the relief of his wife, he relocated the moulding conveyor system to a technician's shop.

He continued to study, frequently visited teaching departments and in 1944 was certified as a Diplomate by the American Board of Anesthesiology. He was discharged from the military with the rank of Lieutenant Colonel in 1946. He became the first full-time anaesthetist in the state of Delaware when he was appointed director of the anesthesia department at Delaware Hospital in Wilmington. He established a school of anesthesia and arranged an affiliation with Jefferson Medical College so that medical students could rotate through a private practice setting.

Anaesthetic techniques for rigid bronchoscopy did not provide satisfactory conditions with adequate pulmonary ventilation for the bronchoscopist to make an unhurried and thorough examination of the bronchial tree. He set out to find a general anaesthetic technique that was safe and effective to relieve patients from the emotional trauma and physical discomfort of rigid bronchoscopy under local anaesthesia. He solved the problem by applying the Venturi principle. He directed a fast-flowing jet of gas down the bronchoscope, parallel to its long axis, so that negative pressure would create the Venturi effect and entrain room air. The resulting pulmonary inflation pressure depended on the driving pressure and the diameters of the jet and the bronchoscope.

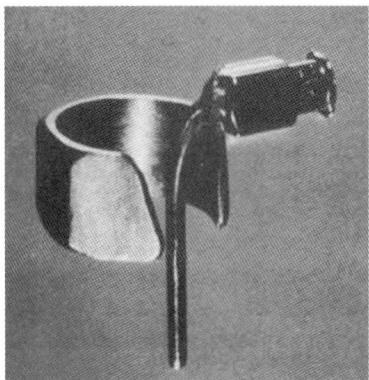

Figure 2. Original injector for Hollinger bronchoscope; collar tapered to fit neck of bronchoscope. (Reproduced with kind permission from the Wood Library–Museum of Anesthesiology, Park Ridge IL, USA.)

Sanders improved his 'jet injector' by soldering a steel intravenous needle to a clip, in order to attach the injector to the proximal end of a Jackson bronchoscope and subsequently to other bronchoscopes (Figure 2). He then placed a simple toggle switch in the pressure line to permit on–off cycling of pulmonary ventilation. He gave the first public demonstration of his injector on 27 September 1966 at the annual meeting of the Academy of Anesthesiology and published details the following year. He generously provided prototypes for colleagues to conduct clinical trials at their own institutions. Several investigators favoured the jet injector technique when comparing it with other general anaesthetic techniques for bronchoscopy. They also described variations and improvements.

The jet ventilation technique soon found other applications. Wolfgang Spoerel in London, Ontario used a plastic intravenous catheter through the cricothyroid membrane for jet ventilation in emergency upper airway obstruction. The technique was adapted for suspension laryngoscopy with the introduction of the short, cuffed Carden endotracheal tube, which incorporated a jet injector tube. Within a decade of Sanders's introduction of the jet principle for conventional pulmonary ventilation, the potential of high-frequency jet ventilation was recognized, investigated and applied to a variety of neonatal, surgical and intensive care clinical situations.

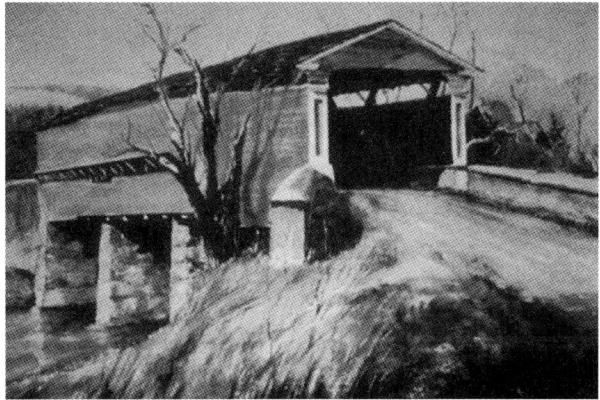

Figure 3. Covered bridge in Delaware backcountry (watercolour). (Reproduced with kind permission from the Wood Library–Museum of Anesthesiology, Park Ridge IL, USA.)

Sanders never patented his devices, nor did he seek reimbursement or royalties from their subsequent commercial production and marketing. His creativity outgrew his finances and, in 1965, he founded the Anesthesia Research Foundation under the aegis of the Delaware Academy of Medicine, and recruited generous private and corporate benefactors.

Sanders loved the sea and the science of navigation and regularly sailed on Chesapeake Bay. His other main hobby was landscape painting. He began painting in the 1950s after a spell in hospital for peptic ulcer disease. He painted mostly outdoor scenes from the countryside of Pennsylvania and Delaware, and the coast of Maine where he spent his summer vacations. He used watercolour (Figure 3) or acrylic in his early works and later preferred egg tempera. He received awards for his paintings at the American Society of Anesthesiologists annual meeting and some of his canvasses hang in the Delaware Art Museum and in Wilmington's Hotel Dupont.

Acknowledgement

Portrait photograph reproduced with kind permission from the Wood Library–Museum of Anesthesiology, Park Ridge, IL, USA.

Further reading

Buckley JJ. Richard Douglas Sanders, M.D. Anesthesiologist, inventor, painter (1906–1977). In: Fink BR, Morris LE, Stephen CR (Eds) *The history of anesthesia third international symposium*. Park Ridge, IL: Wood Library–Museum of Anesthesiology, 1992: 72–7.

Sanders RD. New endotracheal instruments. *Anesthesiology* 1947; 8: 57–61.

Sanders RD. Two ventilating attachments for bronchoscopes. *Delaware Medical Journal* 1967; 39: 170–6.

SCHIMMELBUSCH MASK

Curt Schimmelbusch (1860–1895)

Open methods of administering ether and chloroform were used from the beginning of anaesthesia. Crawford Long gave ether on a towel in 1842 and William Morton saturated his handkerchief with ether to anaesthetize Eben Frost in his dental office on 30 September 1846. Although Morton used a sea sponge in a glass inhaler for his first public demonstration of ether anaesthesia at Massachusetts General Hospital on 16 October 1846, he wrote to the *Lancet* in June 1847 that he had abandoned the inhaler and was using only the sponge. In 1849, John Collins Warren, the Boston surgeon who performed the first operation under ether, administered ether 'freely on a sponge or cloth'. Simpson's open method for chloroform was to gather up a handkerchief

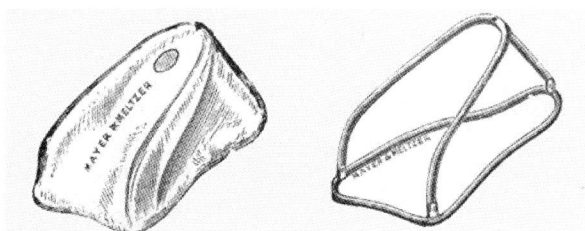

Figure 1. Skinner's frame for chloroform. (Reproduced with permission from *Anaesthetics their uses and administration*, 6th edn, H.K. Lewis & Co, 1920: 270.)

or towel into a cuplike form, pour one or two teaspoonfuls of chloroform into the hollow and place the open end over the patient's nose and mouth. The cloth was held an inch or so from the face for the first few inspirations and then lowered onto the face.

Thomas Skinner, a general practitioner and obstetrician from Liverpool, designed the first wire frame for administration of open drop chloroform in 1862. He covered it with domett, a loosely woven cotton–flannel material (Figure 1), and dropped chloroform onto the upper surface. The obstetrician, surgeon or anaesthetist could conveniently carry the device under his top hat.

Curt Schimmelbusch of Berlin designed the only wire-frame open drop mask that is familiar, at least by name, to present-day anaesthetists (Figure 2). He designed it in 1890 for administering chloroform, ether or

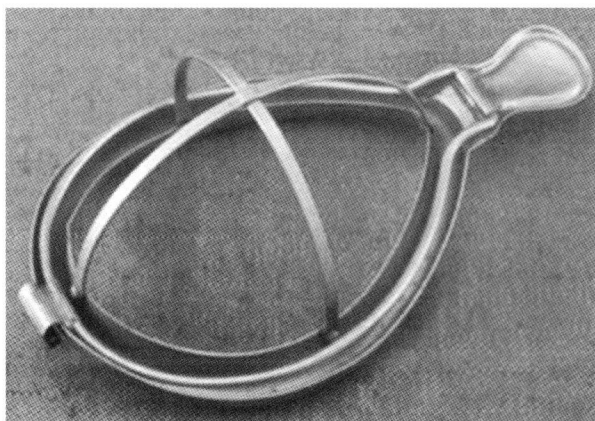

Figure 2. Schimmelbusch mask. (Reproduced with kind permission from the Association of Anaesthetists of Great Britain and Ireland.)

mixtures such as ACE (alcohol, chloroform, ether) when he was an assistant to the surgeon Ernst von Bergmann in Berlin. The mask has a trough-shaped oval rim, with longitudinal and transverse semicircular strips of metal to support the layer of cloth. The trough was designed to prevent excess chloroform from running onto the patient's face and causing blistering. For chloroform, a single layer of cloth was stretched over the frame

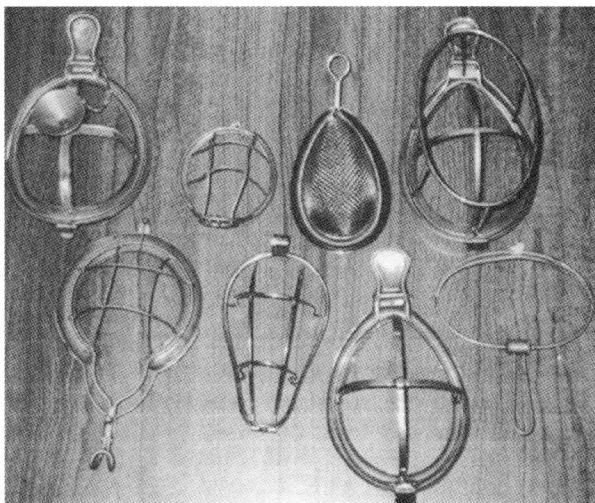

Figure 3. Wire-frame masks. (Reproduced with permission from *A short history of anaesthesia*, Butterworth-Heinemann, 1996: 52.)

and held in place by the hinged rim. For ether, an outer cover of waxed cloth was added. The wire frame could be sterilized by steam and fresh clean cloth was used for each patient.

The Schimmelbusch mask was well-established for several decades. Many modifications were made, including the addition of gas channels for the insufflation of oxygen, gas and vapour mixtures, and even for carbon dioxide from a 'sparklet' bulb. Military surgeons used it in the First and Second World Wars, mostly with chloroform. It continues to be used in smaller hospitals in countries where ether is available and other forms of vaporizer are not available. Schimmelbusch's original mask was still available in 1991 in the catalogue of a reputable German instrument maker and also from Indian manufacturers. Schimmelbusch's mask was comparable to Esmarch's set for chloroform anaesthesia.

Many other anaesthetists and surgeons designed wire-frame masks in the latter half of the 19th century and early part of the 20th (Figure 3). They include John Murray in 1868 (Middlesex Hospital, London), Gustave Jouillard in 1877 (Geneva, Switzerland), Theodore Kocher c. 1890 (Bern, Switzerland), Walter

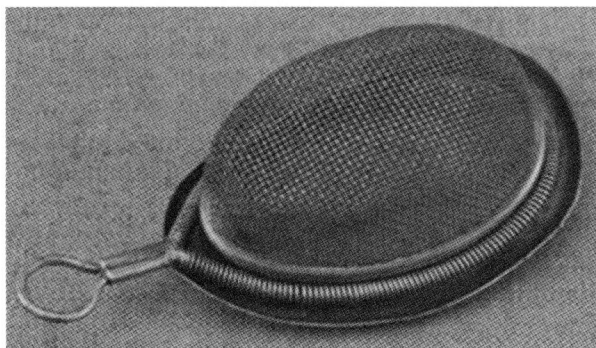

Figure 4. Yankauer mask. (Reproduced with kind permission from the Association of Anaesthetists of Great Britain and Ireland.)

Tyrell *c.* 1890 and Harold Low *c.* 1910 (St Thomas's Hospital, London), and Sidney Yankauer in 1910 (Mount Sinai Hospital, New York).

The Yankauer wire-frame mask (Figure 4) was popular in North America. It was similar to the Schimmelbusch mask in having a gutter to prevent overspill of liquid anaesthetic, but substituted wire mesh for the semicircular wires that supported the gauze. Sidney Yankauer (1882–1932) was an ear, nose and throat specialist and pioneer bronchoscopist who designed many surgical instruments. Anaesthetists are now more familiar with his Yankauer suction tip that is available on nearly every anaesthetic machine and is also used by oral and ear, nose and throat surgeons.

Further reading

Anonymous [Obituary]. Dr. S. Yankauer dies at age of 50. *New York Times* August 28, 1932: page 25 (col 3).

Skinner T. Anaesthesia in midwifery: with new apparatus for safer induction with chloroform. *British Medical Journal* 1862; 2: 108.

Thomas KB. *The development of anaesthetic apparatus.* Oxford, UK: Blackwell Scientific Publications 1975: 249–61.

T.H. SELDON MEMORIAL LECTURE

Thomas Henry Seldon (1905–1991)

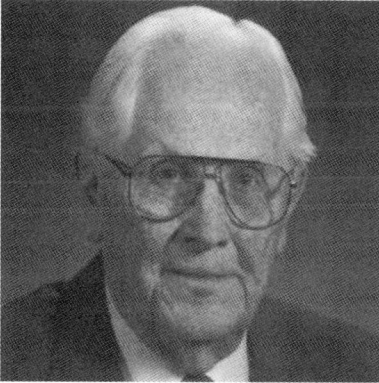

Harry Seldon was born in 1905 in Exeter, Ontario. He graduated MD from Queen's University Medical School in Kingston, Ontario in 1929. After his internship at the Western Hospital in Toronto, Ontario (1929–30), he was a private general practitioner for six years in Sharbot Lake, Ontario.

In April 1936, Seldon moved to Rochester, Minnesota with his wife and infant daughter to become a Fellow in anaesthesia under John Lundy at Mayo Graduate School of Medicine. In 1940, he received a master of surgery degree from the University of Minnesota for his thesis *The Effect of General Anesthetic Agents on Small Blood Vessels* and was appointed to the clinic staff as a consultant in anaesthesia. In 1941, he was certified as a specialist by the American Board of Anesthesiology and was appointed instructor in anesthesia at Mayo Graduate School of Medicine. He was promoted through assistant and associate professor to become a full professor in 1963.

In the early part of his career he was closely involved with blood banking and expanded on Lundy's pioneering efforts. He published over 30 articles on blood transfusion and blood substitutes during the 1940s. He developed a busy blood bank at the Mayo Clinic and was a founding member of the American Association of Blood Banks. He served as its president in 1950 and liaised between them and the American Society of Anesthesiologists (ASA). He was appointed chief of the whole blood programme for the State Civil Defense, Health, Medical and Special Weapons Defense Service in 1960 and was chairman of the ASA committee on blood and blood products in 1968–69.

Seldon was elected to the board of trustees of the International Anesthesia Research Society (IARS) in 1948. When he volunteered for the editorship of its journal, *Current Researches in Anesthesia and Analgesia* in 1954 he inherited a rather feeble publication. He improved and developed it until it became one of the leading anaesthesia journals, commonly referred to as the 'yellow peril' because of the colour of its cover. What began as a hobby became an all-consuming passion. In 1957, he successfully requested that the board of trustees change the title to *Anesthesia and Analgesia – Current Researches* (Figure 1) for easier referencing and to enlarge its historical pocket size to a 7 × 10 inch format. He selected material that was useful and relevant for the practising

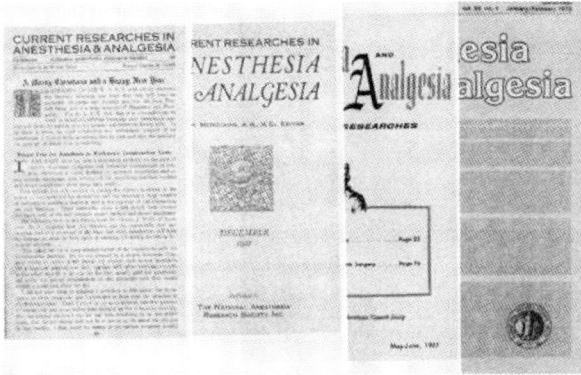

Figure. (Left to right) *Anesthesia and Analgesia* 1922, 1957, 1979. (Reproduced with kind permission from the Wood Library–Museum of Anesthesiology, Park Ridge II, USA.)

anaesthetist and insisted on attractive presentation. He added personal touches to the scientific articles by including a small portrait photograph and brief biographical sketch of each leading author. He also published biographical and academic tributes to current leaders in anaesthesia, including several from countries other than the USA, under the title 'We Salute ...'.

One of his hallmarks was the gentle and friendly manner in which he educated authors and critics without hurting their feelings. He ran a column of 'Office Hints' from 1961 to 1969. His titles suggest that the hints would be as useful now as they were 40 years ago. Here are some examples:

To file or not to file	Don't procrastinate
Building goodwill	Help with medical terms for the secretary
Introducing a speaker	Requesting a favour
Use your dictionary	A sentence should contain one thought
Courteous, friendly phraseology	Write, revise and rewrite

Seldon was a prolific author who wrote more than 100 journal articles from 1939 to 1972. His main interests in addition to blood transfusion were related to regional anaesthesia, including continuous caudal and spinal anaesthesia, sympathetic blocks for treatment of peripheral vascular disease, pharmacology of general anaesthetic agents, management of trauma and shock and the use of powdered red blood cells to stimulate wound healing. He continued as full-time editor of *Anesthesia and Analgesia* for a further seven years after he retired from the staff of Mayo Clinic in 1970.

Seldon was one of three International Anesthesia Research Society representatives on the organizing committee for the proposed World Federation of Societies of Anaesthesiologists (WFSA) in 1953. Although the ASA was not a founder member of the WFSA, and did not join until 1960, he edited the *Proceedings of the First World Congress of Anaesthesiologists* that was held in Scheveningen in The Netherlands in 1955.

Seldon was one of the founders of the Minnesota Society of Anesthesiologists and was its second president. He was elected to Honorary Fellowship of the Faculty of Anaesthetists of the Royal College of Surgeons of Ireland in 1972. He was a member of the Academy of Anesthesiology, the American Association for the History of Medicine and the North Central Chapter American Medical Writers Association of which he was president in 1972.

Table 1. T.H. Seldon lecturers and lecture titles

Year	Lecturer	Title
1983	H. Jeremy C. Swan	Hemodynamic monitoring of the cardiovascular system.
1984	Edmond I Eger (II)	Nitrous oxide – a drug of the past.
1985	M.T. 'Pepper' Jenkins	Standards for excellence.
1986	J. Alfred Lee	Excellence achieved.
1987	John W. Severinghaus	Oximetry: origins, observations and outlook.
1988	Frank K. Standaert	Anesthesia, science and art.
1989	Thomas N. James	A cardiogenic hypertensive chemoreflex.
1990	Arthur S. Keats	Anesthesia mortality in perspective.
1991	Nicholas M. Greene	Anesthesia journals: the backbone of the specialty – past, present, future.
1992	Jerome H. Modell	Anesthesiology: pacesetter or follower?
1993	Lawrence J. Saidman	Relationships between anesthesiology and industry: a mixed blessing.
1994	Joseph C. Gabel	A conception of the future where opportunities prevail.
1995	Harry H. Bird	Health care reform and the politics and policies of limits.
1996	David C. Sabiston, Jr	The development of surgery of the coronary circulation.
1997	James F. Arens	An anesthesiology career: halothane to desflurane.
1998	Robert K. Stoelting	Anesthesiology – a medical specialty with unique challenges.
1999	Edward D. Miller	What path should anesthesiology follow in the 21st century?
2000	John P. Kampine	Challenges to anesthesia practice and theory in the 21st century.
2001	Ronald D. Miller	The role of publications in the future of anesthesia.
2002	Sten G.E. Lindahl	Discoveries: good for mankind.

He was a leader in the Presbyterian Church, a skilled woodworker, displayer of honestly earned trophy fish and an enthusiastic proponent of various civic organizations.

The T.H. Seldon Memorial Lecture is given at the annual congress of the International Anesthesia Research Society (Table 1).

Acknowledgement

Portrait photograph reproduced with kind permission from 'Art to Science' by K. Rehder, P. Southorn and A.D. Sessler.

Further reading

Anonymous. We salute . . . T.H. Seldon, M.D. *Anesthesia and Analgesia* 1972; **51**: 586-7.

Craig DB, Martin JT. Anesthesia and Analgesia: seventy-five years of publication. *Anesthesia and Analgesia* 1977; **85**: 237-47.

Seldon TH. Anesthesia and Analgesia – 50 years of publication. *Anesthesia and Analgesia* 1971; **50**: 571-7.

SELLICK MANOEUVRE

Brian Arthur Sellick (1918–1996)

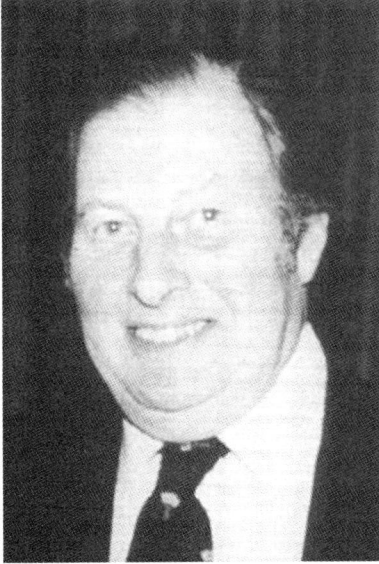

Brian Sellick was born in Dorking, Surrey in 1918, towards the end of the First World War. He was educated at Caterham School, where he played rugby for the first fifteen and at the Middlesex Hospital, London, where he gained his MRCS and LRCP in 1941. He was appointed junior resident anaesthetist and, with Peter Dinnick as senior resident anaesthetist, gave most of the emergency anaesthetics at the hospital during the Blitz. He explained years later that they had only been able to cope because 'surgeons were much quicker in those days!' He was senior resident anaesthetist from 1942 to 1944 and obtained the Diploma in Anaesthetics in 1943.

He served as a specialist anaesthetist in the Royal Naval Volunteer Reserve in the Far East and in Australian waters. After demobilization, he was appointed to the honorary consultant anaesthetic staff of the Middlesex Hospital in 1946 and soon afterwards to both Harefield Hospital and Royal Masonic Hospital. These posts were not salaried until the introduction of the National Health Service in 1948, so he also gave anaesthetics at King Edward VII Hospital for officers and at various sanatoria that treated the post-war epidemic of tuberculosis.

Sellick was one of Britain's early cardiac anaesthetists. In 1956 he visited Henry Swan's clinic in Denver, Colorado to observe the use of hypothermia. He introduced a modified technique at the Middlesex, using extracorporeal cooling on a water-cooled circulating blanket while an intravenous line was inserted and temperature probes positioned. The patient was then put into a cold bath at 15–17°C to which ice was added to cool it down to 8–10°C. Minimal anaesthesia with relaxants and ether were used to vasodilate the patient and accelerate cooling to c. 30°C oesophageal temperature. This allowed circulatory arrest for 8 to 10 minutes to close atrial secundum defects, but was not long enough for repair of atrial primum defects involving the mitral and tricuspid valves and the upper ventricular septum. The following year he reported 32 cases without mortality, attributing that success to teamwork led by the cardiologist Evan Bedford and the surgeon (later Sir) Thomas Holmes Sellors. Sellick was considered not only the leading British expert, but also the European expert in hypothermic anaesthesia.

In 1961, Sellick went to the Mayo Clinic to learn how to use the Mayo–Gibbon vertical screen oxygenator. The Ministry of Health funded three machines for the Middlesex Hospital, Harefield Hospital and the National Heart Hospital. Sellick trained anaesthetists and technicians in their use and maintenance and the Middlesex team ultimately operated on over 400 secundum defects with only one death.

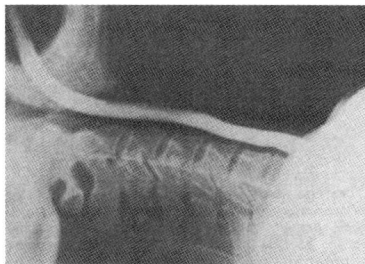

Figure 1. Lateral X-ray of the neck showing soft latex tube in upper oesophagus distended with contrast material. (Reproduced with kind permission from *Lancet* 1961; **2**: 404–6, Elsevier Science.)

Sellick's contributions to cardiac anaesthesia have passed into history but his name lives on because of Sellick's manoeuvre to prevent pulmonary aspiration of gastric contents during tracheal intubation. His seminal 1961 paper in the *Lancet* shows lateral X-rays of the neck

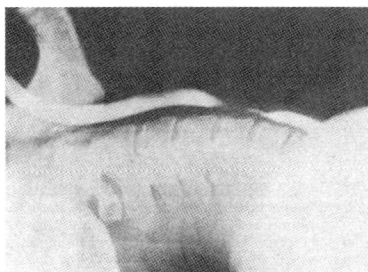

Figure 2. Obliteration of oesophageal lumen by extension of neck and cricoid pressure at the level of C5 vertebra. (Reproduced with kind permission from *Lancet* 1961; **2**: 404–6, Elsevier Science.)

with the oesophagus containing a latex tube filled with contrast medium to a pressure of 100 cm water. Cricoid pressure obliterated the oesophageal lumen and would prevent gastric contents from reaching the pharynx. (Figures 1 and 2). He advocated preoperative passage of a nasogastric tube to empty the stomach as much as possible and its removal before induction of anaesthesia. He recommended light cricoid pressure during preoxygenation, followed by intravenous barbiturate and muscle relaxant and firm application of cricoid pressure (Figures 3 and 4).

'Cricoid pressure must be exerted by an assistant. Before induction, the cricoid is palpated and lightly held between the thumb and second finger; as anaesthesia begins, pressure is exerted on the cricoid cartilage mainly by the index finger. Even a conscious patient can tolerate moderate pressure without discomfort but as soon as consciousness is lost, firm pressure can be applied without obstruction of the patient's airway. Pressure is maintained until intubation and inflation of the cuff of the endotracheal tube is complete. During cricoid pressure the lungs may be ventilated by intermittent positive pressure without risk of gastric distension.'

Sellick recognized that the 'old-fashioned' inhalational induction in the supine or lateral position with head-down tilt had some advantages because if vomiting occurred, it usually did so in light levels of anaesthesia when protective airway reflexes were still present. He criticized use of the sitting position to prevent aspiration because this would predispose to cardiovascular collapse in seriously ill patients and would actually facilitate aspiration if vomiting occurred. He offered cricoid pressure as a third option but warned that it should not be used to control active vomiting because the oesophagus might be damaged by vomiting under high pressure.

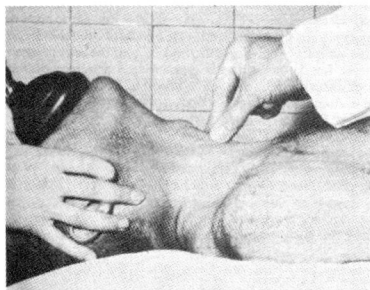

Figure 3. Extended neck and application of cricoid pressure. (Reproduced with kind permission from *Lancet* 1961; 2: 404–6, Elsevier Science.)

He summarized the effectiveness of cricoid pressure in 26 high-risk cases. No regurgitation occurred in 23 of them (laparotomy for intestinal obstruction – 17, gastrectomy for pyloric stenosis – 3, oesophagoscopy of the cardia – 2, forceps delivery – 1). In the remaining three cases, the pharynx filled with gastric contents when the cricoid pressure was removed after intubation, illustrating the effectiveness of the technique for those three cases. He changed what was a frightening and dangerous induction of anaesthesia to a safer and more controlled procedure.

Sellick was elected Fellow of the Faculty of Anaesthetists of the Royal College of Surgeons in 1953. He served on the Board of the Faculty from 1962 to 1978 and was vice-dean from 1972 to 1974. He gave the Sir Frederic Hewitt lecture of the Faculty of Anaesthetists at the Royal College of Surgeons in 1975. He was Hickman Medallist of the Royal Society of Medicine in 1993 and was awarded the Gold Medal of the College of Anaesthetists in 1989.

He retired in 1978 to the Kingsbridge area of Devon where he became chairman of the South Hams Society for 10 years. He was a member of the local history society and an active theatre- and concert-goer. He enjoyed his garden and working in wood and was a regular member of the congregation of Stokenham church. He was a happy, fulfilled man with a great sense of humour whose laughter was always full of glee.

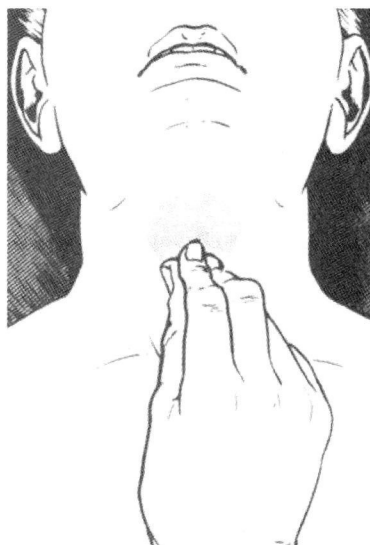

Figure 4. Sellick's diagram for applying cricoid pressure. (Reproduced with kind permission from *Lancet* 1961; 2: 404–6, Elsevier Science.)

Acknowledgement

Portrait photograph reproduced with kind permission from the Association of Anaesthetists of Great Britain and Ireland.

Further reading

Pallister WK [Obituary]. Brian Arthur Sellick MB, BS, FRCA, FFARCS, DA 13 June 1918 to 13 July 1996. *Anaesthesia* 1996; **51**: 1194–5.

Sellick BA. A method of hypothermia for open-heart surgery. *Lancet* 1957; **1**: 443–6.

Sellick BA. Cricoid pressure to control regurgitation of stomach contents during induction of anaesthesia. *Lancet* 1961; **2**: 404–6.

SEVERINGHAUS ELECTRODE

John Wendell Severinghaus (1922–)

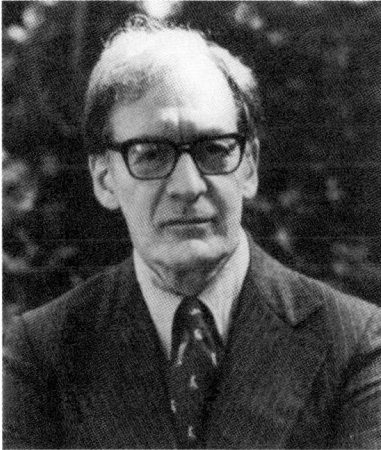

John Severinghaus was born in Madison, Wisconsin in 1922. He is the son of Elmer L. Severinghaus who was professor of medicine at the University of Wisconsin and was President Roosevelt's first Goodwill Ambassador to South America in 1941. He took an undergraduate degree in physics at Haverford, a Quaker College near Philadelphia, Pennsylvania from 1939 to 1943, and he designed radar test equipment at the Massachusetts Institute of Technology (MIT) radiation laboratory during the Second World War. He studied medicine at the University of Wisconsin in Madison and Columbia University in New York City from 1945 to 1949 to prepare for a career in biophysics research. He constructed, sold and published descriptions of the first electrophrenic respirators to several anaesthesia departments while he was still a student.

Severinghaus published the first measurements of the rate of uptake of nitrous oxide during anaesthesia in 1952, during his anaesthesia residency with Robert Dripps at the University of Pennsylvania. He also collaborated with Julius Comroe (1911–84) at the Cardiovascular Research Institute of the University of California, San Francisco (UCSF), and with Robert Forster in studies of dead space in the lung and the pharmacological responses of the carotid body hypoxic chemoreceptors. From 1953 to 1958, he served in the US Public Health Service at the National Institutes of Health as chief of anaesthesia research and as the US government's expert representative on the National Research Council's anaesthesia advisory council. He studied human hypothermia, introduced the term 'alveolar dead space' and developed extremely accurate blood pH monitoring methods.

Richard Stow, a physical chemist at Ohio State University in Columbus, described his invention of a CO_2 electrode at an American Physiologic Society meeting in 1954. He had covered a bulb-shaped pH electrode with a rubber membrane, with a salt solution or distilled water under the rubber. Stow could not make it stable enough for research or clinical use but Severinghaus was in the audience and immediately realized a way to stabilize it by adding sodium bicarbonate to the trapped electrolyte. He suggested this to Stow who replied that the bicarbonate would buffer the solution and eliminate the signal, but agreed that Severinghaus was free to test the idea.

One day of trial showed Severinghaus that his idea worked – bicarbonate both doubled and stabilized the signal. From 1954 to 1956, he and his

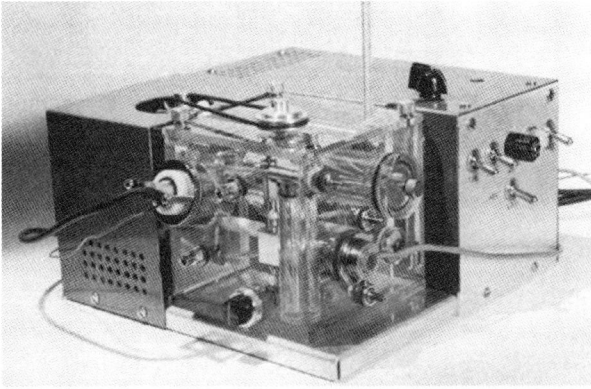

Figure 1. The earliest commercially available blood-gas system, which was demonstrated at the Ciba Symposium in December 1958. (Reproduced with permission from *The history of blood gases, acids and bases,* Munksgaard International Publishers Ltd, Copenhagen, Denmark, 1986.)

technician Freeman Bradley designed, constructed, modified, perfected and tested the CO_2 electrode and used it in their research on pulmonary physiology, especially during hypothermia. In 1956–57, during a second year of anaesthesia residency with Stuart Cullen at the University of Iowa, he designed and built the first blood-gas analysis system. He mounted his CO_2 electrode with a Clark O_2 electrode in a thermostated water bath. The Clark electrode cuvette contained a miniature stirring paddle that was needed for accuracy with the large cathode of this early electrode. One of Severinghaus's early home-made instruments is now in the Smithsonian museum. The first commercial model became available in 1958 (Figure 1), and the paper that described the system was among bioscience's most quoted references in the 1960s. Severinghaus moved to UCSF in 1958 to join Comroe.

Severinghaus took a sabbatical in Copenhagen, Denmark from 1964 to 1965 to learn blood–brain barrier ion transport techniques from H.H. Ussing. Poul Astrup (1915–2000) and Ole Siggaard Andersen had developed accurate thermostated pH analysis and an equilibration method for estimating blood PCO_2 levels with help from the Danish Radiometer Company in Copenhagen. Astrup was trying to create a nomogram to correct PO_2 for the effects of temperature and pH on the oxygen dissociation curve. Knowing that these corrections applied in a logarithmic way to PO_2, Severinghaus designed a blood-gas slide rule with a log PO_2 scale sliding against saturation. The slide rule had settings for pH and temperature and he arranged for its manufacture and distribution by Radiometer. He added scales for the Henderson–Hasselbalch equation, computing base excess, blood pH, PCO_2 and PO_2 temperature corrections, converting gas volumes to either BTPS or STPD at altitudes up to 5500 metres and for reading the true O_2 fraction from expired gas O_2 and CO_2 concentrations.

In order to obtain accurate data for both the human oxygen dissociation curve and the temperature and Bohr effects, he joined Astrup in a group in Aarhus, Denmark. The group consisted of Severinghaus, F.J.W. Roughton of Cambridge and I. Fatt of the University of California, Berkeley, and together they attempted to define the extreme upper and lower ends of the oxygen dissociation curve. In 1979 he published a decade's worth of data defining the standard human curve, Bohr effect variations and a modified Hill equation describing the oxygen dissociation curve. That simple equation remains the most accurate of all published attempts.

Severinghaus is now Emeritus Professor of Anesthesia at UCSF and a senior staff member of the Cardiovascular Research Institute. He continues his research at UCSF, with interests in the biochemical causes of high altitude cerebral oedema, the theory of the limits of oxygen delivery to muscle cytochrome during maximum work, methods of testing human hypoxia responses and instrumentation in anaesthesia.

Severinghaus received the Borden Undergraduate Award in 1949 and the Bicentennial Silver Medallion and Joseph Mather Smith Prize from Columbia University in 1967. He was named UCSF Faculty Research Lecturer in 1981 and received the first ASA Award for Excellence in Research in 1986. He was elected to Fellowship of the Faculty of Anaesthetists of the Royal College of Surgeons in 1975; Doctor of Medicine Honoris Causa at the 500th anniversary of the University of Copenhagen in 1979; and Honorary Fellowship of the Royal College of Anaesthetists in 1989. The Radiometer Company of Copenhagen funded a Radiometer–John W. Severinghaus Anesthesia Research Fellowship and a laboratory at UCSF.

He married Elinor Peck, a Wellesley graduate and artist-educator, in 1948. They have four children and have lived in Ross, California since 1958, where they continue their interests in Democratic politics and a Unitarian Fellowship. Severinghaus is a keen gardener, back-packer, biker and skier. He now struggles with corporate management of his leased local hospital as a member of the public Marin Healthcare District Board, hoping to restore quality health care.

Acknowledgement

Portrait photograph reproduced with kind permission from the Wood Library–Museum of Anesthesiology, Park Ridge, IL, USA.

Further reading

Astrup P, Severinghaus JW. *The history of blood gases, acids and bases.* Copenhagen: Munksgaard, 1986.

Severinghaus JW. Simple accurate equations for human blood O_2 dissociation computations. *Journal of Applied Physiology* 1979; **46**: 599–602.

Severinghaus JW, Bradley AF. Electrodes for blood PO_2 and PCO_2 determination. *Journal of Applied Physiology* 1958; **13**: 515–20.

SIR JAMES YOUNG SIMPSON
MEMORIAL LECTURE

James Young Simpson (1811–1870)

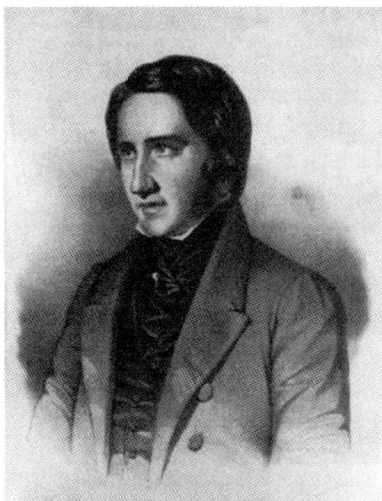

James Simpson was born in 1811 in Bathgate (Figure 1), near Edinburgh in Scotland. He added the name Young after he became a doctor, one explanation being that he appeared youthful and was known to his friends as 'Young Simpson'. He was the seventh son of David Simpson, who was a baker and whose wife was the dominant partner in the business as well as the family. The family all made sacrifices for James, the brightest son, so that he could be well educated and go to university.

Simpson entered Edinburgh University at the age of 14 and learned Greek, Latin and mathematics in his first year. He enrolled as a medical student in his second year and was awarded a bursary of £10 per year. He had an intensely critical mind and was not afraid to challenge the established ideas of his teachers. He graduated in 1830, one month before his 19th birthday and became a LRCSEd.

He spent some months assisting in general practices in Falkirk and Bathgate. He then returned to Edinburgh, completed an MD thesis *Death from Inflammation* in Latin and became assistant to the professor of pathology. Simpson immersed himself in the study in the neglected field of obstetrics and gynaecology. He also began to teach classes outside of the university, to participate in meetings of societies and to write for journals. In 1835 he visited leading medical centres in London, Paris and Belgium, and he published his presidential address to the Royal Medical Society in German and other languages. In 1840, still only 29 years old, he canvassed vigorously for the chair of midwifery. Edinburgh city council, whose members elected

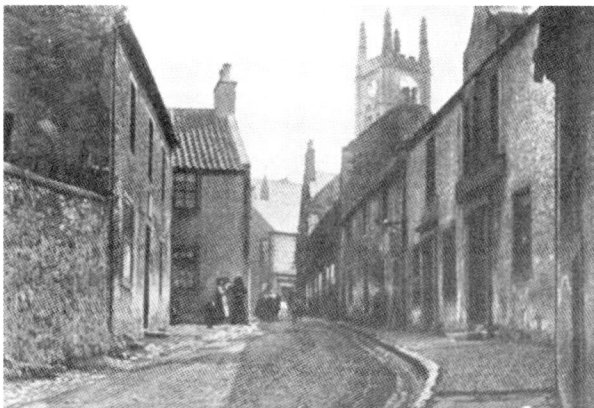

Figure 1. Main Street, Bathgate. Simpson was born in the house in the left foreground. (Reproduced from *Simpson and Syme of Edinburgh*, E. and S. Livingstone, 1969: 144.)

their university professors, chose Simpson by one vote.

Simpson had tremendous energy, working and writing at all hours of the day and night. He had great charm, but also entered enthusiastically into any debate with his medical colleagues and university academics. He was well prepared for the controversy that ensued when he introduced and promoted ether and chloroform for pain relief in childbirth.

Robert Liston performed a leg amputation under ether at University College Hospital, London on 21 December 1846 and immediately wrote to the Edinburgh surgeon, James Millar, who lived next door to Simpson. Simpson went to London at the end of December to visit Liston and to hear the news first-hand. Although Simpson was concerned that ether might stop uterine contractions, cause convulsions or damage the baby, he administered it on 19 January 1847 to a woman with a contracted pelvis. The woman's previous labour had lasted four days and the baby had eventually been extracted in pieces. Simpson administered ether for 20 minutes, turned the infant and delivered the limbs and trunk. Delivery of the head was extremely difficult and the child died. However, the mother 'quickly regained full consciousness and talked with gratitude and wonderment of her delivery and her insensibility to the pains of it'.

On the same day, Simpson received the letter stating his appointment as Queen's Physician in Scotland. He wrote to his brother that he was; 'far less interested in [the appointment] than in having delivered a woman this week without any pain while inhaling sulphuric ether. I can think of naught else'. He published a full report on using ether in natural labour as well as for forceps or operative deliveries in the Edinburgh *Monthly Journal of Medical Science* in March 1847. He soon faced opposition on various grounds from other authoritative obstetricians. Those who opposed it on medical grounds feared adverse consequences to the mother or child. Simpson refuted these claims by collecting data in 1848 from colleagues whose experience totalled more than 800 cases. Those who opposed it on moral grounds likened its effects to those of alcohol, claiming that it caused 'lascivious thought'. To those who said it was 'unnatural', Simpson suggested that travelling by ship or by stagecoach instead of swimming or walking was equally unnatural. He wrote a well-argued pamphlet (Figure 2) to answer religious opposition, which appears not to have come from the Church as an organization, but from individual patients, doctors or clerics.

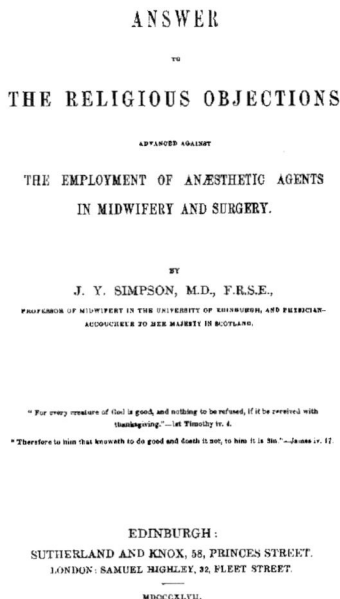

ANSWER

TO

THE RELIGIOUS OBJECTIONS

ADVANCED AGAINST

THE EMPLOYMENT OF ANÆSTHETIC AGENTS
IN MIDWIFERY AND SURGERY.

BY

J. Y. SIMPSON, M.D., F.R.S.E.,

PROFESSOR OF MIDWIFERY IN THE UNIVERSITY OF EDINBURGH, AND PHYSICIAN-
ACCOUCHEUR TO HER MAJESTY IN SCOTLAND.

"For every creature of God is good, and nothing to be refused, if it be received with thanksgiving."—1st Timothy iv. 4.
"Therefore to him that knoweth to do good and doeth it not, to him it is Sin."—James iv. 17.

EDINBURGH:
SUTHERLAND AND KNOX, 58, PRINCES STREET.
LONDON: SAMUEL HIGHLEY, 32, FLEET STREET.

MDCCXLVII.

Figure 2. Title page of Simpson's pamphlet in answer to the religious objections to the use of anaesthetic agents in childbirth and surgery.

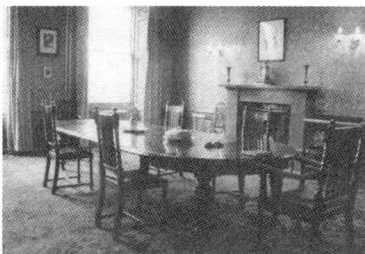

Figure 3. The dining table in Discovery Room at Simpson House, 52 Queen Street, Edinburgh. (Reproduced from Simpson House, Edinburgh.)

Simpson immediately began looking for an agent that provided a more rapid induction, was pleasant to inhale and was more potent so that only a small bottle would need to be carried up flights of stairs in a patient's home. He and his medical friends tested many volatile liquids in the autumn of 1847. David Waldie, a pharmacist in Liverpool Apothecaries Hall, suggested that chloroform might meet Simpson's requirements. Simpson and his colleagues Matthews Duncan and George Keith inhaled chloroform in Simpson's dining room on the evening of 4 November 1847. All three fell unconscious under the dining room table (Figure 3), and on awakening, Simpson's first thought was that 'This is far stronger and better than ether ... '.

Simpson first used chloroform on 8 November 1847 in an obstetrical case; 'on a pocket handkerchief rolled up into a funnel shape'. His first pamphlet on chloroform, acknowledging Waldie's contribution in a footnote, appeared on 15 November, by which date Simpson had successfully administered it for three surgical operations at the Edinburgh Royal Infirmary.

Simpson contributed to the history of archaeology and was president of the Society of Antiquaries in Scotland in 1861. He received a knighthood in 1866 and was given the freedom of the City of Edinburgh. By the time of his death, Simpson was one of the best-known and most influential physicians in Europe. More than 30,000 mourners lined the streets of Edinburgh for his funeral.

The Church of Scotland now owns his house at 52 Queen Street in Edinburgh (Figure 3) and maintains the 'discovery room' unchanged. A statue of Simpson stands on Princes Street in Edinburgh and there is a Simpson memorial plaque in Westminster Abbey. Simpson's Hotel in Edinburgh's old town was originally opened in 1879 as the Edinburgh Royal Maternity and Simpson Memorial Hospital. Simpson Maternity Pavilion is now part of Edinburgh Royal Infirmary. The first James Young Simpson gold medal of the Royal College of Surgeons of Edinburgh was awarded in 1965. The recipient also delivers the Simpson memorial lecture – this rotates between an obstetrician, an anaesthetist, a surgeon and a physician. A Simpson memorial plaque was dedicated in St. Giles Cathedral in Edinburgh in September 1997 to mark the 150th anniversary of chloroform.

Acknowledgement

Portrait photograph reproduced from Simpson House, Edinburgh.

Further reading

Farr AD. Religious opposition to obstetric anaesthesia: a myth? *Annals of Science* 1983; **40**: 159–77.

Shepherd JA. *Simpson and Syme of Edinburgh*. Edinburgh, UK: E. and S. Livingstone, 1969.

Simpson M. *Simpson the obstetrician*. London, UK: Victor Gollancz Ltd, 1972.

JOHN SNOW MEMORIAL LECTURE

John Snow (1813–1858)

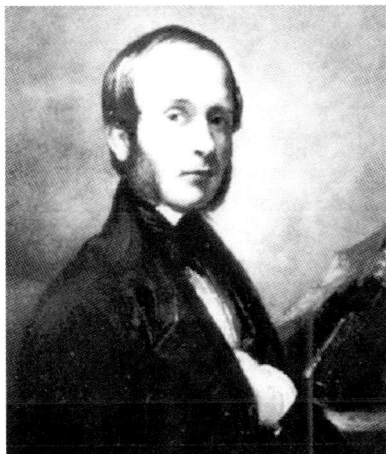

John Snow was born in 1813 in York, Yorkshire, the eldest son of a farmer. He was educated at a private school in York until he was 14, when he began a five-year apprenticeship with William Hardcastle, a surgeon in Newcastle upon Tyne. During his apprenticeship he became a vegetarian and decided to abstain from alcohol. This lasted for most of his life. During the cholera epidemic of 1831–32, Hardcastle sent him to provide care at the nearby Killingworth colliery even though he was still unqualified. After his apprenticeship, he worked as an assistant at Burnop Field near Newcastle and at Pateley Bridge in Yorkshire.

In the summer of 1836, Snow walked 200 miles (300 km) to London to enrol at the Hunterian School of Medicine in Great Windmill Street and later at Westminster Hospital. He gained the MRCS and LSA in 1838 and set up practice in the Soho district of London. He continued to study and obtained his MB, BS from the University of London in 1843, the higher degree of MD by thesis in 1844 and LRCP in 1850.

He regularly attended the meetings of the Westminster Medical Society. In 1841, Snow presented a paper: *On asphyxia, and on the resuscitation of stillborn children* in which he described a device for artificial respiration in the newborn. The device consisted of two syringes fixed side-by-side, each with two valves. When the pistons were raised, one cylinder filled with air from the lungs through an oral tube while the other filled with fresh air. When the pistons were depressed, the first cylinder emptied its exhaled air to the atmosphere and the second delivered the same volume of fresh air through a nasal tube to the lungs.

The first ether anaesthetic in England was administered on 19 December 1846 by James Robinson (1813–62), a dentist in Gower Street, London for extraction of a molar tooth. Snow visited Robinson on 28 December to see him remove a tooth painlessly under ether. Snow began to experiment on animals and himself and he gave his first anaesthetic to a patient in January 1847. Within months, Snow became England's leading anaesthetist. He described his first ether inhaler in the *Lancet* on 30 January, and his definitive model in mid-1847 (Figures 1 and 2). When James Simpson introduced chloroform in Edinburgh in November 1847, Snow

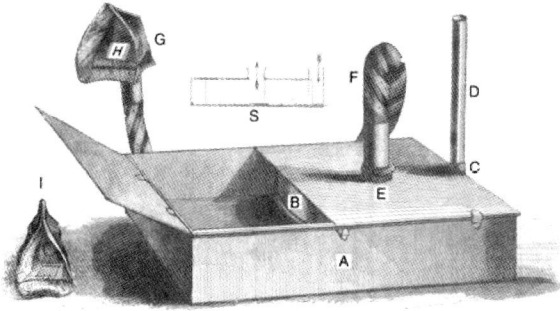

Figure 1. Snow's ether inhaler. A, box of japanned tin or plated copper for storage of breathing tube and mask, or water bath when in use. B, movable spiral ether chamber. F, elastic tube about three feet long. G, facemask. (Reproduced with kind permission from the Wood Library-Museum of Anesthesiology, Park Ridge IL, USA.)

soon changed to chloroform and designed a cylindrical chloroform vaporizer (Figure 3).

There was no scientific base for anaesthesia in 1846–47, and Snow began to lay the foundations. He applied his knowledge of physics to the design of vaporizers. He established the relationship between blood concentrations of anaesthetics and depth of anaesthesia; he experimented with ether and chloroform in birds and frogs; he discussed the clinical use of chloroform in extremes of age, hysteria, epilepsy, pregnancy and pulmonary disease; and he looked at possible causes of death under chloroform. He tested closed-circuit ether on himself, using potassium hydroxide in a to-and-fro closed system to absorb carbon dioxide.

Snow administered anaesthetics for London's leading surgeons in the main operating sessions at St. George's and other London hospitals, and in private practice in the patient's home or lodgings, the surgeon's premises and sometimes in London hotels. He had an extensive private practice with West End dentists as well as his general practice.

Snow administered chloroform to Queen Victoria at the births of Prince Leopold on 7 April 1853 and Princess Beatrice on 14 April 1857. He gave the Queen 'chloroform à la reine', 10–15 drops intermittently on a handkerchief for 53 minutes, and the 'blessed chloroform' met with the Queen's warm approval. Although this event has often been quoted as ending religious opposition to pain relief in childbirth, it was not widely publicised and it now appears that religious opposition had all but disappeared five years earlier.

Snow's second claim to fame came from his epidemiological studies during the 1848–49 and 1854 outbreaks of cholera in England. One school believed that cholera spread through the miasma or environment, the other thought it was contagious. Snow believed from his Killingworth colliery days that it was transmitted by contaminated food, hands and clothing but that contaminated water was the most important source. He proved that it was water-borne during the 1848–49 epidemic. His door-to-door inquiries

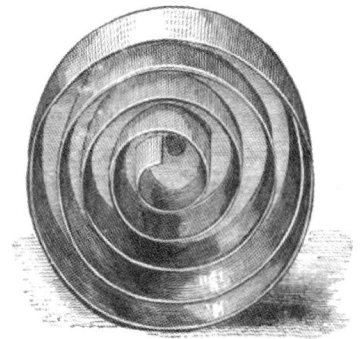

Figure 2. Spiral ether chamber. (Reproduced with kind permission from the Wood Library-Museum of Anesthesiology, Park Ridge IL, USA.)

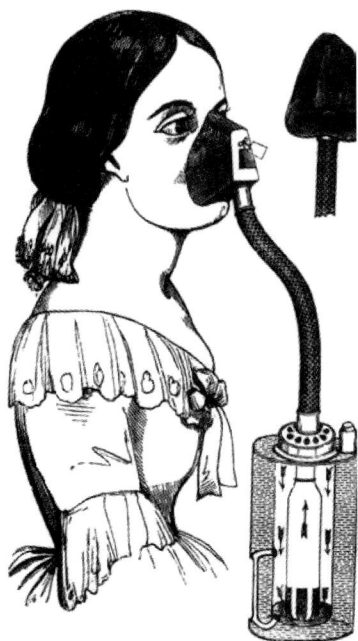

Figure 3. Snow's chloroform inhaler. (Reproduced with kind permission from the Wood Library-Museum of Anesthesiology, Park Ridge IL, USA.)

in south London revealed a much higher incidence in houses whose water company drew sewage-contaminated water from the River Thames compared with those supplied by a company that drew water from several miles upstream. During the 1854 epidemic, Snow made door-to-door inquiries in the Broad (now Broadwick) Street area of Soho, where 578 deaths occurred in 10 days. Almost all the deaths occurred in families that lived near the Broad Street pump or obtained water from it. Snow persuaded the parish council that this was the source of the outbreak and they took his advice to remove the pump handle.

Snow published *On the Inhalation of Ether in Surgical Operations* in 1847, a series of papers titled *On Narcotism by the Inhalation of Vapours* between 1848 and 1852, *On the Mode of Communication of Cholera* in 1855 and *On Chloroform and Other Anaesthetics* posthumously in 1858. He suffered from tuberculosis and kidney disease and died of a stroke at the age of 45 while he was completing the book. Snow's casebooks were transcribed and edited by Richard Ellis (1937–95) who added an introduction and index.

The Association of Anaesthetists of Great Britain and Ireland inaugurated the John Snow Medal for distinguished services in 1947 and the John Snow memorial lecture at the annual scientific meeting in 1958. Eminent individuals from other professions as well as from medicine have given the lecture; and only five anaesthetists have given it. The John Snow public house (Figure 4) stands on the corner of Broadwick Street and Lexington Street, a few metres from a replica of the Broad Street pump. The John Snow Society at the Royal Institute of Public Health was founded in 1993 and John Snow International, founded in Boston, Massachusetts has public health projects in over 20 developing countries. Snow's tombstone is near the north entrance to Brompton Cemetery in London.

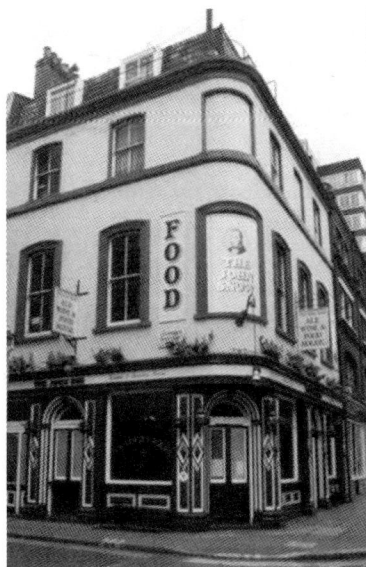

Figure 4. John Snow public house in Soho, London. (Reproduced with kind permission from the Association of Anaesthetists of Great Britain and Ireland.)

Acknowledgement

Portrait photograph reproduced with kind permission from The London School of Hygiene and Tropical Medicine.

Further reading

Ellis RH (Ed.). *The case books of John Snow.* London, UK: Wellcome Institute for the History of Medicine, 1994.

Shephard DAE. *John Snow anaesthetist to a Queen and epidemiologist to a nation.* Cornwall, Prince Edward Island, Canada: York Point Publishing, 1995.

Snow J. *On chloroform and other anaesthetics.* London: John Churchill, 1858. (Reprinted in 1988 by the Wood Library–Museum of Anesthesiology, Park Ridge IL, USA.)

PULMONARY ARTERY
(SWAN-GANZ) CATHETER

Harold Jeremy C. Swan (1922-)
and William Ganz (1919-)

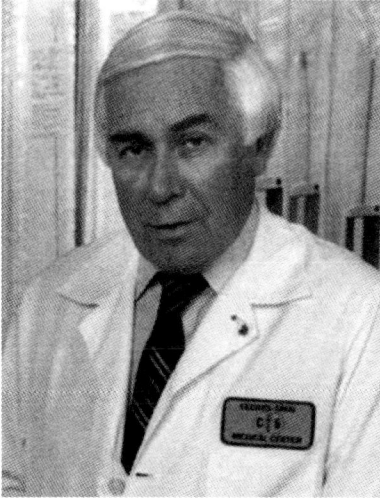

Jeremy Swan

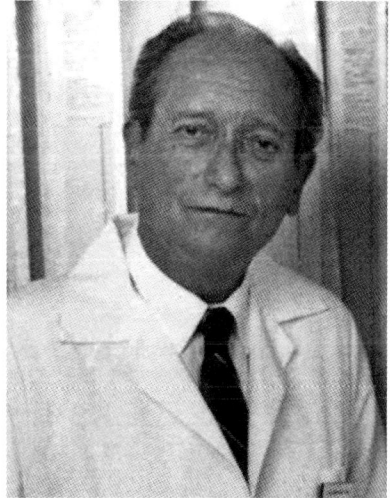

William Ganz

Jeremy Swan, born in Ireland, was a medical student with the late Derek Wylie (1919–98) and Harry Churchill-Davidson at St Thomas' Hospital in London, England between 1939–45. After completing a PhD in human physiology in 1951 under the late Henry Barcroft FRS, he left England for a two-year appointment at the Mayo Clinic in Rochester, Minnesota. He actually remained there for 14 years before becoming chief of cardiology at Cedars Sinai Medical Center in Los Angeles, California and professor of medicine at the University of California, Los Angeles in 1965.

William Ganz, born in Czechoslovakia, escaped the Nazi persecution of the early 1940s. He received his MD degree from Charles University, Prague in 1947 and attained a senior position at the Cardiovascular Institute in Prague. In 1967 he joined Swan's department at Cedars Sinai as an established scientist with a special interest in thermodilution.

Right heart catheterization (RHC) was just emerging in 1950. It provided an understanding of the pathophysiology of congenital and acquired heart disease and proved basic to the development of surgical correction of congenital malformations and valvular stenosis. It was 'the key in the lock' for clinical cardiology, which enabled important new quantitative measurements of cardiac function to be made. Swan became expert in the technique and an enthusiastic and well-published investigator. However, early techniques required patients to be transported to special laboratories equipped with fluoroscopy machines and a variety of measuring devices. Standard cardiac catheters could cause vascular or cardiac perforation and subendocardial haemorrhage. They were inevitably associated with significant ectopy and rarely with ventricular fibrillation.

Cedars Sinai was a large community hospital that served many elderly patients with atherosclerosis and acute myocardial infarction. Little was known about the haemodynamic consequences of myocardial ischaemia and infarction in humans, and knowledge was also limited in animal models. RHCs had been attempted in the acute phase of infarction in conventional laboratory facilities under fluoroscopic control, but reports of prolonged ventricular tachycardia using stiff catheters and serious adverse outcomes, particularly in the sicker patients, were disturbing. Swan's earlier experiences at Mayo were confirmed. It was essential to achieve safe and rapid RHC in the critical care unit without transferring the patient to a formal fluoroscopy facility.

When Swan was an instructor in physiology at St Thomas' Hospital Medical School in 1950, he had become acquainted with Ronald Bradley, a BSc student. Bradley later described the insertion of fine Sylastic tubes percutaneously into the jugular vein in man, and allowing them to float passively into the right ventricle and pulmonary artery. Swan now attempted Bradley's approach in several patients in the intensive and coronary care units at Cedars Sinai. He had limited success in reaching the pulmonary artery and an unexpectedly high incidence of ventricular ectopy. The breakthrough came in the autumn of 1967. A woman with congestive heart failure was given 20 minutes of unsuccessful manipulation of a Bradley-type catheter without complaint, and then she asked, 'Is my heart too big?'

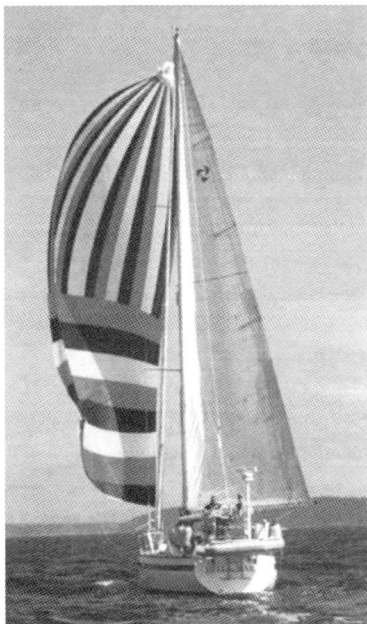

The next day was hot and nearly windless. Swan was with his young children on the beach at Santa Monica when he noticed a sailboat with a large spinnaker (Figure 1) making good progress in spite of light winds. The analogy of the situation to the large heart the night before was clear and the solution seemed evident. A soft catheter of high flexibility with an effective floatation device might pass into the pulmonary circulation consistently, rapidly and without manipulation.

Figure 1. Yacht flying a spinnaker. (Image courtesy of N.C. Watson.)

Swan had acted as consultant to American–Edwards Laboratories who manufactured the Starr–Edwards heart valve and the Fogarty extraction catheter. Edwards was not interested in designing and developing Swan's proposed sail or parachute on a catheter. David Chonette, vice-president of development, suggested that they should test the principle with a balloon catheter that would require minimal investment. Some months later, six hand-fabricated flexible balloon floatation catheters were delivered. Swan and Ganz placed the first catheter in the right atrium of a dog. They inflated the balloon

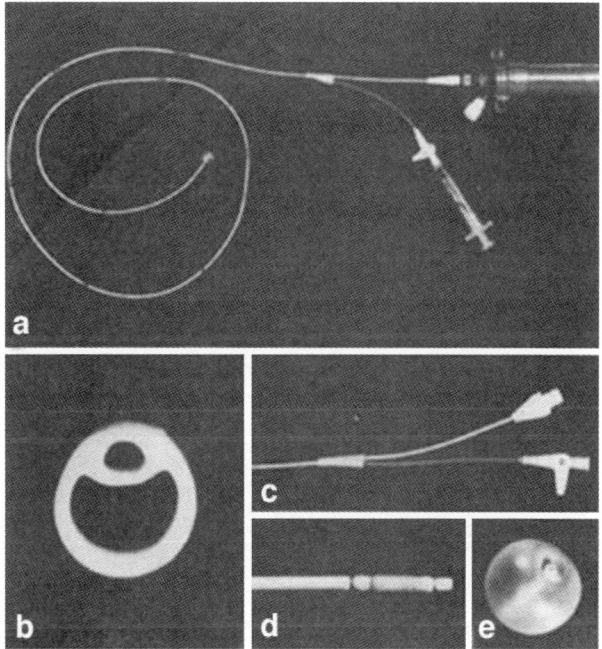

Figure 2. Construction of the pulmonary artery catheter. a) catheter attached to strain-gauge manometer. b) minor inflation lumen and major blood sampling and pressure recording lumen. c) colour coded connector for 1mL and one-way stopcock. d) deflated balloon. e) catheter tip with balloon inflated. (Reproduced from *New England Journal of Medicine* 1970; 283: 447–51. Copyright ©1970 Massachusetts Medical Society. All rights reserved.)

and the catheter immediately disappeared from the fluoroscopic screen without showing right ventricular or pulmonary artery pressures. In one systole, flowing blood and right ventricular contraction had transported the balloon to the pulmonary artery wedge, the 'PA occluded' position. On deflation, the shaft of the catheter immediately returned to the right atrium.

After brief additional experience in the animal laboratory, they used the device for human RHC with and without fluoroscope, with equally gratifying results. The effectiveness of right heart and pulmonary artery catheterization without fluoroscopy or catheter manipulation was proven within the week, and near absence of ectopy during passage of the catheter was a bonus. Federal Device Legislation and Institutional Review Boards did not exist at that time, so they proceeded directly to bedside catheterization in the coronary care unit. Ganz's practical experience in thermodilution later led to the incorporation of a thermistor into the catheter shaft and the development of bedside measurement of cardiac output. Their first paper, published in the *New England Journal of Medicine* on 27 August 1970, became one of the most quoted references over the next two years. The fundamental design of the device described in 1970 (Figure 2) is essentially unchanged after 32 years.

There is no question of its value in the diagnostic catheterization laboratory or in the evaluation of new procedures and drugs in the cardiovascular system. Anaesthetists and critical care specialists use it as an important adjunct during and after surgery in a variety of critically ill patients. The most debated application of the pulmonary artery catheter is the management of critically ill non-surgical patients outside the operating theatre. The procedure must be planned to provide certain specific pre-defined information, relevant to the clinical or research question. Swan has stated that haemodynamic monitoring has little to offer a patient in the absence of an effective therapeutic plan. If the root cause of an illness or disorder cannot be eradicated or modified, or if no intervention is considered to be effective, then haemodynamic monitoring has no place in the management of such patients.

Among their numerous awards, Swan received the Thomas H. Seldon Award of the International Anesthesia Research Society in 1983 and Ganz received the Distinguished Scientist Award of the American College of Cardiology in 1992.

Further reading

Bradley RD. Diagnostic right-heart catheterisation with miniature catheters in severely ill patients. *Lancet* 1964; 2: 941–2.

Cournand AF. Control of the pulmonary circulation in man with some remarks on methodology. In: *Nobel Lectures. Physiology and Medicine (1942–1962) vol. 3.* Amsterdam: Elsevier, 1964: 529–42.

Swan HJC, Ganz W, Forrester J, Marcus H, Diamond G, Chonette D. Catheterization of the heart in man with use of a flow-directed balloon-tipped catheter. *New England Journal of Medicine* 1970; 283: 447–51.

TRENDELENBURG POSITION

Friedrich Trendelenburg (1844–1924)

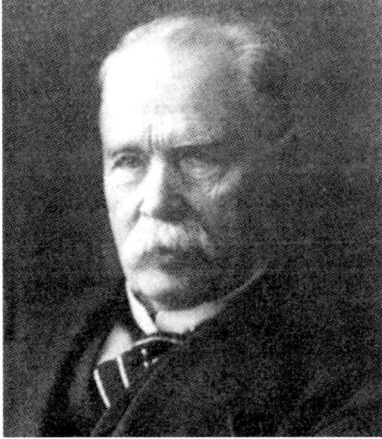

Friedrich Trendelenburg was born in 1884 in Berlin, Germany, the son of Adolf Trendelenburg who became a professor of philosophy. His mother was a teacher and they educated him at home until he was 10 years old. He then attended the Joachimsthal Gymnasium and was the top student when he completed his studies. He was still only 17, so his father sent him to Scotland to the family of a Glasgow publisher to give German lessons. A professor friend of Adolf Trendelenburg allowed Friedrich to sit in on anatomy classes and Joseph (later Lord) Lister's clinical lectures.

Trendelenburg took his medical training at the University of Berlin where he graduated MD in 1866. He was an assistant to the professor of surgery, Bernhard von Langenbeck, from 1868 to 1874 when he was appointed surgeon at the Friedrichshain Hospital in Berlin. He progressed up the professional and academic ladder and was appointed professor of surgery successively at the Universities of Rostock in 1875, Bonn in 1882, and Leipzig in 1885 (Figure 1) – where he remained until 1911.

Trendelenburg prevented the aspiration of blood and debris into the trachea by employing a tracheostomy for major operations on the head and neck in which bleeding into the mouth or pharynx might occur. He anaesthetized the patient and then performed a tracheostomy through which he introduced a metal cannula with a tampon or an inflatable double-walled cuff of India rubber. The cannula was then connected to Trendelenburg's cone via a long flexible tube. The cone was covered with a layer of flannel on to which the anaesthetic was dripped. Fresh air could be drawn in through a ring of holes below the rim of the cone.

The link between Trendelenburg's name and the

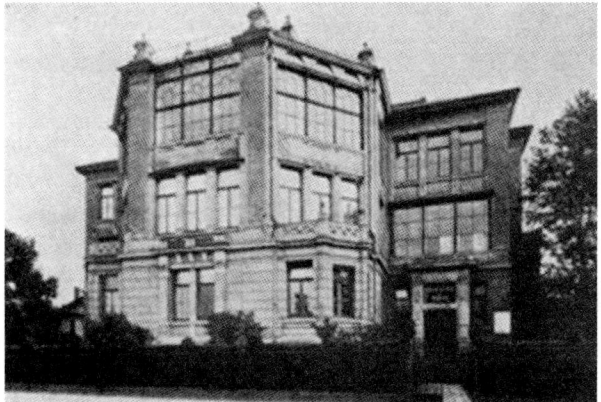

Figure 1. The Surgical Institute, Leipzig where Trendelenburg worked. (Reproduced with permission from *Notable Names in medicine and surgery, 4th edn*, H.K. Lewis and Co, 1983: 225.)

steep pelvis-up, head-down tilt for pelvic surgery is serendipitous. The position had long been used to relieve acute urinary retention. Celsus, in the 1st century CE, and others in the 7th and 10th centuries suggested an inclined position for hernia repair. Later surgeons found that a head-down position facilitated suprapubic cystotomy. In his autobiography, Trendelenburg described his first use of the elevated pelvic position during his Rostock years from 1875 to 1882. He found it useful in surgery for bladder stones, strangulated hernia and gynaecological surgery, especially transvesical repair of vesicovaginal fistula. It was Willy Meyer, Trendelenburg's assistant in Bonn and later a well-known New York surgeon, who publicised the Trendelenburg position in 1885.

The classic Trendelenburg position of 30–45 degree head-down tilt (Figure 2) required some means of preventing the patient from sliding down the operating table. At first, an assistant was needed to support each leg. Later, he built an operating table with padded shoulder braces.

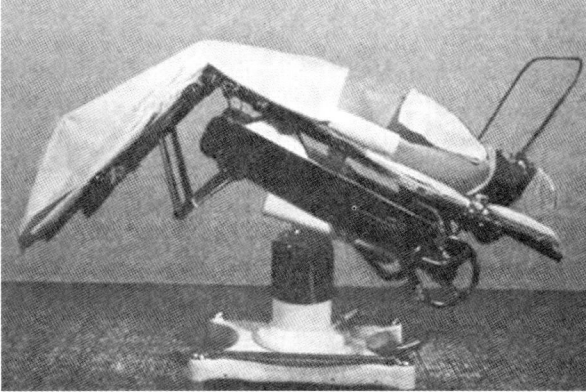

Figure 2. Trendelenburg position. (Reproduced with permission from *Principles of Anesthesiology, 2nd edn*, Lea and Febiger, 1976: 160.)

Wristlets fixed to the table have been used but they may stretch the brachial plexus by the drag of the patient's weight, or cause ischaemia of the hand. In 1953, Langton Hewer (1896–1986), an anaesthetist at St Bartholomew's Hospital, London described a contoured antistatic rubber mattress to support the Achilles tendons, lumbar spine and neck. This prevented a patient from slipping, even at 45 degrees. If the patient was exceptionally heavy, he recommended fitting precautionary shoulder rests that did not actually touch the patient. Brachial plexus palsy had been reported from pressure by shoulder pieces, especially if placed close to the neck, and was more likely if one or both arms were abducted. With the better operating conditions provided by muscle relaxants and positive pressure ventilation over the past 50 years, 10–15 degrees tilt is adequate and the full Trendelenburg tilt is no longer necessary.

During the First World War, the Trendelenburg position was used in the treatment of shock, the rationale being that improved venous return from the lower limbs improved cerebral circulation. Gaston Labat, a pioneer of regional anaesthesia, believed that the Trendelenburg position averted the danger of reduced cerebral perfusion from vasodilatation in the lower half of the body and retarded respiratory failure after induction of spinal anaesthesia. He recommended the position if there was pallor of the patient's face, whether or not this was associated with shallow breathing. Nausea and vomiting were said to be more frequent with the Trendelenburg position because the weight of the abdominal organs caused the diaphragm to contract more strongly. This would increase the negative intrathoracic pressure and dilate the oesophagus.

Trendelenburg was a leader in the major advances of surgery in the second half of the 19th century and described many new operations. He did exceptional work in plastic surgery, congenital dislocation of the hip, surgery of blood vessels and gynaecology. His name is given to the test for incompetence of the valves of veins in the thigh, although the British surgeon Benjamin Brodie (1783–1862) had described the same test in 1846. The Trendelenburg name is also given to a test to confirm shortening of a leg from congenital dislocation of the hip or non-union of a fracture of the femur.

In 1907, he described a surgical approach to pulmonary embolectomy that he had worked out in sheep. His first and only clinical case, in 1908, was a 70-year-old woman who collapsed six days after a fracture of the femoral neck. Trendelenburg took eight minutes to reach the hospital and only five minutes from incision to opening the pulmonary artery. He had no method of artificial ventilation to counteract the pneumothorax under open drop ether and the patient died. However, his pupil Martin Kirschner (1879–1942) of Griefswald and later of Heidelberg performed a successful pulmonary embolectomy in 1924.

Trendelenburg and von Langenbeck founded the German Society of Surgeons, and Trendelenburg was elected president in 1898. He regretted that most doctors lacked interest in history. He believed that; 'Today always rests on the foundations of Yesterday, and it is a matter of the highest interest to trace the gradual development.' He spent the closing years of his life at Nikolassee in Germany and his autobiography was published just before he died from carcinoma of the lower jaw.

Acknowledgement

Portrait photograph reproduced from *Notable names in medicine and surgery, 3rd edn*, H.K. Lewis and Co., 1959: 138.

Further reading

Bernstein AM, Koo HP, Bloom DA. Beyond the Trendelenburg position: Friedrich Trendelenburg's life and surgical contributions. *Surgery* 1999; **126**: 78–82.

Ellis H. *Bailey and Bishop's notable names in medicine and surgery, 4th edn*. London, UK: H.K. Lewis and Co, 1983: 224–5.

Wangensteen OH, Wangensteen SD. *The rise of surgery from empiric craft to scientific discipline*. Minneapolis, MN: University of Minnesota Press, 1978.

TUOHY NEEDLE

Edward Boyce Tuohy (1908–1959)

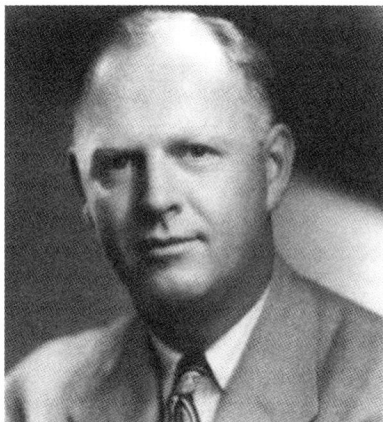

Edward Tuohy was born in 1908 in Duluth, Minnesota. He attended Duluth High School and gained a Bachelor of Science from the University of Minnesota in 1929. He graduated in medicine in 1932 from the University of Pennsylvania in Philadelphia and interned at Roosevelt Hospital and New York Hospital in New York City and Ancker Hospital in St Paul, Minnesota. He entered the Mayo Clinic in Rochester, Minnesota as a fellow in medicine in 1933, but changed to anaesthesia in 1935. He was appointed to the staff as a consultant later that year and in 1936 he became the first anaesthetist in the USA to defend a masters of surgery thesis.

Continuous spinal anaesthesia was first described in 1906 by Henry Dean, a surgeon in London, England but the technique did not become popular. William Lemmon, a professor of surgery at Jefferson Medical College of Philadelphia, Pennsylvania revived the technique in 1940. He had a special operating table with a rubber mattress that was five inches thick with a notch to accommodate the needle (Figure 1). His equipment was similar to that of Dean. He used 17- or 18-gauge malleable spinal needles 2.5–3.5 inches (6.25–8.75 cm) long that were made of German silver. He filled a 10 mL glass syringe with 10% procaine, placed it by the patient's head and connected it via a stopcock to the hub of the needle by about 36 inches (90 cm) of very hard, narrow bore (2 mL capacity) rubber tubing. The technique was credited with reducing the mortality from abdominal wounds from 46 to 12.5% in one American unit during the Second World War.

Tuohy liked being able to give fractional doses for long cases, but found Lemmon's technique to be complicated. Lumbar puncture was difficult because the malleable needle bent easily and sometimes the bevel of the needle pushed but did

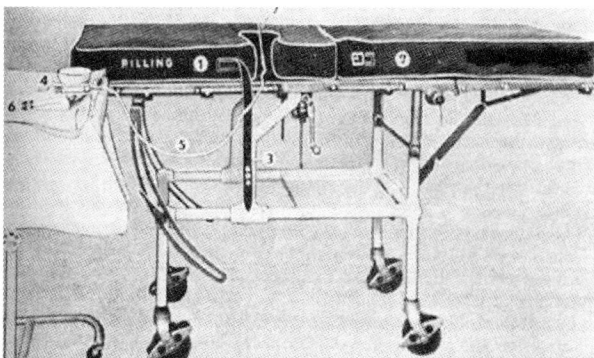

Figure 1. Lemmon mattress and equipment for continuous spinal anaesthesia. (Reproduced from *Foundations of anesthesiology, vol II*, Charles C Thomas, 1965: 885.)

not puncture the dura and arachnoid. To avoid dislodging the needle, two or three assistants were needed to turn patients from the left lateral to supine position. Tuohy's idea of using a

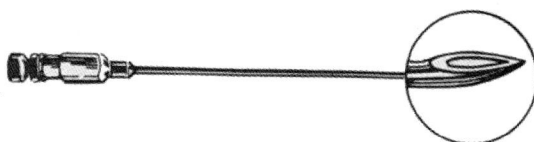

Figure 2. Tip of Tuohy needle. (Reproduced from *Anesthesia and Analgesia* 1966; **45**: 514–19, with permission from Lippincott Williams & Wilkins.)

ureteral catheter for continuous spinal anaesthetics came from others who had already described its use for continuous caudal anaesthesia in 1943, and its earlier use for continuous lumbar subarachnoid drainage for meningitis in 1935. In 1944, he described his alternative technique of passing a size 4 ureteral catheter *through* a 15-gauge spinal needle instead of Lemmon's *end-to-end* attachment of rubber tubing to the hub of the needle. He advanced the catheter 4–5 cm into the subarachnoid space and then removed the needle. When the initial dose of procaine had been injected, the catheter was taped to the patient's side and the 10 mL syringe near the patient's shoulder was attached using a rubber adapter or a 22-gauge needle. The technique was more complicated than a single-shot spinal, so he recommended it only for difficult hernia repairs, laparotomies, biliary tract surgery and lengthy orthopaedic surgery on the lower limbs.

Tuohy first mentioned the 15-gauge needle with a Huber point (Figure 2), manufactured by Becton Dickinson, in 1945. Tuohy claimed no originality for the design, but drew attention to advantages of its lateral opening. This prevented any possibility of plugging with tissue when the stylet was in place, and the closed bevel enabled the anaesthetist to direct the catheter either cephalad or caudad as desired. It was not until 1949 that M.M. Curbelo of Havana, Cuba who had watched Tuohy using the Huber-tipped needles for continuous spinal anaesthesia and Charles Flowers in Baltimore independently described their use of the 'Tuohy' needle for continuous epidural anaesthesia.

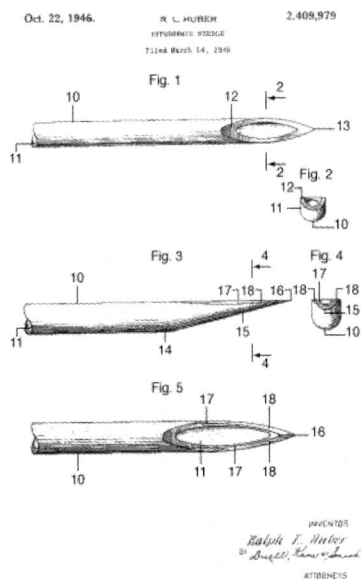

Figure 3. Diagram of tip of hypodermic needle in Huber's patent application. The bevel is closed and the orifice lies parallel to the shaft of the needle. (Reproduced with kind permission from the Wood Library–Museum of Anesthesiology, Park Ridge IL, USA.)

The distinctive tip was not designed by Tuohy, but by Ralph L. Huber (1890–1953) who was a dentist and inventor in Seattle, Washington. Huber omitted to describe his closed bevel design in the medical literature and Joseph Eldor in Jerusalem, Israel recently discovered that Huber applied for US patent No. 2,409,979 on 14 March 1946 (Figure 3). This was a continuation in part of his copending application, filed on 11 March 1943, for a hypodermic needle. He described the needle as one with a perfectly circular body and a tubular bore. After cutting through the tube near the tip at an angle of 15–30 degrees, the end portion is bent to provide a cut face parallel to the axis of the needle and in line with one straight outer edge of the body. This fits Tuohy's 1945 description of the Huber tip of his spinal needle. The original design of the Tuohy needle has undergone many modifications by blunting and alteration of the radius of curvature of the tip, addition of wings to the hub and centimetre markings to the shaft.

Tuohy became professor of anesthesiology and head of the department of anesthesiology at Georgetown Medical Center in Washington DC (1947–52) and clinical professor of anaesthesiology, University of Southern California Medical School in Los Angeles from 1952. He was president of the American Society of Anesthesiologists in 1957, having been given number 248 when it became a national society in 1936. He died from a stroke at the early age of fifty.

Acknowledgement

Portrait photograph reproduced with kind permission from 'Art to Science' by K Rehder, P Southorn and AD Sessler.

Further reading

Eldor J. Huber needle and Tuohy catheter. *Regional Anesthesia* 1995; **20**: 252–3.
Schorr MR. Needles: some points to think about part II. *Anesthesia and Analgesia* 1966; **45**: 514–19.
Tuohy EB. Continuous spinal anesthesia: a new method utilizing a ureteral catheter. *Surgical Clinics of North America* 1945; **25**: 834–40.

WATERS CIRCUIT

Ralph Milton Waters (1883–1979)

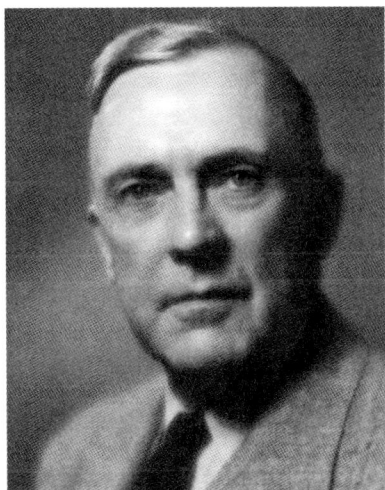

Ralph Waters was born in 1883, the only son of a pioneer family in the village of North Bloomfield in northeast Ohio. Before the age of seven, he rode his black pony Juby with his dog Rover at his heels as he herded cows and sheep on the farm. The family moved a few miles north to Austinburg where Waters attended the Grand River Academy. He graduated in the liberal arts from Adelbert College of Case Western Reserve University in Cleveland in 1907 and graduated from Case Western Medical School in 1912. During his years as a medical student, he also worked in other hospitals as an orderly. This may have contributed to the practical commonsense he showed in medical matters.

After an internship at the German Hospital in Cleveland, Waters took over a general medical practice in the Mississippi valley town of Sioux City, Iowa. Within a few months the local surgeons were calling upon him, with increasing frequency, to provide anaesthesia for their patients. He gradually limited his practice to anaesthesia and, after two to three years, he began to develop new ideas about this neglected field. One of these ideas led to his creation of a successful 'downtown anesthesia clinic' in 1916, with operating room and adjacent recovery area, nearly half a century before the resurgence and proliferation of the current non-hospital and day surgery facilities.

Waters became known outside his local area for the design and promotion of the new and economical to-and-fro carbon dioxide absorption system in the early 1920s. He interposed the Waters canister (containing soda lime granules) between the mask and breathing bag to remove carbon dioxide from the rebreathed gases (Figure 1). In 1915, Dennis Jackson (1878–1930), associate professor of pharmacology in St Louis, Missouri had described a closed-circle system with caustic liquid alkali for use on laboratory animals. Waters preferred the to-and-fro system to the circle because it minimized potential leaks and he could have the canister and breathing bag on the pillow close to the patient's head. This

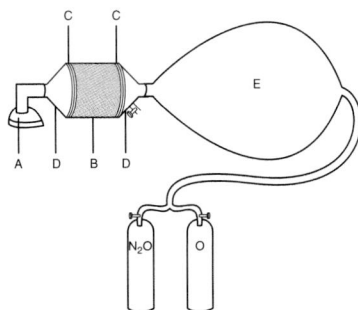

Figure 1. Waters circuit 1924. (A) mask with rubber cushion. (B) soda lime canister 3.5 inches diameter and 4 inches long. (C) wire gauze dams. (D) cone-shaped ends; stop-cock for sampling carbon dioxide. (E) rebreathing bag. (Reproduced from *Anesthesia and Analgesia* 1924; 3: 20–2, with permission fromLippincott Williams & Wilkins.)

made it easy to observe and assist respiration, rather than having to look and reach back to the machine. However, his correspondence with the Foregger Company in the mid to late 1920s reveals his insistence that a circle absorption system should also be available. The circle system eventually became the more popular mode. The closed circuit was economical, conserved heat and minimized anaesthetic pollution of the operating theatre. In later years Mrs. Waters laughingly took some credit for the introduction of the closed system into anaesthesia because she had protested against Waters coming home from work smelling like an ether pot!

The closed carbon dioxide absorption system, originally introduced for ether, attained its greatest use in the two decades following Waters's introduction of cyclopropane, which was expensive and explosive. Cyclopropane eventually went out of favour in the late 1950s and early 1960s as halothane and other non-flammable volatile agents became available. At the same time, manufacturers produced vaporizers that were primarily designed for high-flow systems and were inaccurate at low flows. In recent years, with the advent of anaesthetic agent monitors, there has been a resurgence of interest in low-flow anaesthesia that Waters did so much to promote.

Waters was appointed assistant professor of surgery in charge of anaesthesia at the University of Wisconsin at Madison in 1927. Six years later, in 1933, he was appointed the first full professor of anesthesia in Madison – the first position of its kind. He established the first truly academic programme for training anaesthetists, enlisting basic science colleagues in physiology and pharmacology and initiating research. In less than a decade, Madison became a 'Mecca' in the world of anaesthesia. Waters visited Robert Macintosh in Oxford in 1936, where he inspired interest in John Snow, the English pioneer whom he greatly admired. Macintosh was elected to the newly endowed chair of the Nuffield Department of Anaesthetics in 1937 and returned the visit to see Waters's department in action. These two great leaders had regular correspondence over the next 30 years, which was a benefit to anaesthesia on both sides of the Atlantic.

Waters was actively involved in the founding of the American Board of Anesthesiology in 1938 and served as president of its board of directors. He introduced and investigated new agents, and reinvestigated chloroform in its centenary year. He designed the Waters metal oropharyngeal airway with a side tube for insufflation or suction (Figure 2), cuffs for endotracheal tubes, the Wisconsin folding laryngoscope and equipment for oxygen therapy and resuscitation.

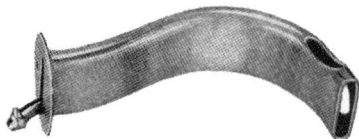

Figure 2. Waters insufflation or suction airway c. 1930. (Reproduced with kind permission from the Wood Library-Museum of Anesthesiology, Park Ridge IL, USA.)

Waters's most important contribution was undoubtedly the establishment of the postgraduate academic programme of education and research for physicians in anaesthesia at the University of Wisconsin, which became the model for subsequent training programmes worldwide. This led to a change in perception of anaesthesia from that of merely a technical exercise to that of dedicated care by a specialist physician before, during and after an anaesthetic. Many of Waters's trainees, the 'Aqua-alumni', from Madison became the second generation of department chairmen, who in turn trained many of those of the third generation shown in the 'Waters tree' (Figure 3). Waters retired to Florida in 1949, where he remained until his death at the age of 96.

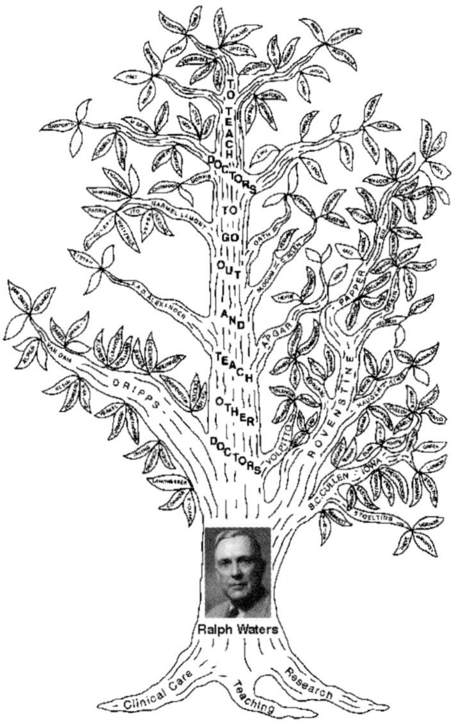

Ralph Waters received honours in Europe as well as America. The Section of Anaesthetics of the Royal Society of Medicine and the Association of Anaesthetists of Great Britain and Ireland elected him to Honorary Membership during his visit to England in 1936. He was Hickman Medallist of the Royal Society of Medicine in 1944, and was elected to one of the first Honorary Fellowships of the Faculty of Anaesthetists of the Royal College of Surgeons of England, in 1948. The King of Sweden awarded him the Order of the Vasa, First Class, in 1947 in recognition of him teaching the first four anaesthetists

Figure 3. Waters tree showing second generation (branches) and third generation (leaves) of anaesthetists who had Waters ancestry. (Reproduced with kind permission from the Wood Library–Museum of Anesthesiology, Park Ridge IL, USA.)

in Sweden – all of whom trained in Madison. He was president of the American Society of Anesthesiologists in 1945 and received its Distinguished Service Award in 1946. His department in Madison has established a Ralph M. Waters visiting professor programme and the Midwest Anesthesia Conference sponsors an annual Ralph M. Waters award and lecture.

Acknowledgement

Portrait photograph reproduced with kind permission from the Wood Library–Museum of Anesthesiology, Park Ridge, IL, USA.

Further reading

Gillespie NA. Ralph Milton Waters: a brief biography. *British Journal of Anaesthesia* 1949; 21: 197–214.

Waters RM. Clinical scope and utility of carbon dioxide filtration in inhalation anesthesia. *Anesthesia and Analgesia* 1924; 3; 20–2.

Waters R.M. The downtown anesthesia clinic. *American Journal of Surgery – Anesthesia Supplement* 1919; 33: 71–73.

WATERTON LAKES NATIONAL PARK

Charles Waterton (1782–1865)

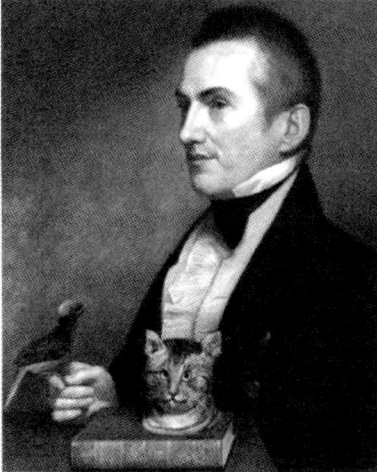

Charles Waterton was born in 1782 at Walton Hall, near Wakefield in Yorkshire. He was known as the 'Squire of Walton Hall' and became one of England's best-known 19th century naturalists and taxidermists. He was educated at Stonyhurst College in Lancashire by Jesuit priests, with whom he kept up correspondence and visits throughout his life. In 1804, Waterton left England to manage family estates in Demerara, in what is now Guyana.

He gave up management of the estates in 1812 and set off from Stabroek, now Georgetown, on the first of four 'wanderings' in South America. The objectives of his three-month expedition by canoe accompanied by six savages, were to collect the strongest samples of curare he could find and to reach the inland frontier post of Portuguese Guiana. The party proceeded up the Demerara River for about 400 miles, portaged across to the Essequibo River, followed one of its tributaries and portaged again into a tributary of the Rio Branco to arrive at Fort San Joachim.

Waterton's enthusiasm to study curare seems to have come from an evening he and an uncle spent with Sir Joseph Banks, president of the Royal Society [of London for the Improvement of Natural History Knowledge] in London, in probably about 1800. After dinner they discussed foreign lands. the 'Indian poison' and how the natives used it in hunting. Sir Joseph said that he was a great traveller and that he was not convinced that curare was strong enough to kill larger animals. Charles Waterton was a keen naturalist, an astute observer and he loved challenges.

About half way up the Demerara River, at an Indian habitation, Waterton obtained his first sample of curare:

> 'A small quantity of the wourali [curare] poison was procured. It was in a little gourd. The Indian who had it, said that he had killed a number of wild hogs with it, and two tapirs. Appearances seemed to confirm what he said; for on one side it had been nearly taken out to the bottom, at different times, which probably would not have been the case, had the first or second trial failed.'

Waterton tested its strength in the thigh of a medium-sized dog. Within four minutes the dog began to stagger, lay down and was dead in 15 minutes. He noticed that its heart continued to beat for several minutes after the rest of the body was motionless. A curare-tipped blowpipe arrow (Figure 1) killed a fowl in five minutes.

He collected more samples at various points on the expedition and finally tested it on a large, well-fed ox. He used three wild hog arrows (Figure 2), one into each thigh and the third into the extremity of the nostril. The curare began to take effect in four minutes:

'The ox set himself firmly on his legs and did not move until the fourteenth minute. He tried to walk, staggered and fell. He breathed hard and emitted foam from his mouth, then he gradually became weaker and in a minute or two more his head and forelegs stopped moving. His heart continued beating faintly for several more minutes but in twenty-five minutes from the time of being wounded he was quite dead.'

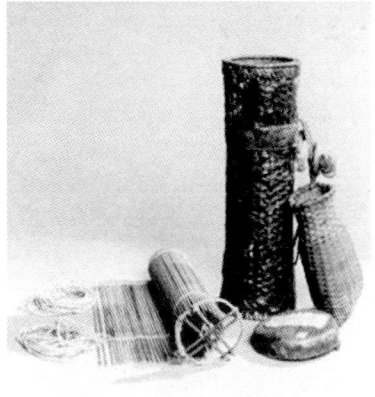

Figure 1. Waterton's quiver and blowpipe arrows. (Image reproduced with kind permission from Wakefield M.D.C. Museums and Arts.)

Waterton concluded that the fowl died in five minutes and the ox in 25 minutes because he had given proportionately more curare to the fowl.

He described how the Macushi Indians, who made the most potent curare, simmered vines and two bulbous plants to produce thick syrup and then tested its strength on arrows. They could shoot blowpipe arrows 300 feet through their smooth 10-foot-long blowpipes to kill birds and small animals.

Waterton asked the Indians if there was an antidote. They told him of pouring sugar cane juice or rum down the throat of an animal or submerging a wounded animal up to its mouth in water. He tried these remedies several times and they always failed. He added that it was 'supposed by some, that wind, introduced into the lungs by means of a small pair of bellows, would revive the poisoned patient, provided the operation be continued for a sufficient length of time.'

Waterton brought blowpipe arrows, a quiver, arrowheads and a block of curare back to England and these are now in Wakefield Museum. In 1814, after he had recovered from a severe bout of malaria, he tested the effectiveness of artificial respiration on a curarized she-ass with the surgeon Sir Benjamin Brodie, and Mr. Sewell of the London Veterinary College. They administered curare in the shoulder

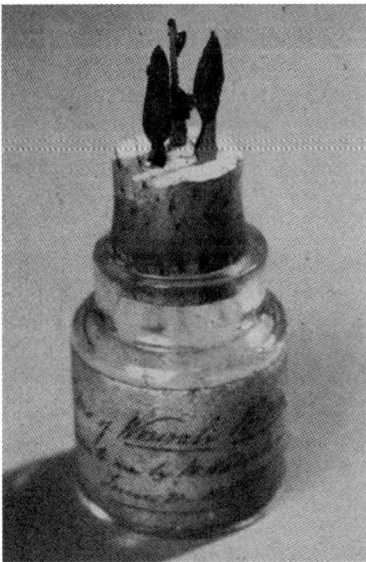

Figure 2. Wourali-tipped arrowheads. The label reads 'Spikes of Wourali Poison given to me by Mr. Waterton June 20, 1839 T. G. W.' (Image reproduced with kind permission from Wakefield M.D.C. Museums and Arts.)

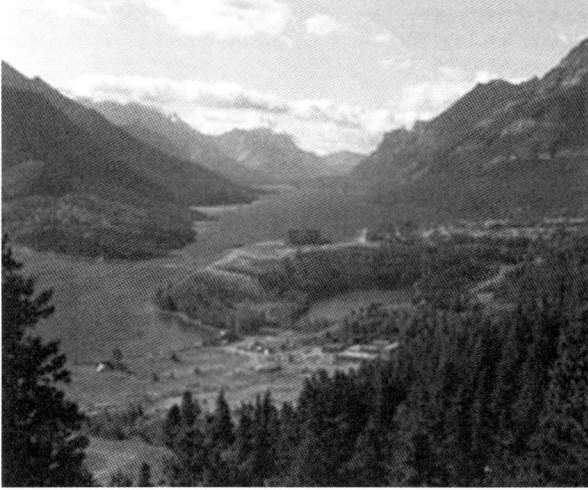

Figure 3. Waterton Lakes National Park, Canada.

region, then performed a tracheotomy and ventilated its lungs with a pair of bellows for two hours. Waterton recorded that this 'saved the ass from final dissolution; she rose up, and walked about; she seemed neither in agitation or pain. She looked lean and sickly for about a year but began to mend the spring after.' He named the donkey Wooralia and took her to Walton Hall where she lived in retirement for 25 years. When she breathed her last on 15 February 1839, he published her obituary in the *St. James Chronicle.*

Waterton devoted much of the remainder of his life to establishing the world's first nature reserve at Walton Hall and to natural history and taxidermy. His home on the Walton Hall estate is now the Waterton Park Hotel.

Waterton Lakes National Park in southern Alberta lies on the Canada–USA border. Charles Waterton never saw the lakes that were named in his honour in 1858 by Thomas Blakiston, a member of the Palliser Expedition (1857–59) who, like Waterton, was a traveller, ornithologist, and taxidermist. The park is noted for its magnificent scenery (Figure 3), variety of plant life and habitat for deer, moose, elk and bears. In 1932, the park was joined with Glacier National Park in Montana to form the Waterton-Glacier International Peace Park, the first international peace park in the world.

Acknowledgement

Portrait photograph repoduced with kind permission from the National Portrait Gallery, London.

Further reading

Edginton B. *Charles Waterton: a biography.* Cambridge, UK: The Lutterworth Press, 1996.

Maltby JR. Charles Waterton (1782–1865): curare and a Canadian national park. *Canadian Anaesthetists' Society Journal* 1982; **29**: 195–202.

Waterton C. *Wanderings in South America, the Northwest of the United States and the Antilles in the Years 1812, 1816, 1820 and 1824.* London, UK: Mawman, 1825.

WHITACRE SPINAL NEEDLE

Rolland John Whitacre (1909–1956)

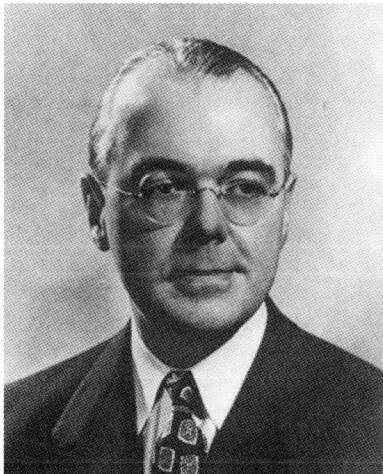

Rolland Whitacre was born in 1909 in Vandergrift, Pennsylvania. He received his premedical training at the University of Pittsburgh, Pennsylvania from 1927 to 1929, and graduated in medicine from Hahnemann Medical College in Philadelphia, Pennsylvania in 1933. He served his internship at Huron Road Hospital in Cleveland, Ohio and became the first full-time anaesthetist in Cleveland. He founded the department of anesthesiology at Huron Road Hospital in 1935 and under his direction it became one of the largest and best-known teaching departments in the country. He was certified as a specialist by the American Board of Anesthesiology in 1939, the year after it was founded.

Whitacre is best known for the pencil-point spinal needle that he and his colleague James Hart described in the *Journal of the American Medical Association* in 1951. Whitacre designed the needle and Hart, who went on to practice in Sandusky, Ohio, helped with its clinical evaluation. Whitacre and Hart got the idea from a paper written in 1926 by H.M. Greene of Portland, Oregon, who sharpened an ordinary 22-gauge spinal needle to a rounded tip, and removed the cutting edges of the bevel. Greene believed that a rounded tip would separate rather than cut or tear the dural fibres and he had only two postspinal headaches in 250 consecutive punctures. Whitacre and Hart asked the Becton Dickinson Company to make a 20-gauge needle with a solid tip (like a finely sharpened pencil point) with the opening on the side of the needle, just proximal to the solid tip (Figure 1). Becton Dickinson manufactured the needle and named it the Whitacre needle.

In 1950, the reported incidence of postspinal headache was approximately 10%. This varied with diagnostic standards applied to headaches due to spinal tap. At Whitacre's hospital, typical postspinal headache occurred in 103 patients in a series of 2070 consecutive spinal punctures, or an incidence of 5% when a 20-gauge short-bevel needle was used. After the pencil-point needle was adopted, 69 headaches developed in 3489 spinal taps, an incidence of 2%, and were usually less severe and shorter lasting.

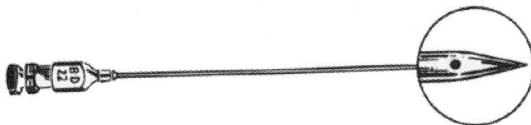

Figure 1. Whitacre needle c. 1951. (Reproduced from *Anesthesia and Analgesia* 1966; 45: 514–19.)

The early Whitacre needles had a very small orifice so that aspiration and injection were difficult. The orifice could be blocked by tissue because the stylet did not occlude it and the reusable needle was difficult to sharpen. Becton Dickinson's disposable Whitacre needle had a larger, oblong orifice. Obstetrical anaesthetists' emphasis on prevention of post-spinal headaches in the 1980s led to renewed interest in pencil-point spinal needles that are now produced by several manufacturers. The important features are believed to be that the orifice should be near the tip, neither large enough to allow multi-compartment injection and weakening of the tip, nor so small that its cross-sectional area is less than that of the lumen of the needle shaft. The Whitacre needle has persisted for 50 years, and has one of the most enduring needle-tip designs.

Whitacre was recognized internationally for pioneering many of the major clinical developments in his field. He was an associate editor of *Anesthesiology* from 1946 and a member of the editorial board of *Current Researches in Anesthesia and Analgesia*. He also incorporated the monthly case history material of the Ohio Anesthesia Study Commission with a summary of all published material about anaesthesia in *Anesthesia Digest*, which he edited and published at his own expense. He guided anaesthesia study commissions in Ohio and elsewhere in his eagerness to find and eradicate the causes of deaths under anaesthesia.

Whitacre was a participant in discussions for a world federation of anaesthesia societies. The five-member Interim Committee from Canada, Belgium, France, Great Britain and Ireland, and Sweden was established in Paris in 1951. Eleven additional members joined in 1953. These included Whitacre from Cleveland, Harry Seldon of Rochester, Minnesota and William Friend of Akron, Ohio. These three joined Harold Griffith of Montreal in June 1953 to fly to Europe to attend a meeting of the Interim Committee in Brussels, Belgium and to see as much as possible of France, Belgium, England and Scotland. Griffith was chairman of the Interim Committee and Whitacre, Seldon and Friend represented the International Anesthesia Research Society. Whitacre and Seldon had never been abroad, and Griffith helped them to make as many professional contacts as possible in the different countries. This meeting eventually led to the formation of the World Federation of Societies of Anaesthesiologists in 1955.

Rolland Whitacre held many high offices before his early death from a sudden heart attack at the age of 46. He was executive secretary and a member of the board of trustees of the International Anesthesia Research Society from 1945; president of the American Board of Anesthesiology; president of the American Society of Anesthesiologists in 1950; chairman of the Section on Anesthesiology of the American Medical Association in 1953 and president of the Academy of Anesthesiology from its birth in 1952 until 1955. He was given the Distinguished Service Award of the American Society of Anesthesiologists posthumously in 1956.

Acknowledgement

Portrait photograph reproduced with kind permission from the Wood Library–Museum of Anesthesiology, Park Ridge, IL, USA.

Further reading

Anonymous [Obituary]. Rolland J. Whitacre, M.D. *Anesthesia and Analgesia* 1956; **35**: 145–7.

Griffith HR. Plans for a world federation of anaesthesiologists. In: Maltby JR, Shephard DAE (Eds). Harold Griffith his life and legacy. *Canadian Journal of Anaesthesia* 1992; **39 Suppl (1)**: 88–91.

Hart JR, Whitacre RJ. Pencil-point needle in prevention of postspinal headache. *Journal of the American Medical Association* 1951; **147**: 657–8.

Wood Library–Museum of Anesthesiology

Paul Meyer Wood (1894–1963)

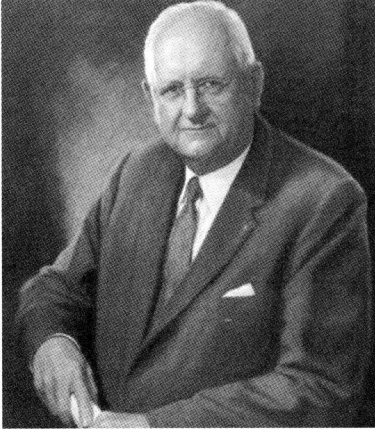

Paul Wood was born in 1894 in Frankfort, Indiana. His father wrote a doctorate thesis on hypnosis and taught psychology and his mother taught language and art. Their home library had more than 14,000 volumes. As a young boy he used old orange crates for bookcases and set up his own lending library with a card for each of his classmates. He decided on a medical career by the time he was 11 years old, and began to collect and catalogue old textbooks and interesting medical items. He studied medical sciences, colour photography and chemistry at Notre Dame College in South Bend, Indiana and graduated from Columbia College in New York in 1917. He interrupted his medical studies to organize and serve in an ambulance company in Italy in the First World War and was decorated by the Italian Government with the Croce de Guerra. He graduated in medicine from Columbia University in 1922, served with the Grenfell Medical Mission in Newfoundland and Labrador for one year and interned at Roosevelt Hospital in New York City in 1923–24.

After declaring to a fellow intern that anaesthesia and obstetrics were both so messy and stupid that he would never go into them, he accepted an appointment as director of obstetrical anesthesia at Fifth Avenue Hospital! He learned how to administer anaesthetics from Paluel Flagg, Gaston Labat and other leading New York City anaesthetists. From 1928 to 1956 he was a consultant at other hospitals in New York State and New Jersey, and he taught dental anaesthesia to dental residents. He was assistant clinical professor of anesthesia at New York Medical College for 17 years.

He joined the New York Society of Anesthetists (NYSA) in 1925 and, with guidance from Frank McMechan, he began his many years of organizational work in anaesthesia. He was secretary of the New York Society from 1928 to 1943, and promoted its transformation into the American Society of Anesthetists (ASA) in 1936 (renamed American Society of Anesthesiologists in 1945). He also guided the merger of the original American Society of Regional Anesthesia with the ASA. He proposed certification at the 1931 Congress of Anesthetists and put together the American Board of Anesthesiology in 1937.

In 1932, during an illness that was thought to be a coronary occlusion, he established the NYSA–ASA Library–Museum in his house at 131 Riverside Drive in New York City by adding his own equipment and books to those previously donated by James Gwathmey, Tom Buchanan, Frederick Erdmann and others. In 1933, the pharmaceutical company of E.R. Squibb and Sons built a skyscraper at 745 Fifth Avenue, NYC and invited scientific groups to use a large, purpose-built meeting room. Buchanan was a friend of the president of Squibb and helped Wood to obtain rent-free quarters for the Library–Museum. The spacious area soon housed the first headquarters for the ASA, followed by the American Board in 1938 and the business office of *Anesthesiology* in 1940.

The NYSA–ASA Library–Museum committee, formed in December 1937, expected the Library–Museum to be entirely supported by voluntary contributions. In 1938, the ASA changed its constitution to allocate 10% of its membership fees to the Library–Museum as an educational, non-profit organization. Wood and the committee chairman catalogued textbooks, journals and museum pieces. The Library–Museum was open two evenings a week from 7 pm to 10 pm with a librarian in attendance. In 1940, it received the first Cotton–Boothby gas machine and an 1847 edition of John Snow's book on ether. By 1942, the Library–Museum had accumulated more than 800 volumes.

The ASA moved its headquarters to rented offices in Chicago in 1947. Limited funds made it impossible to find adequate space for the Library–Museum as well, so it remained in New York, moving to a building at 137 West 11th Street that was owned by St Vincent's Hospital. When differences of opinion arose within the Australian Society of Anaesthetists in 1948, the Australian anaesthetist Geoffrey Kaye gave part of his collection to the Library–Museum. In 1949, the ASA Board of Directors voted that a non-profit corporation be formed, to be known as the Paul M. Wood Library and Museum, and that the ASA donate funds from the dues of active members for its maintenance. The purpose of the corporation was to 'collect, preserve and make available to the profession and the lay public, writings, publications, apparatus and other materials pertaining to the special field of anesthesiology.' The New York State Board of

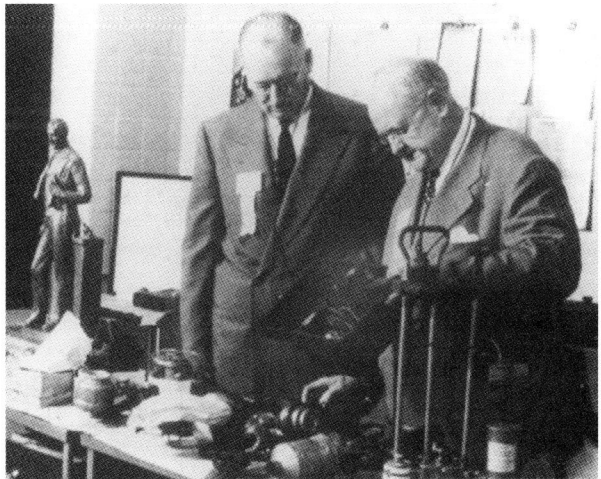

Figure 1. WLM president, left, with WLM librarian-curator Paul Wood preparing to move the Wood Library–Museum from New York to Park Ridge. (Reproduced with kind permission from the Wood Library–Museum of Anesthesiology, Park Ridge IL, USA.)

Regents granted a provisional charter on 21 July 1950 and an absolute charter on 29 February 1952. Paul Wood was the founder and first curator of the Wood Library–Museum of Anesthesiology.

Further financial problems arose in 1953 and an appeal for funds failed. In 1954, the board gratefully accepted an offer from Richard Foregger Sr (the anaesthesia equipment manufacturer) of temporary storage space for most of the material in a boathouse at Roslyn, Long Island. It was not until 1963 that the ASA provided space in the building in Park Ridge, Illinois for the Wood Library–Museum. Sadly, although Wood oversaw its development and the transport of books and artefacts (Figure 1) from New York City to Park Ridge, he died four months before its dedication. There is plenty of space for the museum, library and offices in the new ASA headquarters building that opened in 1992 (Figure 2), and the staff of full-time librarian, assistant librarian, archivist and secretary enables it to achieve its original objectives. Its Board of Trustees awards two Paul M. Wood Fellowships each year to enable anaesthesia historians to take full advantage of this outstanding facility.

During his lifetime, Paul Wood was honoured with the Silver Cup of the International Anesthesia Research Society, Honorary Membership in the Australian Society of Anaesthetists and the first Distinguished Service Award of the American Society of Anesthesiologists in 1945. The Wood Library–Museum is his living memorial.

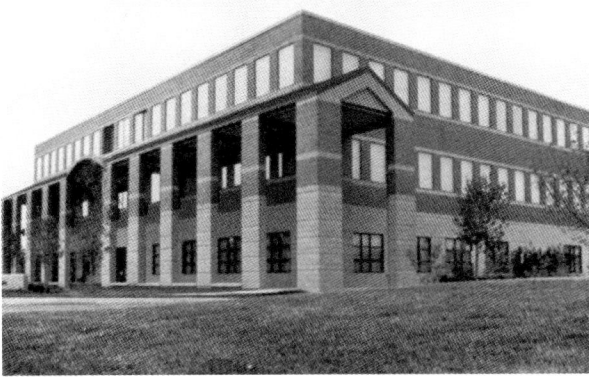

Figure 2. American Society of Anesthesiologists' headquarters building, 1992 Library and WLM offices are located on the top floor, and the museum is in the basement. (Reproduced with kind permission from the Wood Library–Museum of Anesthesiology, Park Ridge IL, USA.)

Acknowledgement

Portrait photograph reproduced with kind permission from the Wood Library–Museum of Anesthesiology, Park Ridge, IL, USA.

Further reading

Anonymous. We salute . . . Paul M. Wood, M. D. *Anesthesia and Analgesia* 1962; **41**: 263–4.

Betcher AM. The Wood Library–Museum of Anesthesiology. *Anesthesiology* 1961; **22**: 618–31.

Sim PP. From Indiana to New York: Dr. Paul Meyer Wood's Hoosier roots. *ASA Newsletter* 1994; **58 (9)**: 8–13.

THE WOOLLEY AND ROE CASE

The Woolley and Roe case, which came to trial in 1953, is one of the most famous medicolegal cases in British anaesthetic history. Albert Woolley and Cecil Roe were the plaintiffs. On Monday 13 October 1947, Malcolm Graham, a consultant anaesthetist in Chesterfield, Derbyshire, gave hypobaric nupercaine spinal anaesthetics to three patients in one day. Roe, aged 45 and healthy, was the first patient on the morning operating list and underwent removal of a semilunar cartilage. The second patient was very ill and had an emergency laparotomy for intestinal obstruction; he died five days later from peritonitis and pneumonia. Woolley, aged 56 years and healthy, had a hydrocoele repaired in the afternoon.

By the following day, Woolley and Roe had developed flaccid paralysis of the legs, anaesthesia from the waist down and complete incontinence. After initial improvement, their symptoms progressed to painful spastic paraparesis. Roe was affected more severely than Woolley, but both were severely disabled. There was no evidence of meningitis in either patient, although the similarity of their conditions strongly suggested a related cause. Whether the very ill third patient developed neurological abnormalities is uncertain. By May 1950, Roe had developed such severe flexor and adductor spasms that his legs and buttocks had to be tied down. A laminectomy revealed a large thick-walled arachnoidal cyst under the laminae of T10–11. Below the cyst, the entire contents of the dural sheath were a solid mass of fibrous tissue with scarcely any identifiable neural elements.

Both men remained severely disabled. Roe had previously been a farm labourer who grew vegetable and flowers and did his own house decorating. After the event, he could wash, shave and feed himself but had severe muscular spasms and no bowel control. Woolley was never able to work again, nor could he pursue his hobbies of gardening and pigeon racing.

The case came to trial in 1953. All allegations against the manufacturers were withdrawn during the trial. Professor Macintosh from Oxford put forward the theory that phenol, in which the ampoules of nupercaine had been immersed to sterilize the exterior, had leaked into the ampoules through cracks that were invisible to the naked eye. The judge accepted this explanation. He pointed out that, although Macintosh now recommended autoclaving everything, in 1947 when the tragedies occurred, a responsible anaesthetist could have been unaware of the potential for antiseptic contamination through invisible cracks in glass. He discounted evidence from two expert witnesses who were not anaesthetists. An eminent surgeon for the defence, Sir Hugh Griffiths, apparently intended to show that the plaintiff's neurological damage was not consistent with the injection of phenol. This upset his counsel who was happy with the phenol theory. An eminent neurologist, Sir Francis Walshe, also rejected the phenol theory, although his belief that spinal anaesthetics were inherently toxic was challenged because Woolley had previously had two uneventful spinal anaesthetics.

The judge found that the plaintiff's claims of negligence failed, both against the hospital and against Graham. The Appeal was dismissed and neither Woolley nor Roe received any compensation.

Although the judge accepted the phenol theory, many anaesthetists including Graham were not convinced. The case resulted in a dramatic decline in the use of spinal anaesthesia in the UK for almost 25 years. Macintosh in Oxford and Alfred Lee in Southend-on-Sea were among the few who used and taught the technique.

Thirty years after the trial, Graham was still convinced that phenol and the 'invisible cracks' were red herrings. He and a colleague had tried to crack the 20 mL glass ampoules and could not do so. The glass either shattered or was undamaged. He was sure he had not given the wrong drug because there were no similar ampoules in the hospital. The only explanation that Graham could suggest was some sort of contamination of the needles and/or syringes. How else could the same thing happen twice, possibly three times, in one day? There had to be a common cause.

There had been reports of similar cases in the USA and Britain around the time of the Woolley and Roe case, also without satisfactory explanation. In 1990, Chris Hutter, a consultant anaesthetist in Nottingham approached the Woolley and Roe puzzle by asking when the local anaesthetic became contaminated. He concluded that contamination of the needles and syringes occurred when they were boiled in a sterilizing pan of the type that was used in British hospitals until the 1960s. The only likely contaminant was an acid descaler that was inadvertently left in the pan in the Monday morning. Graham mentioned that the theatre sister (head nurse) had gone off duty at lunchtime on that day with vomiting and a violent headache. She later had surgery for a pituitary tumour. Water would be added during the day to replace that lost by evaporation. This would dilute the acid and explains why Woolley, having his surgery in the afternoon, was less severely affected than Roe. The pathological changes of adhesive arachnoiditis are consistent with the known toxicology of acid in the spinal fluid. The descaler theory is now generally accepted and it explains why such cases disappeared when single-use disposable needles and syringes became available.

The wedding picture with Roe in a wheelchair (Figure 1) shows the outcome of his spinal anaesthetic. Three years after

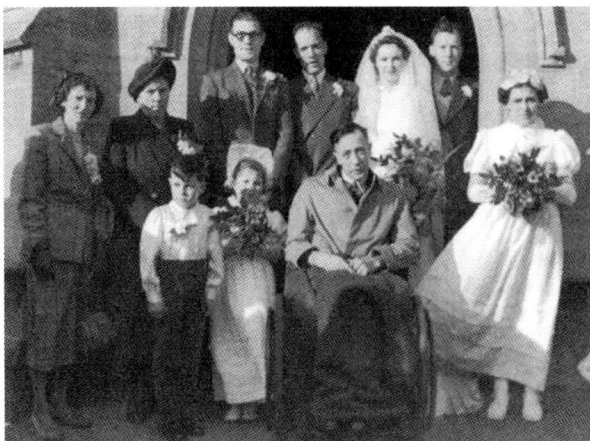

Figure 1. Cecil Roe in a wheelchair at his son's wedding. (Image courtesy of Charles Roe.)

the trial he was admitted to hospital for terminal care. He asked to see Graham, who went with some trepidation. Roe said he wanted to tell Graham how sorry he was for all the trouble he had caused; he had not wanted to bring the case, it was his union. Graham replied that the union was quite right; after all, Roe had come for a simple operation and finished up with his legs paralysed. Graham told him that he had not been given the wrong drug, but explained that he still [in 1956] did not know what went wrong. Roe's response was one of thanks for telling him. In Graham's declining years, Hutter's explanation removed the shadow of suspicion that Graham believed had always hung over him.

Further reading

Cope RW. The Woolley and Roe case. Woolley and Roe versus Ministry of Health and Others. *Anaesthesia* 1954; 9: 249–70.

Hutter CDD. The Woolley and Roe case a reassessment. *Anaesthesia* 1990: 45; 859–64.

Maltby JR, Hutter CDD, Clayton KC. The Woolley and Roe case. *British Journal of Anaesthesia* 2000; 84: 121–6.

Lewis H. Wright Memorial Lecture

Lewis H. Wright (1894–1974)

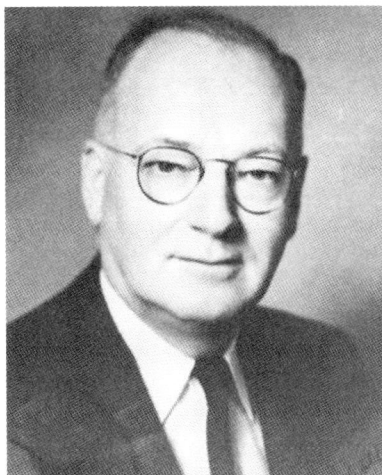

Lewis Wright was born in 1894 in Trail County, North Dakota. He never knew his father who died before he was born. His mother moved to Vermont the next year, where he graduated from high school in 1912. He studied veterinary medicine at Cornell University in Ithaca, New York; Texas A&M University in College Station, Texas; and the University of Nevada in Reno and taught at Georgia Veterinary College in Athens for one year in 1921–22. He graduated in medicine in 1925 from the Medical College of Georgia in Augusta, where he interned and practised obstetrics and anaesthesia for five years. His life then followed an unusual course.

In 1930 he joined the medical department of E.R. Squibb and Sons and began a 32-year role as a roving ambassador of goodwill between the pharmaceutical manufacturer who supplied the drugs and practising anaesthetists who used them. He attended medical conventions in every state, visited hospitals and got to know anaesthetists everywhere. He took time off from Squibb in 1936–37 to complete a full residency in anaesthesia under Emery Rovenstine at Bellevue Hospital, New York City, New York but never undertook much clinical practice. He had a role in the early development of cyclopropane as an anaesthetic agent, but his most significant contribution was the part he played in the introduction of curare into clinical anaesthesia.

Richard Gill (1902–58), an American explorer, made several visits to South America. In 1932, a few days before returning to the USA, he was thrown from his horse and a few days later developed what was subsequently diagnosed as multiple sclerosis. His neurologist, Walter Freeman, advised him that curare might improve his muscle spasticity if a suitable preparation could be found. Gill never accepted the diagnosis and, during a remission in 1938, he and his wife took another trip into the jungles of Ecuador. He brought back 25 pounds (more than 11 kg) of crude curare as the natives prepared it, but he could not find anyone who was interested in trying to refine it. Finally, Squibb accepted it and their chemists prepared an extract that they standardized, using the rabbit 'head-drop' test to measure its potency. One unit was the amount of curare that caused the head to drop and Squibb marketed it as Intocostrin, containing 20 units per millilitre.

In 1938–39, Gill also sent curare to A.E. Bennett, a professor of neurology and psychiatry in Omaha, Nebraska to use in children with spasticity. Bennett's pharmacology colleague standardized the preparation but the clinical results were disappointing. However, it was spectacularly successful in preventing fractures in the recently introduced convulsive therapy in psychiatry.

It was Wright's job to market Squibb's Intocostrin. He was aware of Bennett's work and took samples to Stuart Cullen at the University of Iowa and Emanuel Papper at Columbia University in New York. Cullen was not convinced of the reliability of his experimental work with the Intocostrin, and at Columbia, Papper's two cats developed acute asthmatic attacks and died. Emery Rovenstine, the chairman at Columbia, suggested that the young Papper should try it in man! Papper gave curare to only two patients, both under ether anaesthesia, and they both developed prolonged apnea that required tiring manual artificial ventilation. He suggested to Rovenstine that the drug was too dangerous for clinical practice.

When Wright offered Intocostrin to Harold Griffith in Montreal, Quebec, Griffith administered small doses cautiously under cyclopropane anaesthesia. This was mainly done to provide the surgeon with a more relaxed patient during opening and closing of the abdominal cavity. He and his resident Enid Johnson gave it to their first patient on 23 January 1942 and published their first 25 cases in *Anesthesiology* later that year. The rest is history. It was Lewis Wright's persistent belief in the value of the drug that led to what was one of the greatest advances in anaesthesia since the introduction of ether. He never sought any recognition for his contribution.

Wright served in the US Navy from 1943 to 1946. He was on active service in Australia, New Guinea and other South Pacific Islands, and he waded ashore at Leyte in the Philippines on 'D' Day in October 1944. He then became chief of anesthesiology at the US Naval Hospital in St. Albans, New York, with the rank of commander of the US Naval Reserve. When he resumed civilian status, he continued his connection with clinical anaesthesia at many New York hospitals and joined the faculty of New York Medical College. He became a diplomate of the American Board of Anaesthesiology in 1945.

Wright was actively involved in the New York State Society of Anesthesiologists (NYSSA). His name appeared as a member of various committees at the 1948 NYSSA Post Graduate Assembly (PGA) where he succeeded Rovenstine as PGA general chairman. He was one of the founders of the Wood Library-Museum of Anesthesiology and served as president-emeritus of the Board of Trustees. He was a member of the ASA board of directors for 15 years, and received the Distinguished Service Award of the American Society of Anesthesiologists in 1955.

Lewis Wright and Paul Wood had similar interests in collecting memorabilia and equipment, which they both moved into the Squibb building in New York City when the collections grew too big for their homes. It was Wright's idea that the collection should be incorporated under New York state laws and be named the Wood Library-Museum. He retired in 1962 but always remained a collector. He collected bleeding bowls, lancets, scarifiers, feeding cups, pap boats, nursing bottles – especially those before the days of rubber teats – and anything that pertained to the history of anaesthesia.

The Lewis H. Wright Memorial Lecture is presented during the ASA annual meeting under the auspices of the board of trustees of the Wood Library–Museum (Table 1).

Table 1. Lewis H. Wright lecturers and lecture titles

Year	Lecturer	Title
1967	Chauncey D. Leake	Practical aspects of the history of anesthesia.
1968	Thomas E. Keys	Early pneumatic chemists and physicians.
1969	John S. Lundy	The introduction of sodium pentothal.
1970	David M. Little, Jr	In the beginning (on Horace Wells).
1971	James H. Young	Crawford W. Long, MD – a Georgian innovator.
1972	Leroy D. Vandam	Early American anesthetists.
1973	Peter D. Olch	William S. Halsted and local anesthesia contributions.
1974	Charles C. Tandy	Treasures of the Wood Library–Museum.
1975	Albert M. Betcher	The civilizing of curare.
1976	J. Englebert Dunphy	The contributions of anesthesiology to surgery.
1977	Rod A. Gordon	A capsule history of anaesthesia in Canada.
1978	W. Denis A. Smith	Henry Hill Hickman: quack or anti-quack?
1979	K. Garth Huston, Sr	Gardner Q. Colton: itinerant chemist, 49'er, proponent of anesthesia.
1980	John W. Pender	Contemporaries of Lewis Wright.
1981	William B. Bean	The dangers of precocious discovery: anesthesia and the Civil War.
1982	Betty J. Bamforth	The evolution of modern anesthesiology residency.
1983	Roderick K. Calverley	Arthur Guedel: the life and times of an extraordinary man.
1984	B. Raymond Fink	Leaves and needles: the discovery of local anesthesia.
1985	Richard H. Ellis	Early ether anesthesia: the Anglo–American connections.
1986	Richard J. Wolfe	The first operation under anesthesia: Robert C. Hinkley's interpretation.
1987	Selma H. Calmes	Virginia Apgar: a woman physician's career in a developing specialty.
1988	John W. Severinghaus	Monitors, the patent medicine of anesthesia.
1989	Nicholas M. Greene	Contributions by non-anesthetists to the development of anesthesia.
1990	Thomas B. Boulton	Balancing the anaesthetic.
1991	C. Ronald Stephen	The great triumvirate.
1992	Francis F. Foldes	Impact of muscle relaxants: the role of Lewis H. Wright.
1993	M. T. 'Pepper' Jenkins	Epochs in intravenous fluid therapy.
1994	James E. Eckenhoff	The growth of anesthesiology as viewed by artists and photographers.
1995	Ephraim S. Siker	Anesthesia safety – an evolution.
1996	Joseph F. Artusio, Jr	From symmetrical to asymmetrical.
1997	Donald Caton	Feminists and the early development of obstetric anesthesia.
1998	Steven M. Zeitels	The origin and development of laryngoscopy and laryngology.
1999	Sherwin B. Nuland	Surgery as it was on that day in 1846: before and after.
2000	Peter Safar	On resuscitation medicine in the 20th century.
2001	Dale C. Smith	Anesthetist: argument, attainment and authority, 1870–1920.

Acknowledgement

Portrait photograph reproduced with kind permission from the Wood Library–Museum of Anesthesiology, Park Ridge, IL, USA.

Further reading

Foldes FF. The impact of muscle relaxants on the development of anesthesia and surgery: the role of Lewis H. Wright. *Anesthesia History Association Newsletter* 1993; 11 (4): 1, 4–6.

Gill RC. *White Water and Black Magic*. New York, NY: Henry Holt and Company, 1940.

Smith P. *Arrows of Mercy*. Toronto, Ontario: Doubleday Canada, 1969.

WRIGHT ANEMOMETER

Basil Martin Wright (1912-2001)

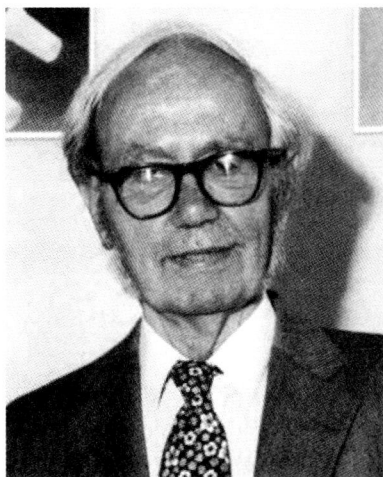

Martin Wright was born in 1912 in Dulwich, London, the second son of the Reverend Basil and Margaret Wright. He showed an unusual interest in the workings of gadgets during his school years at Winchester College, and in what made humans 'tick' during his under-graduate years at Trinity College, Cambridge University. His parents had moved to the nearby parish of Trumpington where he set up a laboratory in the vicarage outbuildings. He took additional physiology studies in his preclinical years at Cambridge, and obtained a first class degree before moving to St. Bartholomew's Medical School in London as an exhibition scholar.

He graduated in medicine and surgery in 1938 and had a busy period of emergency medical service work at the beginning of the Second World War. He volunteered to serve in the Royal Army Medical Corps in 1942 and was seconded to the Medical Research Council unit to investigate tank warfare problems. He then spent five years as a graded pathologist in Sierra Leone and Singapore. In these posts, he designed and made pieces of essential apparatus – some of which were still in use when he returned 40 years later. He attained the rank of Colonel as deputy director of pathology services in South East Asia before he was demobilized in 1946.

The postwar Labour government was concerned about the health of miners, especially in the Minister of Health's constituency in South Wales, and a special Medical Research Council pneumoconiosis research unit was formed at Llandough Hospital near Penarth. Charles Fletcher (1911–95), professor of epidemiology in London, recruited Wright as an experimental pathologist to study dust inhalation. Wright actually concentrated on designing mechanical devices for projects undertaken by his associates. These included Archie Cochrane (1909–88), professor of chest diseases at the University of Wales, after whom the Cochrane Centres for evidenced-based medicine are named.

The only way to measure breathing capacities until 1959 was with a large clumsy spirometer. When asked about the spirometer's suitability for field use, one of Wright's colleagues said, 'You'd be lucky to get it into a field!' Wright introduced his portable peak flow meter in 1959 and it soon became the standard means of assessing respiratory problems, such as asthma and bronchitis. He then invented and produced his hand-held peak flow meter, maximum forced expiratory rate and ventilation meter. More than one million miniature plastic versions of the peak flow meter (Figure 1) have been sold and are found in British medical bags, consulting rooms and the homes of asthmatics.

Wright introduced his idea of the anemometer (Figure 2) at meetings of the Physiological Society and Royal Society in 1954 as 'a cylinder which air enters through a number of tangential jets and drives a very light two-bladed rotor which is connected to a counting train'. It took four years of work to reach perfection. It was original, had virtually linear calibration and was constructed so that although its mechanism was delicate, the complete unit was robust. The British Oxygen Company bought the production rights from the National Development Corporation but the precision work needed to make the meters could only be done by Swiss watch craftsmen. Anaesthetists worldwide found it indispensable at a time when they were using muscle relaxants with few monitors and were becoming involved with intensive care.

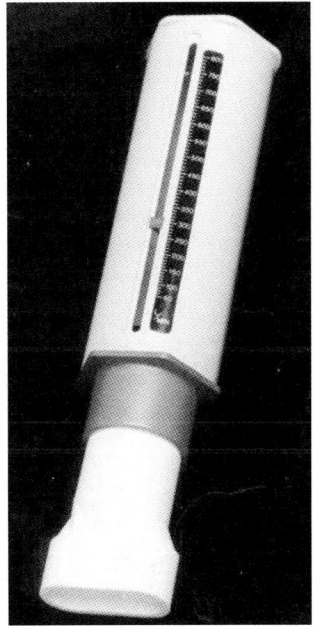

Figure 1. Miniature Wright peak flow meter. (Image courtesy of H.T. Davenport.)

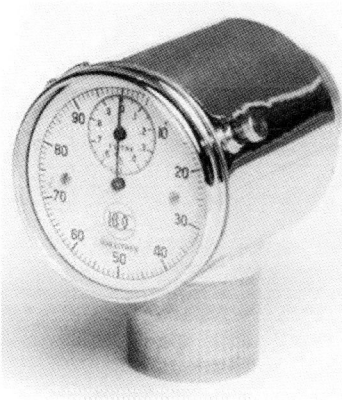

Figure 2. Wright anemometer. (Image courtesy of H.T. Davenport.)

Wright worked full-time on instrument development for 20 years from 1957, first at the National Institute of Medical Research at Mill Hill and then at the new Medical Research Council Clinical Research Centre (Figure 3) at Northwick Park Hospital, Harrow, Middlesex, which opened in 1969. He continued as a visiting worker supported by commercial consultancies for more than 10 years after retirement age, and a further four years as an honorary research fellow at University College Hospital, London. Anaesthetists are familiar with several of his monitoring inventions, but are less likely to recognize those he designed in response to clinicians' requests for monitoring, diagnosis and treatment. These include:

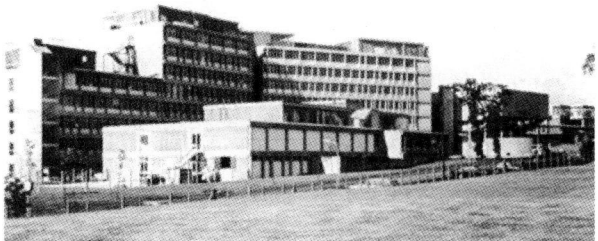

Figure 3. MRC Clinical Research Centre at Northwick Park. (Image courtesy of H.T. Davenport.)

● Monitoring
- oxygen supply failure device
- pollution testing and extraction system
- neonatal apnoea metre
- anaesthetic gas differentiation whistle
- neonatal triggered ventilator
- breath alcohol measurement.

● Diagnostic
- random zero sphygmomanometer
- ataximeter, portable ballistograph
- bed weighing machine
- finger blood pressure measurement.

● Therapeutic
- nebulizer
- cryogenic probes
- drip monitor
- infant incubator Venturi feed
- syringe driver
- safe Heidbrink valve
- watch-driven infuser.

Wright preferred mechanical to electrical devices because they were simpler, more reliable and cheaper, but he faced resistance from some manufacturers and users. His small portable syringe driver and wrist watch infuser had universal application, but their value was only fully recognized for thallassaemia treatment and palliative care. His neonatal apnoea monitor, which he developed in response to two tragic deaths in Northwick Park's special care nursery, was favoured by parents, but dubiously approved by cot death (sudden infant death syndrome) experts.

At the age of 39, Wright married Sheila Smith, publications officer at the Medical Research Council, and they had five children. He could be relied on to mend any broken toy or item of household equipment, many of which he had motorized, yet he was markedly lacking in personal ambition. He cared little about either financial gain or professional advancement, he had no postgraduate qualifications and assiduously avoided committee and administrative work. The Medical Research Council holds the patents on all his inventions and receives most of the royalties flowing from them. He was content to receive a steady income for doing what he enjoyed.

He received a number of design awards and a Queen's Award for Industry for the breathalyser. He was elected to Honorary Fellowship of the Royal College of Physicians and received a Cambridge MD in recognition of his published papers.

Acknowledgement

Portrait photograph courtesy of H.T. Davenport.

Further reading

Anonymous [Obituary]. Martin Wright inventor of simple and elegant medical instruments, including the breathalyser, who found fulfilment not in material rewards but in the work itself. *The Times,* 23 March 2001, p.25.

Byles PH. Observations on some continuously-acting spirometers. *British Journal of Anaesthesia* 1960; **32**: 470–5.

Davenport HT. Dr Martin Wright – an appreciation. *Royal College of Anaesthetists Newsletter* 1998; **41**: 18–19.

WYLIE & CHURCHILL-DAVIDSON'S 'A PRACTICE OF ANAESTHESIA'

The first edition of *A Practice of Anaesthesia*, better known as 'Wylie and Churchill-Davidson', appeared in 1960. It was an instant success and was the 'Bible' for a whole generation of aspiring anaesthetists. Each edition drew in more specialist authors, but it always maintained the essential elements of readability, accuracy and practicality. It was an enormous undertaking, the magnitude of which was probably not lost on 'Miss D' – Jean Davenport, the department secretary who typed and retyped each chapter of each edition without the aid of a computer. It was also published in the USA and was translated into Italian, Polish, Portuguese and Spanish.

William Derek Wylie (1919–1998)

Derek Wylie was born in Huddersfield, Yorkshire where his father was a dental practitioner. He was educated at Uppingham School, Gonville and Caius College, Cambridge and St Thomas' Hospital Medical School, London, graduating in 1943. He intended to become a specialist physician and held junior appointments as casualty officer, house physician and resident anaesthetist.

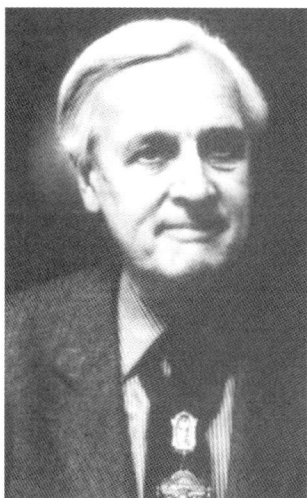

Within two years he obtained the DA and MRCP London. What little anaesthesia training he received came from Michael Nosworthy, a consultant at St. Thomas' and a leader in British anaesthesia. Wylie joined the Royal Air Force Volunteer Reserves in 1945 and served as a physician in England, Palestine and Aden before demobilization in 1947.

St Thomas' offered him a post as honorary anaesthetist shortly before the introduction of the National Health Service (NHS) in 1948, despite his minimal experience in anaesthesia. There was no guarantee of adequate financial assistance if he undertook the training necessary to become a specialist physician so he decided to accept the anaesthetic offer. Before the NHS, the voluntary teaching hospitals made their own rules and St Thomas' clearly thought that Wylie had potential. He quickly brought himself up to date in what was then a very limited specialty. He practised and taught anaesthesia, carried out clinical research with colleagues, lectured in Britain and overseas and wrote many papers.

In the early 1950s he was a member of a committee of four anaesthetists appointed by the Association of Anaesthetists of Great Britain and Ireland to investigate the causes of deaths associated with anaesthesia. This was probably the first national investigation of its kind and it was the direct forerunner of the current national confidential enquiry into perioperative deaths, known as NCEPOD, an independent body that is supported by the associations of anaesthetists and surgeons and their Royal Colleges. Wylie became interested in medical negligence and its prevention. He joined the council of the Medical Defence Union in 1962 and was President from 1982 to 1988. He believed that the union should play a significant part in the prevention of medical problems and initiated publication of the union's own quarterly journal.

Wylie was elected to Fellowship of the Faculty of Anaesthetists of the Royal College of Surgeons in 1957; Royal College of Physicians in 1967; and Royal College of Surgeons in 1972. He served on the board of the Faculty of Anaesthetists from 1960 to 1970 and was dean from 1967 to 1969. He was president of the Section of Anaesthetics of the Royal Society of Medicine, 1963–64 and president of the Association of Anaesthetists of Great Britain and Ireland, 1980–82.

Derek Wylie was a quiet and approachable man who was liked by all grades of staff. He had a liberal philosophy and expressed his firmly held views courteously. He was one of those few people who have held such high office but rarely caused offence and made no enemies.

Harry Cunningham Churchill-Davidson (1922–1995)

Harry Cunningham Churchill-Davidson was born in Camberley, Surrey in 1922 where his father was a general practitioner. He was educated at Charterhouse School and Trinity College, Cambridge where he represented the university at squash and soccer. He completed his clinical studies at St Thomas' Hospital Medical School, which was evacuated to Hydestile, near Godalming in Surrey during the war. He graduated in medicine and surgery in 1945.

Wylie and Churchill-Davidson arrived at St Thomas' department of anaesthesia at almost the same time. Churchill-Davidson rose rapidly through the ranks of registrar and senior registrar to consultant anaesthetist in 1955 at what was then the exceptionally young age of 33. He was also appointed to the staff of the Chelsea Hospital for Women and the Brompton Hospital for diseases of the chest. His 1953 MD thesis on the clinical and pathological features of acute pulmonary collapse exemplified the thoroughness of his clinical investigation.

He had a crusading zeal to impart his knowledge and understanding to others. In 1970 he established a series of lecture courses at St. Thomas' for the FFARCS examinations at a time when formal courses were uncommon.

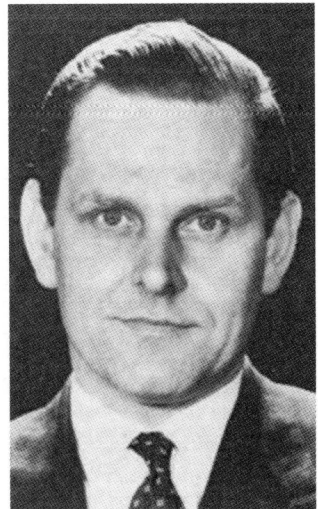

He possessed a flair for acquiring funds for various projects and in 1978 he set up the academic unit in the anaesthetic department. Hardly a month would pass without a St. Thomas' department publication in the anaesthetic journals. He was deeply involved in the study of neuromuscular blockade and published much of the basic work on the subject. A film in the departmental archives shows the young doctors Wylie and Churchill-Davidson administering Flaxedil (gallamine) to each other.

Churchill-Davidson did much to enhance the standing of British anaesthesia abroad. In 1954 he was a Fulbright travelling scholar and visited hospitals throughout the USA. In 1963 he spent one year as visiting professor at the University of California, San Francisco and in 1975 he delivered the Emery A. Rovenstine lecture at the American Society of Anesthesiologists annual meeting. As advisor to the World Health Organization, he taught in South Africa, Kenya and Southern Rhodesia (now Zimbabwe) in 1957–58 and in Venezuela and Bogota in 1971. He served a record term of 24 years on the board of the Faculty of Anaesthetists and was president of the Section of Anaesthetics of the Royal Society of Medicine, 1982–83. He retired from St Thomas's in 1986 after 31 years as a consultant anaesthetist.

Acknowledgement

Portrait photograph of Wylie reproduced with kind permission from the Association of Anaesthetists of Great Britain and Ireland; of Churchill-Davidson reproduced from *Anesthesia and Analgesia* 1961; **40**: 204–5, with permission from Lippincott Williams & Wilkins.

Further reading

WYLIE:

Anonymous [Obituary]. Dr Derek Wylie. *Anaesthesia News* 1998; **137**: 2.

Edwards G, Morton HJV, Pask EA, Wylie WD. Deaths associated with anaesthesia. A report on 1000 cases. *Anaesthesia* 1956; **11**: 263–7.

Wylie WD. 'There, but for the Grace of God … '. *Annals of the Royal College of Surgeons of England* 1975; **56**: 17–80.

CHURCHILL-DAVIDSON:

Anonymous. We salute … Harry Cunningham Churchill-Davidson M.A., M.D., F.F.A.R.C.S. *Anesthesia and Analgesia* 1961; **40**: 204–5.

Churchill-Davidson HC. A philosophy of relaxation eleventh annual Baxter-Travenol lecture. *Anesthesia and Analgesia* 1973; **52**: 495–501.

Mathias JA [Obituary]. Harry Cunningham Churchill-Davidson ('CD'). *British Medical Journal* 1995; **311**: 1636.

Wylie WD, Churchill-Davidson HC. *Wylie and Churchill-Davidson's A practice of anaesthesia, 5th edn.* London, UK: Lloyd-Luke, 1984.

INDEX

Loefgren, Nils, lidocaine (Xylocain) synthesis 76–7
Long, Crawford Williamson 149–150
 Crawford W. Long Medical Museum 117–19
low-flow anaesthetic breathing systems
 analysis of, Mapleson, William Wellesley 132–4
 Waters, Ralph Milton 220
Low, Harold, wire-frame mask 191–2
lumbar puncture
 Bier, August 19
 Lee, John Alfred 115
 Quincke, Heinrich Irenaeus 164–6
 Tuohy, Edward Boyce 216
 Whitacre spinal needle 225–7
Lundquist, Bengt, lidocaine (Xylocain) synthesis 76–7

Macintosh laryngoscope blade 121
Macintosh, Sir Robert Reynolds 120–2
 Nuffield chair of anaesthetics 154–6
 vaporizer devices 56–9
Magill, Sir Ivan Whiteside
 Magill forceps 123–5
 Magill laryngoscope 102
 Magill red rubber tubes 102
maladie de Denborough 46–8
malignant hyperthermia, Denborough, Michael 46–8
Mallampati score, Mallampati, Seshagiri Rao 126–8
Manley, Roger Edward Wentworth
 Manley ventilator 129–30
 Penlon Manley Multivent 130–1
Mapleson D coaxial system, Bain modification 10–12
Mapleson, William Wellesley
 Mapleson breathing systems 132–4
 Mapleson Medal 134
Masked Marvel see Bonica, John Joseph
masks
 nasal mask for dental anaesthesia, Goldman, Victor 72–3
 open drop ether anaesthesia
  Esmarch, Johan Friedrich von 61
  Schimmelbusch, Curt 190–2
 Rendell-Baker-Soucek mask 173–5
 wire-frame masks 190–2
McGill Pain Questionnaire, Melzack, Ronald 135–6
medals
 Hickman, Henry Hill 91–4
 Koller, Carl 105–7
 Mapleson, William Wellesley 134
 Snow, John 205–7
mediastinoscopy, Carlens, Eric 37
medical research ethics, Beecher, Henry Knowles 14–15
medico-legal trial, Woolley and Roe case 231–3

Melzack, Ronald, Melzack and Wall's gate control theory of pain 135–7
Mendelson's syndrome, Mendelson, Curtis Lester 138–40
Meyer, Helge, and Gordh needle 75–7
Miller, Donald, classification of semi-closed breathing systems 133
Miller laryngoscope blade, Miller, Robert Arden 141–3
minimal alveolar concentration (MAC), Eger II, Edmond I 53–5
Minnitt gas and air apparatus, Minnitt, Robert James 103, 144–6
Moch, Meyer, disposable plastic medical equipment 16–18
Morris, William Richard (Lord Nuffield) see Nuffield, Lord
mortality, anaesthetic-related
 Beecher and Todd report 13–14
 malignant hyperthermia, Denborough, Michael 46–8
 Wylie, William Derek 242–3
Morton, William Thomas Green, the ether dome 147–50
motor blockade score, Bromage, Philip Raikes 31–4
mouth gags
 Boyle-Davis gag 26–7
 Ring gag, Ring, Wallace Harold 167
mouth-to-mouth resuscitation
 Flagg, Paluel Joseph 68
 Resuscitube, Berman, Robert Alvin 17
 training manikin, Ruben, Henning 186
Murphy eye, Murphy, Francis John 151–3
Murray, John, wire-frame mask 191
muscarine effects, Ringer, Sydney 177
muscle, anaesthetic effects on, Ringer, Sydney 176–7
muscle disorders, and malignant hyperthermia, Denborough, Michael 46–8
muscle relaxants see neuromuscular blocking agents
museums
 Charles King Collection of Anaesthetic Equipment 101–4
 Crawford W. Long Medical Museum 117–19
 Geoffrey Kaye Museum of Anaesthetic History 98–100
 Wood Library–Museum of Anesthesiology 228–30
myopathies, and malignant hyperthermia, Denborough, Michael 46–8

nalorphine hydrochloride, neonatal asphyxia treatment, Eckenhoff, James Edward 50
nasal intubation, Magill, Sir Ivan Whiteside 123–4
nasal mask, for dental anaesthesia, Goldman, Victor 72–3

nasal tubes, Murphy, Francis John 153
needles
  contamination of, Woolley and Roe case
    231–3
  Gordh intravenous needle 75–7
  Hingson–Edwards caudal needle 95–6
  Lee epidural needle 115
  Oxford Tuohy needle 121–2
  Quincke spinal needle 164–6
  spinal needles 164–6
  Tuohy needle 216–18
  Whitacre spinal needle 225–7
neonates
  apnoea monitor, Wright, Basil Martin 240
  artificial respiration device, Snow, John
    205
  asphyxia treatment, Eckenhoff, James
    Edward 50
  assessment of, Apgar score 4–6
neostigmine effects, Gray, Thomas Cecil 79
neuromuscular blocking agents
  and anaesthetic-related deaths, Beecher
    and Todd report 13–14
  curare
    Griffith, Harold Randall 81–2
    Waterton, Charles 222–4
    Wright, Lewis H 234–6
  gallamine 132, 244
  suxamethonium 46-7, 142
  d-tubocurarine chloride, and Liverpool
    technique 78–80
nitrous oxide–air mixtures, Minnitt gas and
  air apparatus 103, 144–6
nitrous oxide–oxygen apparatus, King,
  Charles 101–2
nitrous oxide–oxygen ether anaesthesia,
  Boyle, Henry Edmund Gaskin 25–7
nitrous oxide–oxygen mixtures
  and diffusion anoxia, Fink, Bernard
    Raymond 63–5
  Hewitt, Sir Frederic William 87–8
non-rebreathing valve
  Fink, Bernard Raymond 63
  Ruben, Henning 184
  Stephen-Slater 185
Nuffield department of anaesthetics 154–6
Nuffield, Lord 154–6
Nunn's Applied Respiratory Physiology,
  Nunn, John Francis 157–9

obstetric anaesthesia
  Apgar, Virginia 5
  Bonica, John Joseph 22–3
  Hingson, Robert Andrew 95–6
  Mendelson, Curtis Lester 138–40
  Simpson, Sir James Young 202–4
obstetric analgesia, Minnitt gas and air
  apparatus, Minnitt, Robert James 144–6
Olovson, Thore, and Gordh needle 75–7
open drop anaesthesia, wire-frame masks 61,
  190–2

ophthalmic anaesthesia, Koller, Carl 105–7
organ transplantation, and definition of
  death, Beecher, Henry Knowles 15
oropharyngeal airway
  Berman, Robert Alvin 16–18
  Foregger company 71
  Guedel oral airway 85–6
  Hewitt, Sir Frederic William 88–9
  Waters, Ralph Milton 220
orotracheal intubation, Mallampati score
  126–8
Oxford inflating bellows, Macintosh, Sir
  Robert Reynolds 120–1
Oxford miniature vaporizer (OMV) 59
Oxford Tuohy needle, Macintosh, Sir Robert
  Reynolds 121–2
Oxford vaporizer
  Epstein, Hans G. 56–7
  Macintosh, Sir Robert Reynolds 120–2
oxygen–ether apparatus, Foregger, Richard
  von 69–70
oxygen generator, Foregger, Richard von
  69–70
oxygen levels, low, survival experiments,
  Pask, Edgar Alexander 160–1
Oxyvent (Glostavent) anaesthetic machine
  131

paediatric anaesthesia
  Apgar score 4–6
  Ayre's T-piece 7–9
  Miller laryngoscope blade, Miller, Robert
    Arden 143
  RAE (Ring, Adair and Elwyn) endotracheal
    tubes 167–9
  Rees, Gordon Jackson 170–2
  Rendell-Baker, Leslie 173–5
paediatric biochemistry, Hartmann, Alexis
  Frank 177–9
pain clinics, Bonica, John Joseph 23
pain lectureships, Bonica, John Joseph 23–4
pain research
  Bonica, John Joseph 23–4
  Melzack, Ronald 135–7
  Wall, Patrick David 135–7
parallel Lack anaesthetic breathing system
  112–13
Pask certificate of honour, Pask, Edgar
  Alexander 160–3
peak flow meter, Wright, Basil Martin 238–9
peer review, and medical research ethics,
  Beecher, Henry Knowles 14–15
pelvic surgery, Trendelenburg position
  213–15
Penlon Manley Multivent, Manley, Roger
  Edward Wentworth 130–1
phantom limb pain
  Melzack, Ronald 136
  Wall, Patrick David 137
pharmacokinetics, Mapleson, William
  Wellesley 132–4